Anxiety Disorders in Adults

Anxiety Disorders in Adults

A Clinical Guide

VLADAN STARCEVIC

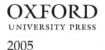

UNIVERSITY PRESS

2005

OXFORD
UNIVERSITY PRESS

Oxford   New York
Auckland   Bangkok   Buenos Aires   Cape Town   Chennai
Dar es Salaam   Delhi   Hong Kong   Istanbul   Karachi   Kolkata
Kuala Lumpur   Madrid   Melbourne   Mexico City   Mumbai   Nairobi
São Paulo   Shanghai   Taipei   Tokyo   Toronto

Copyright © 2005 by Oxford University Press

Published by Oxford University Press, Inc.
198 Madison Avenue, New York, New York, 10016
http://www.oup.com

Oxford is a registered trademark of Oxford University Press

Library of Congress Cataloging-in-Publication Data

Starcevic, Vladan.
Anxiety disorders in adults : a clinical guide / Vladan Starcevic.
p.   ;   cm.
Includes bibliographical references and index.
ISBN 0-19-515606-4
1. Anxiety. 2. Phobias.   I. Title.
[DNLM: 1. Anxiety Disorders—therapy. WM 172 S795a 2005]
RC531.S687 2005
616.85'22—dc22   2004043465

9 8 7 6 5 4 3 2 1

Printed in the United States of America
on acid-free paper

To KK, for patience and understanding

Acknowledgments

This book is a product of many years of clinical work, research and collaboration with colleagues. Although it is difficult to single out among many people who have been influential, helpful and supportive in my professional endeavors, I believe that I will do no injustice by mentioning Professor Eberhard H. Uhlenhuth and Professor Ljubomir Eric. Professor Uhlenhuth (Uhli) has been a dedicated mentor and a reliable friend; he has been consistently supportive, providing me with invaluable feedback and guidance when I needed it most. Professor Eric is "responsible" for sparking my interest in anxiety disorders and for showing me different roads that can be traveled to approach the subject of this book.

I am grateful to Fiona Stevens, Senior Editor at Oxford University Press, for her encouragement and remarkable patience throughout my work on this project.

Preface

Anxiety disorders are common in clinical practice. They often run a chronic course and have an adverse, though often overlooked, impact on the quality of life. Anxiety disorders often co-occur with other psychiatric conditions. This further complicates their course and treatment and leads to greater disability. Despite advances in their diagnosis and treatment, the recognition of anxiety disorders is still unsatisfactory, and many sufferers remain untreated. Others are not treated adequately, respond only partially to treatment, or are treatment-resistant.

Although there has been much interest in the anxiety disorders as well as intense research activity over the last two decades, many issues remain unresolved, particularly in the area of etiology and pathogenesis. Also, the abundance of information and data on the treatment of anxiety disorders often produces conflicting effects, sometimes leaving therapists puzzled as to what treatment approach to use with a particular patient and in a given clinical situation.

This book was conceived mainly out of practical need to present the anxiety disorders as they occur and as they are treated in the "real world." That is, the main purpose of the book is to contribute in a practical way to both understanding and treatment of people with anxiety disorders. The book has been guided by clinical relevance of the problems that it addresses, regardless of whether these problems are of a conceptual and theoretical nature or pertain more to etiological and treatment issues. The book attempts to fill the gap between the textbook-like comprehensiveness and ultrapractical, reductionistic approach of some clinical and treatment guides.

The book is organized around the six main categories of anxiety disorders: panic disorder (with and without agoraphobia), generalized anxiety disorder, social anxiety disorder (social phobia), specific phobias, obsessive-compulsive disorder, and posttraumatic stress disorder. Each of these disorders is presented in a separate chapter, following a uniform style. Thus, each chapter has sections on clinical features of the disorder, the relationship between that disorder and other conditions, assessment (which includes diagnostic issues, assessment instruments, and differential diagnosis), epidemiology, course and prognosis, etiology and pathogenesis, and treatment.

The emphasis of the book is on the phenomenology, etiology, and treatment of anxiety disorders, using a practical approach with frequent reference to clinical examples and scenarios. Thus, clinical features of each disorder are described in some detail, as the knowledge of these features is crucial for recognition and understanding of the underlying psychopathology. Each chapter also presents the most important models of etiology and pathogenesis, which serve as the basis for treatment of the corresponding disorders. Finally, main types of pharmacological and psychological treatment are described in a manner that clinicians will find useful, as the book contains practical tips, descriptions of the relevant therapeutic procedures, and treatment guidelines for use in commonly encountered clinical situations.

The book does not "favor" any type of etiological explanation and treatment, but emphasizes models that have a heuristic and practical value and treatments whose usefulness has been demonstrated. The etiological models and treatments are presented critically, so that the reader can appreciate both their strengths and weaknesses. The book is a project that balances and integrates what is currently known about anxiety disorders and their treatment.

While the treatment approaches are presented mainly from an evidence-based (efficacy) perspective, the book also takes into account various treatment goals for patients, available resources, and applicability of evidence-based treatments to real-life and complex clinical situations (effectiveness perspective). I acknowledge that I have been influenced by movements toward integration within psychological treatments and between pharmacotherapy and psychotherapy. Combined treatments are presented, however, with due consideration of the unresolved issues and caution about their unsatisfactory empirical status.

The book will be most useful to a professional audience, which includes psychiatrists, clinical psychologists, other mental health workers, primary care physicians, other medical specialists, and physicians-in-training. The book may also be of interest to students of medicine and psychology and to a general audience, particularly individuals interested in anxiety and those suffering from anxiety disorders.

Practicing clinicians will benefit from the multifaceted approach to conceptual issues and from practical treatment suggestions that will guide them in their clinical work. Indeed, the important aims of the book are to help clinicians make everyday clinical decisions about diagnosis and treatment and tailor their treatment approaches to the specific needs and characteristics of patients with various anxiety disorders. This is accomplished by describing not only what to do in treatment but also how to do it.

As the book is put to the test before its readers, I hope that it will help clarify some of the salient issues surrounding the anxiety disorders and help the readers feel better equipped to deal with the various challenges posed by anxiety disorders, without sacrificing appreciation of the complexity of these conditions.

Penrith, New South Wales V.S.
Australia

Contents

Anxiety Disorders in Adults

1

Anxiety Disorders: Introduction

Anxiety disorders can be defined as conditions characterized by pathological anxiety that has not been caused by physical illness, is not associated with substance use, and is not part of a psychotic illness. Since pathological anxiety has been postulated as the sine qua non of anxiety disorders, it is important to first make a distinction between pathological and "normal" anxiety. For the sake of clarifying this matter, the terms *anxiety* and *fear* are used here interchangeably (as they both denote a response to a perceived threat and danger), although some hold the view that conceptual differences do exist between them (see also Table 2–21 and Barlow's account of panic attacks in Chapter 2 for further discussion of this issue).

There is broad agreement that pathological and normal anxiety can be distinguished on the basis of the criteria listed in Table 1–1. These criteria cut across all the components of anxiety: subjective, physiological (somatic), cognitive, and behavioral. Although the criteria may seem clear-cut, in practice it may be difficult to draw a precise boundary between pathological and normal anxiety.

It is often assumed that normal anxiety has an adaptive role, because it serves as a signal that there is danger and that measures need to be taken (e.g., a fight or flight response) to protect oneself against that danger; both the danger perceived and the measures taken are considered appropriate

TABLE 1–1. Pathological Anxiety vs. Normal Anxiety

Criteria for Differentiation	Pathological Anxiety	Normal Anxiety
Intensity	Relatively high and/or out of proportion to the situation or circumstances	Relatively low and/or proportionate to the situation or circumstances
Duration	Generally longer lasting or recurrent	Generally shorter lasting
Preoccupation with anxiety	Yes	No
Quality of the experience	Distressing, overwhelming, incapacitating	Unpleasant, but not too distressing or not distressing for a long time
Effects on behavior and functioning	Causes long-standing changes in behavior, impairs functioning	Generally does not affect behavior more than temporarily, does not impair functioning

(i.e., not exaggerated) in normal anxiety. For example, a student who judges herself to be well below the sufficient level of knowledge and thereby risks failing the exam, doubles the effort to catch up with her studies and tries to minimize the risk of failing. In contrast, pathological anxiety pertains to an inaccurate or excessive appraisal of danger; protective measures taken against this danger are way out of proportion to the real threat.

CONCEPTUALIZATION AND CLASSIFICATION

Anxiety disorders were introduced in 1980 as a distinct nosological group in the Third Edition of the *Diagnostic and Statistical Manual of Mental Disorders* (DSM-III; American Psychiatric Association, 1980). Before DSM-III, anxiety disorders were conceptualized as neuroses, and they encompassed four conditions: (1) anxiety neurosis; (2) phobic neurosis; (3) obsessive-compulsive neurosis, and (4) traumatic neurosis. In DSM-III, anxiety neurosis was divided into panic disorder and generalized anxiety disorder, whereas phobic disorder was split into agoraphobia, social phobia (social anxiety disorder), and simple (specific) phobia. In the revision of DSM-III, DSM-III-R (American Psychiatric Association, 1987), agoraphobia was "moved" to the realm of panic disorder, in recognition of the close relationship between the two: agoraphobia rarely occurs without panic attacks or panic disorder.

Anxiety disorders were retained as a distinct nosological group in the subsequent DSM revisions, from the Fourth Edition, DSM-IV (American Psychiatric Association, 1994), to the text revision of DSM-IV, DSM-IV-TR (American Psychiatric Association, 2000). However, the conceptualization and diagnostic criteria for all psychopathological entities within anxiety disorders underwent changes from DSM-III to DSM-IV-TR; the most important of these changes are presented in the chapters on individual disorders below. In DSM-IV-TR, the group of anxiety disorders includes the following diagnostic entities (Table 1–2): panic disorder (with and without agoraphobia), agoraphobia without history of panic disorder, generalized anxiety disorder, social anxiety disorder (social phobia), specific phobia, obsessive-compulsive disorder, acute stress disorder, posttraumatic stress disorder, anxiety disorder due to a general medical condition, substance-induced anxiety disorder, and anxiety disorder not otherwise specified.

Of these conditions, anxiety disorder due to a general medical condition and substance-induced anxiety disorder do not "belong" in the category of anxiety disorders as they are defined more restrictively in this volume. Likewise, these two disorders have a dual status in DSM-IV-R, as substance-induced anxiety disorder has also been classified among substance-related disorders, while anxiety disorder due to a general medical condition has also been classified among mental disorders due to general medical conditions. "Anxiety disorder not otherwise specified" is a residual diagnostic category, for use in those situations when a diagnosis of the specific anxiety disorder cannot be made.

TABLE 1–2. Disorders Included in the Group of Anxiety Disorders in DSM-IV-TR

Panic disorder without agoraphobia

Panic disorder with agoraphobia

Agoraphobia without history of panic disorder

Generalized anxiety disorder

Social anxiety disorder (social phobia)

Specific phobia

Obsessive-compulsive disorder

Acute stress disorder

Posttraumatic stress disorder

Anxiety disorder due to a general medical condition

Substance-induced anxiety disorder

Anxiety disorder not otherwise specified

In the latest version of the *International Classification of Diseases*, ICD-10 (World Health Organization, 1992), anxiety disorders have not been granted a separate, independent status. Instead, they are a part of a large group of disorders termed "neurotic, stress-related and somatoform disorders." Within such a group, anxiety disorders encountered in the DSM system are placed in four subgroups that resemble the pre–DSM-III classification (see Table 1–3). For most anxiety disorders, there are important differences between the way they are conceptualized and diagnosed in the DSM and ICD systems, and these differences are presented and discussed in the chapters on individual disorders that follow. In addition, ICD-10 has included with anxiety disorders conditions that are not present in the DSM system (e.g., mixed anxiety and depressive disorder) and conditions that are in the DSM system but classified elsewhere (e.g., adjustment disorders).

Conceptual, Diagnostic and Classification Issues

Regardless of whether the DSM or ICD conceptualization and classification are adopted, the classification overhauls of anxiety disorders during

Table 1–3. Classification of Anxiety Disorders in ICD-10[a]

Phobic Anxiety Disorders

Agoraphobia without panic disorder

Agoraphobia with panic disorder

Social phobias

Specific (isolated) phobias

Other Anxiety Disorders

Panic disorder (episodic paroxysmal anxiety)

Generalized anxiety disorder

Mixed anxiety and depressive disorder

Obsessive-Compulsive Disorder

Reaction to Severe Stress and Adjustment Disorders

Acute stress reaction

Posttraumatic stress disorder

Adjustment disorders

[a]"Other" and "unspecified" diagnostic categories are excluded, as are subtypes of obsessive-compulsive disorder and adjustment disorders.

the last two decades have resulted in splitting the four pre–DSM-III diagnostic entities into a large number of diagnostic subcategories. Moreover, the diagnostic categories within anxiety disorders have undergone further splitting, so that almost all the categories now have two or more subtypes. The upshot of this trend is a high likelihood for various anxiety disorders and their subtypes to co-occur. Therefore, high rates of co-occurrence among the anxiety disorders—or "comorbidity," as this phenomenon is often referred to—are not surprising. The rarity of pure cases of most anxiety disorders in clinical practice is a logical consequence of this situation. More often than not, however, the high rates of comorbidity do not reflect a genuine co-occurrence of independent disorders, but rather are likely to represent an artifact of the splitting classification trends.

Another issue has arisen from the creation of so many categories of anxiety disorders: the presumed distinctness of many of the anxiety disorders and their construct validity have yet to be confirmed. There have also been calls to halt the proliferation of diagnostic categories and look more for what the individual anxiety disorders share than for the ways in which they differ. The links between anxiety disorders, depression, somatoform disorders, and some personality disorders have been emphasized in an attempt to understand how these apparently distinct forms of psychopathology are related to each other, especially over time (e.g., through a "general neurotic syndrome," Tyrer, 1985; Tyrer et al., 1992). However, these attempts at "lumping" and integration have generally been ignored by the architects of the major classification systems. The splitting trends seem likely to continue, which will have further consequences on how anxiety disorders are conceptualized and classified.

Anxiety disorders are grouped together on the basis of the assumption that pathological anxiety is their common, defining characteristic. But it is not clear that this is the case with all the disorders that are included in the DSM-IV-TR group of anxiety disorders. For example, it can be argued that posttraumatic stress disorder is as much a disorder of memory, a dissociative disorder, or even a condition that should be placed in its "own" class of trauma-related disorders as it is an anxiety disorder (see Table 1–4 and Chapter 7). By contrast, some conditions that are currently not included among the anxiety disorders in DSM-IV-TR (e.g., some forms of hypochondriasis and personality disturbance such as avoidant personality disorder) may be better conceptualized as anxiety disorders. The conceptual and diagnostic dilemmas about specific anxiety disorders are summarized in Table 1–4 and discussed below with regard to individual disorders.

Table 1–4. Conceptual and Diagnostic Dilemmas about Specific Anxiety Disorders

Disorders	Dilemmas
Panic disorder	1. Should panic disorder have a diagnostic primacy over agoraphobia when both are present?
	2. Is agoraphobia always secondary to panic attacks? Can agoraphobia be an entity in its own right or is it merely a subtype of panic disorder?
Generalized anxiety disorder	1. Is generalized anxiety disorder a diagnosis in search of its unique psychopathology? Is it a valid diagnostic category?
	2. Does generalized anxiety disorder really exist in the absence of depression or other anxiety disorders?
Social anxiety disorder disorder	Should the generalized subtype of social anxiety be conceptualized as personality disturbance?
Specific phobia	In view of its heterogeneity, should a specific phobia be split into its current subtypes, as separate diagnostic entities?
Obsessive-compulsive disorder	1. Should obsessive-compulsive disorder be retained among the anxiety disorders or be classified elsewhere?
	2. Are there clinically meaningful subtypes of obsessive-compulsive disorder?
Posttraumatic stress disorder	In view of its complexity and heterogeneity, should posttraumatic stress disorder be placed in its own class of trauma-related disorders? Should it be considered a primary disorder of memory, or as a dissociative disorder?

Etiological Models

The etiological understanding of the anxiety disorders continues to be split into biological and psychological models. There is an increasing need, however, to combine the contributions of these models in an effort to arrive at a more comprehensive understanding of the etiology and pathogenesis of anxiety disorders.

Regardless of the preferred model, conceptualizing the predisposing, precipitating, and maintaining factors can afford better etiological understanding of the anxiety disorders. Also, this is where the main differences between various etiological models can be found: for example, biological models postulate that people are predisposed to develop anxiety disorders because of their genetic makeup, whereas psychological models find this predisposition in early childhood events, in certain personality features, or in the way that the symptoms are perceived and appraised. Whatever the nature of the predisposition, it is "dormant" until the precipitating factors—usually certain life events—"activate" this predisposition, bringing about a disorder. The factors that maintain anxiety disorders are particularly emphasized in behavioral and cognitive models, and these factors are targeted accordingly by the behavioral and cognitive therapies.

No biological model has proved to be unique for any particular type of anxiety disorder, although some models may be relatively more specific for some anxiety disorders. In addition, various biological mechanisms may operate in the same anxiety disorder.

Several types of studies have examined the role of genetic factors in the etiology of anxiety disorders. They include family studies (studies of the first-degree relatives of probands with a particular anxiety disorder), twin studies, and, more recently, genetic linkage studies. No adoption studies of anxiety disorders have been reported. Family studies have been most commonly conducted, with findings of increased rates of specific anxiety disorders in first-degree relatives of probands with the same anxiety disorders being interpreted as a sign of possible genetic transmission. Such findings may also reflect influence of the shared environment on family members. Genetic studies generally suggest that there may be a genetic predisposition for some anxiety disorders in certain patients. It is not yet known, however, what this predisposition entails and what is inherited.

Studies of the neurotransmitter systems in anxiety disorders have largely been propelled by the efficacy of medications that act via the corresponding transmitters. Since several types of medications have been efficacious in several types of anxiety disorders, it is not surprising that many findings suggestive of specific neurotransmitter abnormalities are, in fact, nonspecific for any particular type of anxiety disorder. The only exception to this may be a relative specificity of the serotonin system abnormalities in obsessive-compulsive disorder. It is not clear whether some of the neurotransmitter abnormalities precede the onset of anxiety disorders, whether they are a biological marker, a consequence, or a correlate of these disorders, or whether they are more associated with conditions that co-occur with particular anxiety disorders.

The psychological models of anxiety disorders that are most relevant for clinical practice include behavioral, cognitive, and psychodynamic models. Behavioral models are based on the learning theory and emphasize the crucial role of behaviors such as avoidance in maintaining the disorders. The latter explains the focus on behavior modification in behavior therapy. The behavioral models are often criticized as simplistic, and indeed, they often do not provide a convincing account of the acquisition of fear and origin of anxiety disorders. Behavior therapy has nonethesess been the most successful psychological treatment across all the anxiety disorders, and it should be a part of any pragmatic treatment approach.

Cognitive models of anxiety disorders emphasize the role of specific beliefs and appraisals of threat and of one's ability to cope. These models are becoming increasingly popular, perhaps because they attempt to give a fairly comprehensive account of anxiety disorders and seem credible in doing so. However, cognitive models have generally not been sufficiently tested, and the treatment based on them has yet to demonstrate whether it is as efficacious as behavior therapy. The attractiveness of cognitive models—and cognitive therapy—also lies in their radical dismantling of the psychological mechanisms in anxiety disorders and in their proposition that therapeutic change should occur as a result of changes in the more fundamental patterns of thinking. At the same time, this ambitious proposition may be the reason why cognitive therapy seems less pragmatic and perhaps less applicable to *all* patients with anxiety disorders.

The psychodynamic models of anxiety disorders invoke several concepts that are now often considered controversial, if not untenable. These modes are nonetheless reasonably well placed within the general psychodynamic theory. The main general aspect of psychodynamic models is the proposition that "neurotic" anxiety occurs as a result of intrapsychic conflicts between sexual or aggressive urges and defenses erected against these urges—and, more broadly, that such anxiety signals the existence of certain unconscious processes or phenomena. Therefore, the goal of psychodynamic treatment is that patients gain insight into these unconscious conflicts and resolve them, thus "releasing" the person from anxiety. The efficacy of psychodynamic psychotherapy for anxiety disorders has barely been studied, but it is certainly not the type of treatment that should be or could be routinely offered to patients with these conditions.

TREATMENT

With recent emphasis on evidence-based treatments in psychiatry, clinicians are in a better position to administer treatments that are likely to work. The reality of clinical practice, however, calls for treatment of patients who do not easily match patients on whom various evidence-based treatment guidelines and algorithms are based. The latter usually come from research settings in which randomized, controlled trials have been conducted, and they may have relatively "pure" and uncomplicated forms of psychopathology and are not necessarily representative of patients in the real world. Thus, we have a somewhat paradoxical situation: although there are many evidence-based treatment guidelines and algorithms for anxiety disorders, clinicians are often puzzled as to how to apply them to individual patients or do not apply them at all.

Part of the reason for treatment guidelines and algorithms being difficult to implement is their frequent failure to take into account different treatment goals for different patients. That is, treatment guidelines and algorithms erroneously assume that all patients have the same treatment goals. Because different treatment goals often imply a need for different treatment approaches, it is reasonable to first identify treatment goals and then consider various treatment options for achieving these goals.

Treatment goals for anxiety disorders should be openly discussed with patients and patients should be encouraged to formulate their own goals. Treatment goals may be expressed in many different ways. Typical patient statements, which reflect diverse expectations, are "controlling my anxiety," "getting rid of it," "not having to avoid things," or "wanting my normal life back." Some of these expectations may be rather unrealistic (e.g., "never again feeling anxious," "having full control over my life," "completely eliminating my anxiety"), and when these are identified, it is important to point out to patients that such expectations cannot serve as the basis for formulating treatment goals. Actively engaging patients in formulating their treatment goals and in the treatment decision-making process is fundamental, because the responsibility for the course and outcome of treatment should be shared between patients and therapists. This is the foundation for *collaborative negotiation* between patients and therapists in the treatment process.

All treatment goals for anxiety disorders pertain to reducing the negative impacts of anxiety (Fig. 1–1). The disagreements, particularly among therapists, pertain mainly to how negative impacts of anxiety are to be reduced. Whereas some clinicians prefer to achieve this by suppressing the symptoms of anxiety with a medication, others use different strategies (Fig. 1–1).

It is important to point out that different treatment goals are not mutually exclusive, especially at different stages of treatment. For example, a patient may initially request quick relief of anxiety and the associated physical symptoms, whereas later he or she may want to be free from the fear of anxiety and its symptoms. By the same token, treatment strategies used to achieve these goals are not inherently incompatible, hence a rationale for the use of both pharmacotherapy and cognitive-behavioral therapy, either sequentially or simultaneously, is possible.

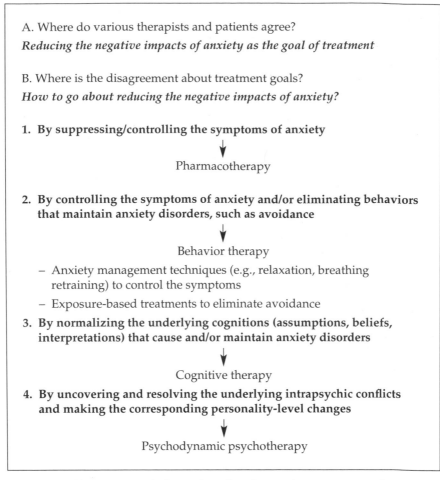

A. Where do various therapists and patients agree?
Reducing the negative impacts of anxiety as the goal of treatment

B. Where is the disagreement about treatment goals?
How to go about reducing the negative impacts of anxiety?

1. **By suppressing/controlling the symptoms of anxiety**
   ↓
   Pharmacotherapy

2. **By controlling the symptoms of anxiety and/or eliminating behaviors that maintain anxiety disorders, such as avoidance**
   ↓
   Behavior therapy
   – Anxiety management techniques (e.g., relaxation, breathing retraining) to control the symptoms
   – Exposure-based treatments to eliminate avoidance
3. **By normalizing the underlying cognitions (assumptions, beliefs, interpretations) that cause and/or maintain anxiety disorders**
   ↓
   Cognitive therapy
4. **By uncovering and resolving the underlying intrapsychic conflicts and making the corresponding personality-level changes**
   ↓
   Psychodynamic psychotherapy

Figure 1–1. Treatment goals for anxiety disorders and treatments used to achieve these goals.

Pharmacotherapy or Psychological Therapy? Or Both?

Ideological battles about the efficacy and usefulness of various treatments in anxiety disorders are still vehemently fought. The profession is no longer divided over the value of psychoanalysis and psychodynamic psychotherapy, as these forms of psychological therapy are not generally regarded first-line treatment for anxiety disorders. The focus has now shifted to pharmacotherapy and cognitive-behavioral therapy, with their relative advantages and disadvantages often being bitterly debated. For example, an anonymous biological psychiatrist, cited in van Dyck and van Balkom (1997), had this to say about cognitive-behavioral therapy: "Exposure is not a real therapy, but the acquisition of a stoic attitude toward symptoms . . . Cognitive therapy [is] a form of indoctrination" (p. 112). Tyrer (1999), in contrast, has made the following statement about the pharmacotherapy of anxiety disorders: "All new drug treatments of anxiety should be regarded as addictive until proved otherwise" (p. 117). Such views do not merely promote a dialogue between various mental health professionals; they also impede progress in our efforts to offer patients more efficacious treatments. Offering patients one type of treatment while denigrating the other does not take into consideration what particular patients need and therefore does not reflect a genuine intent to help; rather, such an attitude reflects the therapist's allegiance to a group within which beliefs about etiology and treatment are shared.

A well-balanced, nondogmatic approach to the choice of treatment of anxiety disorders involves matching treatment goals with treatment modalities (Fig. 1–1). In addition, the clinician should take into consideration short term and long-term treatment effects. Pharmacotherapy usually produces therapeutic effects faster than cognitive-behavioral therapy, it is

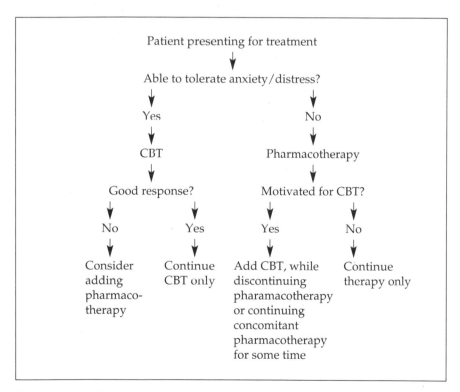

Figure 1–2. Initial and subsequent choice of treatment in anxiety disorders. CBT, cognitive–behavioral therapy.

TABLE 1–5. Factors That Affect Treatment Choice in Anxiety Disorders

Treatment-Related Factors

- Well-established efficacy (short-term efficacy: no advantage for pharmacotherapy or CBT, or may favor pharmacotherapy; long-term efficacy: generally favors CBT)
- Faster onset of therapeutic effects (favors pharmacotherapy)
- General ease of administration (favors pharmacotherapy)
- Wide availability (favors pharmacotherapy)
- Relatively low cost (favors pharmacotherapy; in the long run, this advantage may be lost to CBT)

Disorder-Related Factors

- Greater overall severity of the disorder (the more severe the disorder is, the more likely it is for pharmacotherapy to be used)
- Greater disability caused by the disorder (the more disabled patients are, the more likely it is for pharmacotherapy to be used)
- Presence of other disorders, especially depression (generally favors pharmacotherapy)

Patient-Related Factors

- Specific needs of patients, which determine treatment goals (pharmacotherapy or CBT may be preferred, depending on the treatment goals)
- Ability to tolerate symptoms, anxiety, and distress (the greater this ability is, the more likely that CBT will be used)
- Ability to withstand treatment-associated discomfort (e.g., side effects of medications or deliberate induction of anxiety in the course of CBT)
- Specific attitudes toward medications and psychological treatment (pharmacotherapy or CBT may be preferred, depending on the nature of these attitudes)
- Motivation, "psychological-mindedness," ambitiousness of treatment goals (the greater these are, the more likely that CBT will be used)

Clinician-Related Factors

- Clinician's preferences for or bias against pharmacotherapy or CBT
- Degree of familiarity with pharmacotherapy or CBT

CBT, cognitive-behavioral therapy.

easier to administer, and it is more widely available. But medications usually work in anxiety disorders only for as long as they are taken, and relapse rates following their discontinuation tend to be high. Cognitive-behavioral therapy generally takes longer to work; it is more demanding and less available than pharmacotherapy. Its main advantage, however, is a greater likelihood of producing long-lasting treatment effects that tend to persist after the cessation of treatment, with relatively low relapse rates.

Since most patients with anxiety disorders usually want a relatively quick relief of their anxiety and distress, as well as long-term benefit of the therapy, ideal treatments should be able to produce both short-term and long-term therapeutic effects. In reality, such treatments rarely exist, and the two main treatment options may be offered initially on the basis of the patient's need, or lack thereof, to have anxiety or distress quickly alleviated (Fig. 1–2). Thus, if the patient cannot tolerate anxiety or distress, the usual initial choice of treatment is pharmacotherapy; if the patient is able to tolerate anxiety or distress, cognitive-behavioral therapy may be offered from the beginning of treatment. Later in the course of treatment, these initial choices may be modified depending on the patient's response, but also on the basis of the patient's needs and preferences (Fig. 1–2). The issues arising from combining pharmacotherapy and cognitive-behavioral therapy are addressed in more detail in Chapter 2. In clinical practice, it is usually a combination of factors that is taken into account when treatment decisions are made; these factors and their impact are presented in Table 1–5.

2
Panic Disorder With and Without Agoraphobia

Panic disorder is characterized by two components: recurrent panic attacks and anticipatory anxiety. Panic attacks within panic disorder are not caused by physical illness or certain substances and they are unexpected, at least initially; later in the course of the disorder, many attacks may be precipitated by certain situations or are more likely to occur in them. *Anticipatory anxiety* is an intense fear of having another panic attack, which is present between panic attacks. Some patients with panic disorder go on to develop *agoraphobia*, defined as fear and/or avoidance of the situations from which escape might be difficult or embarrassing or in which help might not be available in case of a panic attack; in such cases, patients are diagnosed with panic disorder with agoraphobia. Those who do not develop agoraphobia receive a diagnosis of panic disorder without agoraphobia. Components of panic disorder are presented in Figure 2–1.

Patients with agoraphobia who have no history of panic disorder or whose agoraphobia is not related at least to panic attacks or symptoms of panic attacks are rarely encountered in clinical practice. The diagnosis of agoraphobia without history of panic disorder has been a matter of some controversy, especially in view of the differences between American and European psychiatrists (and the DSM and ICD diagnostic and classification systems) in the conceptualization of the relationship between panic disor-

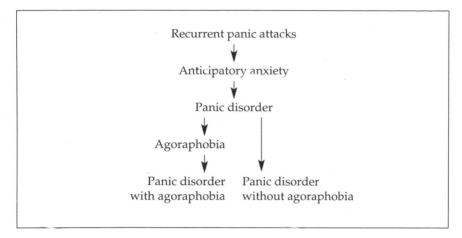

Figure 2–1. Components of panic disorder.

der and agoraphobia. The conceptualization adhered to here is the one derived from the DSM system, as there is more empirical support for it.

CLINICAL FEATURES

Panic Attacks

There is no universal description of a panic attack, because attacks differ in terms of their symptoms and how they are experienced. *Panic attacks* can nonetheless be defined as sudden episodes of severe anxiety that are characterized by physical symptoms and anticipation of dreadful consequences. The affected person typically believes that something horrific is about to happen and often has a tendency to escape right away, perhaps in an attempt to avert such a catastrophe. Panic attacks reach their peak very quickly (within 10 minutes according to DSM-IV-TR) and usually last up to half an hour. After the attack, patients typically feel tired or exhausted. The frequency of panic attacks can vary greatly even in the same patient: from an occasional attack in months or years to dozens of attacks a day.

There are several features that make panic attack a unique experience, and not merely a more severe form of anxiety (Table 2–1). First, panic attacks occur abruptly and, at least initially, they are often described as "coming out of clear blue skies." Second, panic attacks reach the peak of their intensity very quickly. Third, panic attacks are characterized by prominent physical symptoms (e.g., heart racing or pounding, shortness of breath, dizziness), which often dominate the entire clinical presentation. Fourth, patients react to physical symptoms with a sense of a catastrophe,

TABLE 2–1. Distinction Between Panic Attacks and Anxiety

Factor	Panic Attacks	Anxiety
Onset	Abrupt, sudden	More gradual
Reaching peak of intensity of anxiety	Very quickly (maximum 10 minutes)	More slowly
Physical symptoms	Very prominent	Not necessarily prominent
Catastrophizing	Very typical and prominent	Less typical and not prominent
Behavioral response	Immediate escape	Delayed escape, avoidance
Overall duration	Relatively short	Variable, but usually longer

as they believe that something terrible is going to happen to them as a result of their symptoms: they are going to die, lose control, or go mad. Fifth, there is a sense of urgency in the behavioral response to panic attacks; for example, patients have to escape immediately to a place perceived as safe. Sixth, panic attacks do not last very long—often 10–20 minutes—and only rarely is their duration longer than 1 hour; however, the duration of an attack may seem much longer to the sufferers.

The experience of a panic is usually puzzling and frightening, especially when it occurs for the first time. If there is nothing obvious in the person's life circumstances or current situation that might make it possible for him or her to understand the occurrence of a panic attack, as is often the case, the attack is experienced with even more bewilderment. The anxiety reaction precipitated by exposure to an objectively dangerous or life-threatening situation is usually not conceptualized as a panic attack, although it may have many characteristics of a panic attack, except that catastrophizing is not present (see Table 2–1).

It is intriguing to note not only what brings on panic attacks but also which mechanisms are involved in their cessation. Radomsky et al. (1998) have speculated that panic attacks cease because of physical exhaustion, which, in turn, is caused by extreme autonomic hyperarousal. Some patients believe that they can terminate panic attacks by escaping from the situations in which attacks occur or by taking medications that act "very fast." But these are only examples of an illusion of having some control over the attacks. Patients may learn to abort panic attacks by slow breathing if hyperventilation is the main pathophysiological mechanism that triggers the attacks.

Types of Attacks

According to DSM-IV-TR, there are three types of panic attacks: unexpected, situationally predisposed, and situationally bound (Table 2–2).

TABLE 2–2. Types of Panic Attacks According to DSM-IV-TR

	Association with Particular Situations, Objects, or Events	Disorders in which Type of Attacks Is Usually Seen
Unexpected	None	Panic disorder without agoraphobia
Situationally predisposed	Moderately strong (greater likelihood of the attacks occurring on exposure to certain situations, objects, or events)	Agoraphobia (panic disorder with agoraphobia) Less common in social anxiety disorder and specific phobias
Situationally bound	Very strong (attacks occur almost always and immediately on exposure to certain situations, objects, or events)	Social anxiety disorder and specific phobias May also be seen in agoraphobia (panic disorder with agoraphobia)

Unexpected panic attacks occur "spontaneously," which means that the person does not associate their occurrence with any particular situation, object, or event. Of course, that does not mean that such attacks are never triggered by external influences; it is more likely that such influences are just not apparent to the person, and attacks are therefore experienced as occurring "for no reason." Unexpected attacks are typically seen in panic disorder without agoraphobia, especially during initial stages of the condition, before the patient has "learned" to expect panic attacks in certain situations.

Situationally predisposed panic attacks are more likely to occur in certain situations, but they do not occur every time the patient is in that situation; also, the attacks do not necessarily occur immediately upon exposure to that situation. For example, a patient may experience a panic attack after leaving home, but the occurrence of panic attacks cannot be reliably predicted by the patient being in that situation. Sometimes panic attacks do not occur at all, whereas at other times, they may occur hours after the patient has left home. This type of attacks is characteristic of agoraphobia (and panic disorder with agoraphobia), but may also be seen among patients with social anxiety disorder and specific phobias.

Situationally bound panic attacks occur almost always and immediately upon exposure to a certain situation or object or while the patient is anticipating such an exposure. In other words, the exposure or anticipation of exposure almost invariably provokes a panic attack. For example, patients with a phobia of spiders have panic attacks upon seeing a spider or merely thinking that they are going to see a spider in certain situations. Situationally bound panic attacks are typical of social anxiety disorder and specific phobias, but may also be seen in patients with agoraphobia.

These types of panic attacks are phenomenologically very similar and their crucial differentiating characteristic pertains to whether or not they are associated with certain situations, objects, or events. However, some studies (e.g., Klein and Klein, 1989) suggest that in comparison with other types of attacks, situationally bound panic attacks are characterized by fewer respiratory symptoms and less prominent fears of dying, losing control, or going crazy. Also, unlike situational attacks, unexpected attacks seem amenable to suppression by antidepressant medications (Uhlenhuth et al., 2000, 2002).

Because of the unpredictability of the occurrence of unexpected and situationally predisposed panic attacks and difficulty of controlling them by avoidance of the corresponding situations, patients with these types of attacks may be more afraid of them than patients who only have situationally bound attacks.

Physical Symptoms

Although the DSM-IV-TR diagnostic criteria stipulate that any combination of at least four symptoms is sufficient for the diagnosis of a panic attack, it appears that some physical symptoms are more frequent and more typical of panic attacks (Rapee et al., 1990a; Starcevic et al., 1993a; Cox et al., 1994b). Therefore, they could be termed "first-rank" panic symptoms (Table 2–3). These include heart racing (tachycardia) and pounding

TABLE 2–3. Physical Symptoms During Panic Attacks

First-Rank Physical Symptoms, Also Useful for Screening Purposes

Heart racing (tachycardia) and pounding (palpitations)

Dizziness, lightheadedness, or fainting feeling

Shortness of breath

Choking sensations

Other First-Rank Physical Symptoms

Chest discomfort or pain

Sweating

Trembling

Second-Rank Physical Symptoms

Hot and cold flushes

Numbness or tingling sensations

Nausea or upset stomach

(palpitations), dizziness or lightheadedness, shortness of breath, choking sensations, chest discomfort or pain, sweating, and trembling. Of these first-rank symptoms, there are several (heart racing and pounding, dizziness or lightheadedness, shortness of breath, and choking sensations) that could be used for screening purposes. Patients in whom panic disorder is suspected should routinely be asked about these symptoms, because at least one of them is likely to be present during a panic attack. Other physical symptoms are less common and less typical of a panic attack and could be considered "second-rank": hot and cold flushes, numbness or tingling sensations, and nausea or upset stomach.

It has been suggested (Briggs et al., 1993) that panic attacks could be differentiated on the basis of the presence or absence of prominent respiratory symptoms (shortness of breath, choking sensations, hyperventilation). Panic attacks with prominent respiratory symptoms are characterized by chest pain, numbness or tingling sensations, and fear of dying; they are more likely to be unexpected and may respond better to imipramine. In contrast, panic attacks without prominent respiratory symptoms are more likely to be situationally bound and may respond better to alprazolam. The distinction between respiratory and nonrespiratory types of panic attacks has received further support (e.g., Biber and Alkin, 1999; Nardi et al., 2003), but the presence or absence of respiratory symptoms during panic attacks has not yet become a major factor in the selection of medication for panic disorder.

Psychological Aspects

Although there are reports of nonfearful panic attacks, most patients describe panic attacks as being not only unpleasant but also frightening. Such an experience of panic is usually a consequence of the particular (catastrophic) interpretation of physical symptoms occurring during panic attacks. Broadly speaking, there are two types of catastrophes that panic patients anticipate (Table 2–4): one pertains to the physical consequences of an attack and the other to psychological and social consequences. As for physical consequences, patients are afraid that they might die suddenly (usually from a heart attack, stroke, or choking) or that they might collapse, lose consciousness, fall, and/or injure themselves.

The feared psychological and social consequences of panic attacks are reflected in frightening thoughts about losing control, going mad, "making a scene," and/or embarrassing oneself. Panic patients often feel that they do not know what they will be doing during the attack, that they might run aimlessly and "look crazy," that they might say something senseless, scream, or behave in an inappropriate or aggressive manner. Although these consequences of panic do not occur, paradoxically this does not

Table 2–4. Catastrophes Anticipated as a Consequence of Panic Attacks and Related Fears

Physical Consequences

Fear of dying suddenly from

   Heart attack

   Stroke

   Choking

Fear of collapsing, losing consciousness, falling, and/or injuring oneself

Psychological and Social Consequences

Fear of losing control

Fear of going mad

Fear of "making a scene"

Fear of embarrassing oneself

---

diminish patients' beliefs that "something dreadful" will happen. Patients often think that they were "lucky" in the past and that a catastrophe will certainly occur next time.

Patients' ability to concentrate is often diminished during the attacks, and they may feel that they cannot plan or think rationally. This is true to a certain extent, as patients are typically immersed in the frightening experience and may have trouble focusing away from that experience and thinking clearly about other matters. However, their appraisal of their cognitive abilities is distorted in that they are much more able to act rationally than they think they are. In fact, the only "irrational act" to which patients may be prone during a panic attack is leaving suddenly or escaping; when they do that, it may seem somewhat unusual to others, but not "crazy," as patients often think.

Patients tend to feel that their panic experience sets them apart from others; they perceive panic as rather unique, unusual, and/or very difficult to describe. Patients often feel isolated because of panic and are surprised when they learn that other people also have panic attacks. Because panic is usually experienced in this manner, it is not unusual for patients to feel that no one can understand them. This may lead to a feeling that they are beyond the reach of any help. Recurrent panic attacks, accompanied by a feeling of helplessness and a strong sense of being unable to cope, may also undermine patients' hope and lead to demoralization.

Depersonalization and derealization experiences during panic attacks occur in various forms and are experienced with varying intensity. Patients typically state that they feel as if they were not real or as if their personality and identity had changed. In more extreme cases, patients report that they feel detached from their bodies, observing themselves as if they were at a certain distance. Panic patients usually respond to these experiences with fear that they signal a loss of control and onset of madness.

Behavioral Aspects

The most typical behavioral response to a panic attack is escape. Because they feel vitally threatened or fear that they might lose control, panic patients have an urge to "do something" to escape the danger. And, because the danger is usually associated with the situation or a place in which the attack has occurred, patients feel compelled to flee to a place where they would feel safe. Depending on the nature of the underlying fear, that safety may be provided by one's home, or emergency room of a hospital. Safety, comfort, and reassurance are usually sought from family members and friends or from health-care professionals.

Many patients believe that during the attacks they lose the ability to act rationally and are often concerned that their performance will be impaired. This usually does not happen, however. If the panic attack occurs while patients are engaged in some activity—for example, driving—patients react in different ways: some will continue with their activity (even as they feel apprehensive about panic and its symptoms), whereas others will feel that they have to stop, at least for a brief period of time. Only a few patients feel so incapacitated that they are unable to continue driving for prolonged periods of time. Contrary to their expectations, panic patients tend to behave rationally in situations of real danger and do not jeopardize themselves or others by their behavior (e.g., Starcevic et al., 2002).

Panic patients often believe that their attacks are visible to others and are therefore concerned that the panic might reveal their "weakness." But other people are usually not aware that someone is experiencing a panic attack, and may only guess that "something" is happening to patients on those rare occasions when patients' behavior is unusual because of a panic attack (e.g., when they suddenly leave a social situation).

Variants of Panic Attacks

In addition to typical, full-blown panic attacks, there are several variants that either do not meet full diagnostic criteria for panic attacks or have special features. These variants include limited-symptom attacks, nonclinical attacks, nocturnal attacks, and nonfearful attacks (Table 2–5).

TABLE 2–5. Variants of Panic Attacks

Variant	Defining Characteristics
Limited-symptom attacks	Fewer symptoms during panic attacks (less than four according to DSM-IV-TR)
Nonclinical attacks	Panic attacks for which no help is sought
Nocturnal attacks	Panic attacks that occur during sleep
Nonfearful attacks	Fear is not experienced or reported during panic attacks

Limited-Symptom Attacks

Limited-symptom panic attacks are characterized by fewer symptoms—less than four according to DSM-IV-TR. The demarcation on the basis of the number of symptoms, and not on the basis of their severity, is arbitrary; there are patients who have panic attacks with only two or three severe symptoms and patients with full-blown panic attacks who have more than four symptoms of mild intensity. Consequently, patients with limited-symptom attacks may be more disabled than those with the full-blown ones, and except for the number of symptoms, limited-panic attacks may in other respects be identical to full-blown attacks (Katerndahl, 1990). Likewise, limited-panic attacks should be treated in the same way as full-blown attacks are. Limited-symptom attacks usually occur along with full-blown attacks. During the treatment of panic disorder, the appearance of limited-symptom attacks and disappearance of full-blown attacks may indicate improvement, but not a full response. Some patients continue to occasionally experience limited-symptom panic attacks for a long time after their treatment has ceased. The clinical significance of limited-symptom attacks that do not occur as part of panic disorder is not clear.

Nonclinical Attacks

Nonclinical panic attacks have been observed in people who do not seek help for panic. These attacks are quite common in the population and are more frequently encountered among women. In comparison with full-blown panic attacks, nonclinical attacks are less severe and less frequent, they have fewer symptoms, and they are far less often characterized by fears of dying, losing control, and/or going mad (Telch et al., 1989b; Cox et al., 1992). Nonclinical attacks appear in stressful situations, especially when the person's performance and behavior are under scrutiny from others—for example, when taking a test or being examined (Norton et al., 1986). The circumstances under which help is sought for the previously nonclinical panic attacks are not clear. It can be speculated that this occurs when persons become excessively concerned about the attacks and their potential consequences (Telch et al., 1989b).

Nocturnal Attacks

Nocturnal panic attacks usually occur along with panic attacks during the day, but some patients experience mainly nocturnal attacks. These attacks may characterize a more severe form of panic disorder (Labbate et al., 1994), but this view has recently been disputed (Craske et al., 2002). Typically, patients wake up in the midst of an attack, often with intense fear and severe symptoms, particularly shortness of breath and a choking feeling. Nocturnal attacks do not occur during the rapid eye movement (REM) phase of sleep, and are not preceded by dreams or nightmares. Therefore, patients usually do not confuse nocturnal panic attacks with dreams and nightmares. The sleep is usually disturbed as a consequence of nocturnal attacks, and patients often have difficulty falling asleep after such attacks. Patients' memory for the details of nocturnal attacks is usually excellent. Patients with nocturnal panic attacks seem distressed by sleep and other states in which they are not fully vigilant (e.g., relaxation, meditation, hypnotic trance), because of the association between attacks and the state of consciousness in which the attacks usually occur (Craske et al., 2002). These patients are less likely to develop agoraphobia and tend to respond to cognitive-behavioral therapy just as well as other panic patients (Craske et al., 2002).

Nonfearful Panic Attacks

These are a controversial type of panic attacks (Kushner and Beitman, 1990), because they are not characterized by fear, hence the alternative terms "somatic panic," "noncognitive panic," "alexythymic panic," and "masked anxiety." Since there is no reported fear, what qualifies them as panic attacks? Phenomenologically, they look like panic attacks, except for the absence of fear: they are characterized by a sudden surge of physical (usually cardiac) symptoms. Like "regular" panic attacks, nonfearful attacks can be induced by lactate infusions and treated with the same medications (Russell et al., 1991). In view of the nature of their symptoms, patients with nonfearful panic attacks usually seek help from primary-care physicians and various specialists, particularly cardiologists. A recent study (Fleet et al., 2000b) has estimated that 32%–41% of panic disorder patients who seek treatment for chest pain have a nonfearful panic disorder. Panic disorder is recognized in the minority of such patients; without treatment, the prognosis of patients with these panic attacks is relatively poor. The absence of the experience of fear, so typical of "normal" panic attacks, is striking: the question of how physical symptoms occurring during the attacks are processed and interpreted by patients remains open. Perhaps the fear is underreported, deeply repressed, denied, or "somatized," but this is all highly speculative.

Anticipatory Anxiety

Anticipatory anxiety is at least as important as panic attacks for the conceptualization of panic disorder. There are several ways in which anticipatory anxiety can be defined (Table 2–6). Most broadly, anticipatory anxiety (sometimes also referred to as "fear of fear") can be defined as a persistent and almost constant fear of having another panic attack (and/or fear of certain symptoms during the attack). More specifically, this fear pertains to the anticipated consequences of panic attacks. These consequences may be of a physical, psychological, or social nature, with patients typically fearing that they might die, go crazy, or embarrass themselves as a result of panic attacks.

In DSM-IV-TR, anticipatory anxiety is deemed essential for the diagnosis of panic disorder and is conceptualized in the ways referred to above. If the patient does not have these typical features of anticipatory anxiety, DSM-IV-TR makes a provision that there should be a significant and consistent change in the patient's behavior, that is related to panic attacks and reflects anticipatory anxiety. For example, this change can pertain to avoidance of certain situations or undergoing numerous medical investigations.

It is an intriguing question as to why some individuals only experience occasional panic attacks, whereas others are distressed by the anxious anticipation of the attacks more than by the attacks themselves. It can be assumed that persons who develop anticipatory anxiety (and thereby panic disorder) are in some way predisposed to it; for example, this predisposition may involve a belief that anxiety and its symptoms are dangerous (see Etiology and Pathogenesis, below).

TABLE 2–6. Meanings of Anticipatory Anxiety

Persistent and almost constant fear of

    Having another panic attack

    Certain symptoms of panic attacks

    Anticipated consequences of panic attacks:

        Physical consequences (death through a heart attack, stroke, choking, etc.)

        Psychological consequences (loss of control, becoming "crazy," etc.)

        Social consequences (embarrassment, shame, etc.)

As already noted, anticipatory anxiety may be more pronounced among patients with unexpected panic attacks, because the occurrence of such attacks is unpredictable and cannot be prevented by avoidance or other behavioral "maneuvers." Anticipatory anxiety may be overshadowed, however, by avoidance behavior in those patients whose panic attacks are largely predictable, that is, bound to certain situations.

Agoraphobia

Among patients with panic disorder, agoraphobia is seen along the continuum of severity—from very mild cases that do not require immediate treatment and in which phobic avoidance disappears with successful treatment of other components of panic disorder, to severe avoidance, when patients are homebound and treatment has to immediately address the agoraphobic component of illness.

As stated before, *agoraphobia* is defined as the fear and/or avoidance of various situations from which escape might be difficult or embarrassing or in which help might not be available in case of a panic attack. In accordance with this definition, there are two basic themes that link various situations that agoraphobic patients fear and avoid; these themes are related to different means of acquiring a sense of safety (Table 2–7).

The first theme pertains to the fear of being confined or trapped, and the corresponding concern that patients will not be able to escape *immediately* in case of a panic attack. The urge to escape is so strong because panic attacks are perceived as dangerous, and patients may believe that attacks will attenuate or disappear only if they know in advance that they can escape. Therefore, just being able to escape is for many agoraphobic patients of crucial importance and is also the main criterion that distinguishes between "safe" and "unsafe" situations. Indeed, not being able to escape may be the main reason why some agoraphobic patients are afraid of flying or traveling on trains or buses; patients typically state that they

TABLE 2–7. Underlying Themes in Agoraphobic Patients' Thinking and Means of Acquiring a Sense of Safety in Agoraphobia

Underlying Danger-Driven Beliefs	Means of Acquiring a Sense of Safety
It is dangerous to be in a confined place from which immediate escape might be difficult (in case of a panic attack)	Being able to escape immediately
It is dangerous if professional (medical) help is not immediately available (in case of a panic attack)	Being able to access medical help immediately

are more afraid when trains or buses make no stops, rendering their escape, in case of a panic attack, impossible.

The second theme is related to the patients' need to get *immediate* medical help in case of a panic attack. These patients believe that there will be dire consequences if help is not available right away. Therefore, they seek safety through physical proximity to individuals (e.g., doctors) and/or institutions (e.g., hospitals) that might help them. These patients often have to know the location of hospitals before they venture out, and especially if they travel to areas with which they are not familiar.

Three types of situations are generally feared and avoided by agoraphobic patients (Table 2–8). First, there are situations in which patients are

---

TABLE 2–8. Types of Situations Feared and Avoided by Agoraphobic Patients

When Patients Are Alone and/or Outside Their Own Safety Zone

Leaving home alone

Traveling alone

Going far away alone

Driving alone

Staying at home alone

Where It Might Be Physically Difficult or Impossible to Escape (in case of a panic attack)

Crowded places

Trains, buses, and boats in motion

Airplanes during the flight

Controlled-access highways (e.g., freeways, turnpikes, motorways)

Underground railway (subway)

Elevators

Tunnels

Bridges

Where It Might Be Awkward or Embarrassing to Escape (in case of a panic attack)

Restaurants

Social functions

Hairdresser's chair or dentist's chair

Open public places (e.g., streets)

Theaters, cinemas

Shopping malls, department stores

Supermarkets

Standing in line

alone and outside their own safety zone (e.g., traveling far away by themselves). The second type is represented by situations from which it would be physically difficult or impossible to escape (e.g., crowds and trains in motion). Finally, agoraphobic patients may be afraid of situations from which it would be awkward or embarrassing to escape in case of a panic attack (e.g., a social function that a patient would feel an urge to leave immediately).

The unique feature of agoraphobia is the multiple number of situations and/or places that are feared and avoided. Also, patients with agoraphobia tend to avoid more and more situations with the passage of time. The "profile" of the avoided situations may differ greatly from one patient to another and depends on the underlying themes described above. Local circumstances may determine whether patients with agoraphobia exhibit prominent avoidance of situations or places, such as bridges, tunnels, or a subway, and whether they are disabled by such avoidance.

Some situations may be particularly difficult for agoraphobic patients and seem to be avoided at all cost. These are usually the situations in which patients had their first panic attack or in which anxiety symptoms and panic attacks were particularly severe or embarrassing. Among the symptoms that agoraphobic patients fear the most are lightheadedness, fainting feelings, and/or dizziness. Patients usually interpret these symptoms as a warning that they might faint, collapse, fall, and/or lose control, and they feel that the occurrence of these events in public would be particularly embarrassing.

The avoidance of agoraphobic situations may be subtle but still interfere with functioning. For example, patients may avoid traveling on buses or trains only during peak traffic hours and therefore come to work or leave work too early or too late. The avoidant behavior may, to a certain extent, be masked by the presence of a "phobic companion." That is, agoraphobic patients may not exhibit significant avoidance if persons whom they trust and who provide them with a sense of security accompany them. These are usually patients' partners or, less often, family members or friends. The functioning of such patients may be relatively good; for example, they may commute to work every day and hold a job for years if their partners regularly accompany them. The extent of phobic fear then becomes fully apparent when partners are no longer able or willing to accompany patients.

Onset of Panic Disorder

The first panic attack is usually well remembered by patients: it was so different from everything that they had experienced before that it usually remains vivid in patients' memory even many years after its occurrence. However, the first panic attack often does not denote the onset of panic disorder and for this reason the precise onset of the disorder may be more difficult to ascertain.

Although many patients describe their first panic attack as quite sudden and unexpected and deny that there were any events preceding it, often there are prodromal symptoms leading up to the first panic attack and/or significant life events prior to the onset of panic disorder. Chronic worry and anxiety, and even generalized anxiety disorder and hypochondriasis (Fava et al., 1988, 1992; Garvey et al., 1988) have been described as preceding panic disorder. The first panic attack may occur in a variety of contexts and situations, such as interpersonal conflict, traumatic experience, medical illness, physical exertion, excitement and agitation, sexual intercourse, and intoxication with or withdrawal from certain substances (e.g., alcohol, caffeine, amphetamine, cocaine, cannabis).

The circumstances of the first panic attack (particularly the location where it occurred and its intensity) may determine the person's initial response to the attack and whether the person will develop fear of further panic attacks and avoidance of the situations that might remind him or her of the first attack (e.g., Lelliott et al., 1989; Amering et al., 1997). Thus, if the first panic attack was severe and occurred away from home—and particularly in situations from which a quick escape was impossible (e.g., being in a flying airplane) or in which urgent medical help was not available (e.g., while traveling far away from the nearest hospital)—there is an increased risk that the person will become afraid of another panic attack, that such an attack is anticipated outside the home, and that the person will ultimately develop agoraphobia, avoiding many situations outside the home.

RELATIONSHIP BETWEEN PANIC DISORDER AND OTHER DISORDERS

Psychiatric conditions frequently co-occur with panic disorder, especially in clinical settings. Other anxiety disorders, mood disorders, hypochondriasis, and alcohol abuse are most common among these conditions. Various types of personality disturbance are also seen in patients with panic disorder.

The rates of another anxiety disorder co-occurring with panic disorder in clinical populations over a lifetime range between 35% and 93%; the most frequently co-occurring anxiety disorders include generalized anxiety disorder, specific phobias, and social anxiety disorder (deRuiter et al., 1989; Sanderson et al., 1990; Starcevic et al., 1992b). Most of these co-occurring anxiety disorders usually precede the onset of panic disorder, and they can sometimes be considered to predispose to panic disorder.

The relationship between panic disorder and agoraphobia is of particular importance and is discussed in some detail below. In addition, there are significant implications of the relationships between panic disorder on the one hand and generalized anxiety disorder, depression, hypochondriasis, and alcohol-related disorders on the other (Table 2–9). Finally, the relationships between bipolar disorder and panic disorder and between panic disorder and personality disturbance are also reviewed.

Panic Disorder and Agoraphobia

Patients with panic disorder often resort to the avoidance of situations in which they expect to have panic attacks or some symptoms of the attacks. This is the path that leads to agoraphobia. Because agoraphobia is not solely and invariably a consequence of panic disorder, the relationship between panic disorder and agoraphobia has been a source of some controversy. This boils down to the conceptualization of the relationship between panic attacks and phobic fear.

In American psychiatry, as embodied in the DSM diagnostic and classification system (most recently in DSM-IV-TR), panic attack, especially "spontaneous"/unexpected panic attack, is regarded as a qualitatively different "type" of anxiety (Klein, 1981). When both panic attacks and agoraphobic avoidance are present, agoraphobia is seen as a consequence of panic attacks (and panic disorder), whereas agoraphobia itself is defined through panic attacks, or at least, through the symptoms of panic attacks— as the fear of situations in which it would be embarrassing or difficult to escape in case of a panic attack or in which help might not be available, also in case of a panic attack. Therefore, in the DSM system agoraphobia is almost always regarded as part of panic disorder, with panic disorder being the main and primary diagnosis. Agoraphobia does exist as a separate nosological entity (under the name "agoraphobia without history of panic disorder"), but it is rarely diagnosed and often considered spurious (e.g., Horwath et al., 1993).

In contrast, many European psychiatrists and the ICD system (as in ICD-10) postulate that there is a continuum of severity from normal fear through phobic fear to panic attacks. In other words, panic attacks are not seen as being qualitatively different from other types of anxiety, such as phobic or generalized anxiety (Tyrer, 1984), and panic attacks only denote greater severity of anxiety. Therefore, the presence of panic attacks in agoraphobic situations is viewed as an indicator of the severity of phobic anxiety. The main diagnosis in such situations is agoraphobia, hence the

TABLE 2–9. Clinical Implications of the Relationship Between Panic Disorder and Other Disorders

Panic Disorder and Generalized Anxiety Disorder

- Generalized anxiety disorder often co-occurs with panic disorder, but it may be overshadowed by the more dramatic clinical picture of panic disorder and therefore remain unrecognized or missed.

- Chronic worry and anxious apprehension in generalized anxiety disorder sometimes need to be distinguished from anticipatory anxiety in panic disorder.

- Treatment implications are unclear; generalized anxiety disorder may need to be addressed at a later stage of treatment, after some relief has been obtained from panic disorder.

Panic Disorder and Depression

- Many panic patients develop depression and should be closely monitored for any symptoms and signs of depression.

- There are several pathways leading to depression; depression is not just a consequence of the panic-associated demoralization and the feelings of helplessness and hopelessness.

- Both panic disorder and major depressive disorder tend to be more severe when they co-occur than when they appear alone; there is greater impairment in patients who suffer from both conditions; the presence of depression affects negatively the course and outcome of panic disorder, with further complications (e.g., suicide attempts) being more likely.

- Vigorous treatment with antidepressants is needed, along with supportive measures and psychosocial interventions.

Panic Disorder and Hypochondriasis

- Because of the frequent phenomenological overlap, panic disorder and hypochondriasis should be distinguished as much as possible; in most cases, features of hypochondriasis are secondary to panic disorder and abate with successful treatment of panic disorder.

- Panic patients with prominent hypochondriacal features may "attract" some hostility and rejecting behavior, which are otherwise typical of the way patients with hypochondriasis are treated.

Panic Disorder and Alcohol-Related Problems

- It is important to ascertain what role, if any, alcohol-related problems might have played in precipitating panic attacks (e.g., through withdrawals); diagnosis of panic disorder is not warranted if panic attacks occur only during alcohol withdrawals.

- "Self-medicating" with alcohol may occur in panic patients.

- Benzodiazepines should be avoided (or used only with extreme caution) in patients with current or past alcohol-related problems.

ICD-10 diagnostic categories of agoraphobia with or without panic disorder. According to ICD-10, a diagnosis of panic disorder can be made only in the absence of phobic disorders.

There has been some support for both views, but the strength of evidence favors the DSM position. Thus, most studies suggest that panic attacks precede agoraphobia in the vast majority of patients (e.g., Thyer and Himle, 1985; Uhde et al., 1985; Aronson and Logue, 1987; Franklin, 1987). Also, agoraphobic patients are usually not afraid of agoraphobic situations as such, but are much more concerned about the physical symptoms of anxiety and their potential consequences (Buglass et al., 1977; Hallam and Hafner, 1978; Franklin, 1987). Moreover, unlike other phobias, where avoidance is likely to prevent phobic fear, avoidance in agoraphobia does not necessarily prevent panic attacks (Hallam, 1978). In most cases, agoraphobia can be conceptualized as an attempt to avoid certain physical symptoms (particularly dizziness), sudden loss of control, or full-blown panic attacks, which patients believe are more likely to occur in certain places and situations.

In examining the relationship between panic disorder and agoraphobia from the perspective of panic disorder being a chronologically and con-

TABLE 2–10. Risk factors for developing agoraphobia among patients with panic disorder

---

Female gender

Cognitive factors

   Expectation that panic attacks will occur in certain situations (Craske et al., 1988; Rapee and Murrell, 1988; Adler et al., 1989; Telch et al., 1989a)

   Exaggerated expectation of negative social consequences of panic attacks (Telch et al., 1989a)

   Exaggerated expectation of negative consequences of panic attacks in certain specific situations (Franklin, 1987; Noyes et al., 1987a; Craske et al., 1988; Fleming and Faulk, 1989)

   Prominent fear of dying or "going crazy" during panic attacks

   Marked belief that one is not able to cope with panic attacks (Craske et al., 1988; Mavissakalian, 1988; Telch et al., 1989a; Clum and Knowles, 1991)

More prominent lightheadedness and dizziness during panic attacks (Noyes et al., 1987a; Telch et al., 1989a)

Occurrence of the first panic attack outside of the person's "safety zone" (e.g., far away from home, in a public place) (Lelliott et al., 1989; Amering et al., 1997)

Prominent dependency or dependent personality disorder (Kleiner and Marshall, 1987)

Embarrassment about having a panic attack (Amering et al., 1997)

Prominent social anxiety or social anxiety disorder (Rapee and Murrell, 1988)

---

ceptually primary condition, the following main question arises: why do some panic patients go on to develop agoraphobia, whereas others do not? The research to date has identified several risk factors (Table 2–10) for developing agoraphobia among patients with panic disorder. The single most important risk factor is being female: women are three to four times more likely to develop agoraphobia than men, and there may be various cultural, psychological, and biological reasons for this (see Epidemiology and Etiology and Pathogenesis, below). In addition to female gender, it appears that various beliefs and expectations about panic attacks and panic symptoms play a crucial role in predisposing panic patients to agoraphobia (Franklin, 1987; Noyes et al., 1987a; Craske et al., 1988; Mavissakalian, 1988; Rapee and Murrell, 1988; Adler et al., 1989; Fleming and Faulk, 1989; Telch et al., 1989a; Clum and Knowles, 1991). Agoraphobia seems to be predicted by these cognitive factors better than it is by the severity and frequency of panic attacks (Clum and Knowles, 1991). Although agoraphobia can appear at any time in the course of panic disorder, it typically develops in the first year following the onset of panic disorder.

Panic Disorder and Generalized Anxiety Disorder

Generalized anxiety disorder co-occurs fairly frequently with panic disorder, in up to 68% of panic disorder patients. Generalized anxiety disorder is usually diagnosed as a secondary condition, when panic disorder is the main reason for seeking help and treatment. However, generalized anxiety disorder often occurs before panic disorder, but because of the nature of generalized anxiety disorder (see Chapter 3), patients tend to seek help only after a condition such as panic disorder or depression has complicated its course. Generalized anxiety disorder and panic disorder may also occur at approximately the same time, or generalized anxiety disorder follows panic disorder.

Clinical experience suggests that it may be more difficult to treat panic disorder co-occurring with generalized anxiety disorder, but there are no studies to clearly support this impression.

Panic Disorder and Depression

Depression is often seen as a complication of panic disorder, especially in the context of agoraphobia (Thompson et al., 1989; Ball et al., 1994) and a long-standing and more severe panic disorder. In some cases, major depressive disorder and panic disorder develop at approximately the same time, while in the minority of patients, major depressive disorder precedes the onset of panic disorder. It is estimated that between 24% and 88% of patients with panic disorder have at least one major depressive episode in their lifetime (Breier et al., 1984; Lesser et al., 1988).

Such a common co-occurrence of panic disorder with depression has important implications in that panic patients need to be monitored for any symptoms and signs of depression and adequately treated if they develop depression. This is particularly significant in view of findings that both major depressive disorder and panic disorder tend to be more severe when these two conditions co-occur (Breier et al., 1984; Andrade et al., 1994; Grunhaus et al., 1994). The impairment in patients who suffer from both panic disorder and depression is greater than that in those who suffer from either condition alone (Scheibe and Albus, 1994); moreover, the presence of depression affects negatively the course and outcome of panic disorder (Scheibe and Albus, 1994). Finally, the risk of suicide seems to be increased when major depressive disorder co-occurs with panic disorder (e.g., Cox et al., 1994; Warshaw et al., 2000).

Depression cannot be reliably prevented by antidepressant medication, and benzodiazepines may actually induce depression. Inasmuch as some cases of depression develop as a consequence of the panic-associated demoralization and the feelings of helplessness and hopelessness, vigorous treatment of panic disorder and the consequently improved functioning may help in the prevention of depressive episodes.

Panic Disorder and Hypochondriasis

Because of the phenomenological and behavioral overlap between panic disorder and hypochondriasis (preoccupation with physical symptoms, persistent concerns about having a serious physical disease, seeking medical reassurance but apparently rejecting it at the same time, undergoing numerous medical investigations), it may be difficult, though certainly not impossible, to distinguish them (see Differential Diagnosis, below). From the cognitive perspective, the most conspicuous similarity between panic disorder and hypochondriasis is that both are based on catastrophic misinterpretation of innocuous bodily sensations and symptoms (Salkovskis and Clark, 1993).

The relationship between panic disorder and hypochondriasis is complex. Hypochondriasis can be a secondary feature of panic disorder, and many patients (45%–50%) with panic disorder exhibit significant hypochondriacal features (Starcevic et al., 1992a; Benedetti et al., 1997; Furer et al., 1997). These hypochondriacal features then diminish or disappear upon successful treatment of panic disorder. Less often, panic disorder and hypochondriasis coexist, with neither condition considered principal or chronologically primary. Hypochondriasis was also reported to precede panic attacks in some patients (Fava et al., 1990). To better understand the relationship between panic disorder and hypochondriasis, the crucial step is to ascertain whether hypochondriacal features (e.g., excessive bodily preoccupation, disease fear, disease suspicion) are better accounted for by panic disorder—that is, whether they occur primarily during panic attacks and/or as part of anticipatory anxiety.

Panic Disorder and Alcohol Abuse and Dependence

Alcohol abuse and alcohol dependence have been associated with panic disorder in 13%–43% of patients with panic disorder (Otto et al., 1992; Starcevic et al., 1992b; 1993b; Kessler et al., 1997). Alcohol-related problems can precede the onset of panic attacks and can also play a role in the etiology of panic disorder by precipitating panic attacks during withdrawals from alcohol (see Assessment, below). Alcohol abuse and even alcohol dependence can also develop in the course of panic disorder, as a result of patients' attempts to "self-medicate" and thus alleviate their symptoms and anxiety. However, this latter scenario happens less often than in patients with social anxiety disorder and posttraumatic stress disorder.

Bipolar Disorder and Panic Disorder

The relationship between bipolar disorder and panic disorder was discovered relatively recently. This is likely to be a consequence of low rates of the co-occurring bipolar disorder among patients who present for treatment of panic disorder as their principal condition. Hence, findings about the relationship between these two conditions come mainly from studies of patients with primary bipolar disorder.

    The lifetime prevalence of panic disorder among patients with bipolar disorder is approximately 20% (Chen and Dilsaver, 1995; McElroy et al., 2001). Higher rates of the co-occurring panic disorder have been reported in bipolar disorder patients with psychotic features (Pini et al., 1999) and in patients with bipolar depression (Pini et al., 1997). It appears that the link between bipolar disorder and panic disorder has a stronger genetic component (Mackinnon et al., 1997). The presence of panic disorder and panic symptoms in patients with bipolar disorder has been associated with more severe depression, more suicidality, and delayed response to treatment (Frank et al., 2002). The co-occurrence of panic disorder and bipolar disorder may also have implications for treatment in that mood stabilizers, particularly valproate, may be efficacious in the treatment of panic disorder (e.g., Baetz and Bowen, 1998).

Panic Disorder and Personality Disturbance

The relationship between panic disorder and personality disturbance is important because of the implications that it may have for the understanding of psychopathology of panic disorder and for its treatment. Most personality disorders and personality traits that have been found in patients with panic disorder are nonspecifically associated with panic disorder. That is, the same or similar types of the personality-level psychopathology have been found in patients with other anxiety disorders and depression.

The percentage of panic disorder patients who have personality disorders varies from one study to another, and is estimated at 40%–65% (Reich and Troughton, 1988; Brooks et al., 1989; Diaferia et al., 1993; Blashfield et al., 1994). This high prevalence of personality disturbance may be an overestimate from the low threshold for making diagnoses of personality disorders. Predictably, most common among these personality disorders are DSM Cluster C ("anxious, fearful"; avoidant and dependent), followed by Cluster B ("emotional, dramatic"; histrionic) personality disorders (Diaferia et al., 1993); occasionally, Cluster A ("odd, eccentric") personality disorders are found among patients with panic disorder.

There are several possibilities for interpreting the relationship between panic disorder and personality disturbance (Starcevic, 1992). Certain personality disorders, particularly those from the DSM Cluster C, may predispose to panic disorder, but even when they appear to do so there is no evidence that this predisposition is specific for panic disorder. Therefore, it is practically impossible to estimate the likelihood of a person developing panic disorder on the basis of that person having a particular type of personality disturbance. At least some changes in personality functioning, if not personality disorders, may be better conceptualized as a consequence of panic disorder, particularly when panic disorder has been severe, accompanied by agoraphobia, lasting for a long time and/or with an early onset (e.g., in adolescence). For example, some patients with chronic, severe panic disorder with agoraphobia become extremely insecure and dependent, lose self-esteem, or exhibit extensive social withdrawal and isolation; this pattern may seem identical to that of dependent and/or avoidant personality disorders. Other patients become hypervigilant, extremely sensitive in interpersonal situations, mistrustful, and suspicious, traits that may resemble paranoid personality disorder.

Regardless of whether certain personality traits and disorders clearly precede the onset of panic disorder or are more likely to be understood as a consequence of panic disorder, their presence usually implies a less favorable prognosis of panic disorder, with a greater likelihood of various problems in the course of treatment and generally poorer outcome of treatment (e.g., Green and Curtis, 1988; Chambless et al., 1992; Hoffart and Martinsen, 1993). These problems include issues such as fluctuating motivation for treatment, secondary gain, compliance with pharmacotherapy and specific behavioral tasks, and "sabotaging" one's own treatment. However, a successful treatment of panic disorder may sometimes lead to a significant decrease in certain personality traits (e.g., Mavissakalian and Hamann, 1987); in those cases, such traits are far more likely to be a consequence of panic disorder. Some studies (e.g., Dreessen et al., 1994) do not support the notion that personality disorders are usually associated with poorer response to treatment of panic disorder.

ASSESSMENT

Diagnostic Issues

Diagnostic criteria for panic disorder in DSM-IV-TR are relatively straightforward. There are essentially four components of the diagnostic conceptualization of panic disorder according to DSM-IV-TR. Two of these are nonspecific (requirements that features of panic disorder result in substantial impairment in functioning and that panic attacks are not caused by a physical condition or a psychoactive substance). The other two components pertain to the presence of recurrent, unexpected panic attacks and anticipatory anxiety for at least 1 month. To qualify for the diagnosis of panic disorder, most panic attacks have to be unexpected, but some are situationally predisposed or even situationally bound, especially in panic patients who also have agoraphobia. If most panic attacks are currently situationally predisposed or situationally bound, there has to be a history of unexpected attacks at the beginning of the disorder. Otherwise, the diagnosis of another anxiety disorder is more likely, as DSM-IV-TR stipulates that a diagnosis of panic disorder is warranted if its features cannot be better accounted for by social anxiety disorder, specific phobias, obsessive-compulsive disorder, posttraumatic stress disorder, and separation anxiety disorder. In other words, for the diagnosis of panic disorder to be made, panic attacks must not be a part of another psychiatric condition.

The relationship between panic disorder and agoraphobia is also of diagnostic importance. As already noted, in the DSM system agoraphobia is conceived of as a complication of panic disorder or a condition secondary to panic disorder—hence the diagnosis of panic disorder with agoraphobia. According to ICD-10, by contrast, the simultaneous presence of panic disorder and agoraphobia suggests that agoraphobia is a primary condition, and this combination is accordingly designated "agoraphobia with panic disorder." Moreover, ICD-10 imposes a diagnostic hierarchy in that a diagnosis of panic disorder is precluded by the simultaneous presence of phobic disorders or major depressive disorder. The different approaches by DSM-IV-TR and ICD-10 to the relationship between panic disorder and agoraphobia are presented in more detail in Relationship Between Panic Disorder and Other Disorders, above.

It is important to keep in mind that panic attacks and anticipatory anxiety can be overshadowed by avoidance behavior in patients with severe agoraphobia. In such patients, even if panic attacks are successfully "prevented" by avoidance, the fear of panic attacks does not vanish and can be found underneath extensive avoidance behavior.

The diagnosis of panic disorder first depends on the correct assessment of panic attacks. It is worth emphasizing that panic attacks should not be designated as such if they occur only on exposure to life-threatening situations. The most important features of panic attacks are their sudden, abrupt occurrence, very rapid culmination of their intensity, prominent physical symptoms, and catastrophic elaboration of these symptoms. It is usually not difficult to ascertain symptoms that patients experience during panic attacks. However, some patients may focus on one or two dominant and/or the most distressing symptoms (e.g., heart racing and shortness of breath), whereas for comprehensive assessment, patients need to be specifically asked about the presence of other panic-associated symptoms.

Sometimes anticipatory anxiety needs to be differentiated from anxious anticipation and worries that pertain to issues other than panic attacks. As presented in Clinical Features (above), anticipatory anxiety pertains strictly to panic attacks, even when it is conceptualized via changes in behavior, and its duration in DSM-IV-TR is at least 1 month.

There are two crucial steps in establishing the presence of agoraphobia: (1) ascertaining the type and number of situations that patients fear and/or avoid, and (2) asking patients about the reasons for avoidance. Agoraphobia is present if panic patients fear and/or avoid at least two distinct agoraphobic situations, and avoidance (or phobic fear) has to be clearly related to panic attacks. According to DSM-IV-TR, avoidance behavior is not a sine qua non for the diagnosis of agoraphobia; it can also be diagnosed if patients endure agoraphobic situations with great distress and/or fear that they will experience a panic attack or anxiety symptoms in those situations, or if they enter agoraphobic situations only when they are accompanied by the trusted other(s).

Assessment Instruments

The recognition that panic disorder is a multifaceted condition has led to a construction of two instruments for separate assessments of different components and aspects of panic disorder (e.g., panic attacks, anticipatory anxiety, agoraphobic avoidance, health-related concerns, disability). These instruments are the Panic Disorder Severity Scale (Shear et al., 1997) and the Panic and Agoraphobia Scale (Bandelow, 1995; 1999). Both are designed to be used by clinicians, but there are also patient, self-report versions. The use of these instruments allows clinicians to make a more objective, formal assessment of panic disorder and its components, and to monitor both global and specific changes in the course of treatment. In addition, several specific self-report instruments and assessment procedures can be used for the three main components of panic disorder (panic attacks, anticipatory anxiety, and agoraphobic avoidance) to complement clinician-based assessment.

Since retrospective recording of panic attacks is not reliable because of the possible memory bias, panic attacks are best monitored prospectively, in a diary format. A typical panic diary provides information on the frequency and severity of panic attacks, situations in which they occur, and other triggers that may precipitate the attacks. In addition to this "basic" panic diary, more detailed information about panic attacks may be obtained by asking patients to also record the symptoms, thoughts, and feelings that they experience during panic attacks, as well as the duration and type (unexpected or expected) of each attack.

There are two useful instruments for assessing various aspects of anticipatory anxiety. The first one is the Agoraphobic Cognitions Questionnaire (Chambless et al., 1984), which is used to assess the frequency of thoughts about negative (catastrophic) consequences of anxiety and panic. The other instrument is the Anxiety Sensitivity Index (Reiss et al., 1986), which measures the fear of symptoms of anxious arousal.

The Mobility Inventory (Chambless et al., 1985) is suitable for assessment of the degree of avoidance of typical agoraphobic situations. The distinct advantages of this instrument are its comprehensiveness and separate assessment of avoidance when patients are alone and when they are accompanied.

Differential Diagnosis

Differential diagnosis of panic disorder is important and complex for several reasons. First, because of the episodic occurrence of largely physical symptoms, diagnostic work-up of panic disorder includes a consideration of several physical (medical) conditions. Second, panic attacks are often seen in the course of other psychiatric disorders and it is therefore important to ascertain whether panic attacks are better conceptualized as part of another psychiatric condition. Finally, when panic disorder is complicated by agoraphobia, several disorders should be considered in the differential diagnosis of agoraphobia.

Medical Differential Diagnosis of Panic Disorder
In comparison with the general population and patients without panic disorder, patients with panic disorder are more likely to have certain physical conditions. Also, panic disorder occurs relatively often in several nonpsychiatric disorders. These include thyroid dysfunction (Lindemann et al., 1984), mitral valve prolapse (Margraf et al., 1988), asthma (Yellowlees et al., 1987, 1988; Shavitt et al., 1992), chronic obstructive pulmonary disease and other respiratory illnesses (Zandbergen et al., 1991; Spinhoven et al., 1994), vestibular dysfunction (Jacob et al., 1996; Asmundson et al., 1998), irritable bowel syndrome (Walker et al., 1990, 1995; Lydiard et al., 1993; Kaplan et al., 1996; Lydiard 1997), other gastrointestinal syndromes (Lydiard et al., 1994), and various allergies (Ramesh et al., 1991).

A large number of physical diseases and conditions can cause panic attacks (Table 2–11). Of these, the most clinically relevant are hyperthyroidism, cardiac arrhythmias, vestibular dysfunction, mitral valve

TABLE 2–11. Physical Conditions That Can Cause Panic Attacks

More Clinically Relevant (in terms of higher frequency of association with panic attacks)

Hyperthyroidism (or less commonly, hypothyroidism)

Cardiac arrhythmias (e.g., paroxysmal atrial tachycardia)

Vestibular dysfunction

Mitral valve prolapse

Complex partial (temporal, psychomotor) epilepsy

Hypoglycemia

Less Clinically Relevant (in terms of lower frequency of association with panic attacks)

Hypoparathyroidism, hyperparathyroidism

Pheochromocytoma

Pulmonary embolus

Electrolyte disturbances

Cushing's syndrome

Menopause

prolapse, complex partial (temporal, psychomotor) epilepsy, and hypo-glycemia. Not all panic patients need to undergo extensive diagnostic test-ing for all these conditions, and organic work-up in panic patients can be conceptualized as a sequential three-step process (Table 2–12). First, all panic patients should undergo routine physical examination and labora-tory testing, including thyroid function tests. Second, if patients complain repeatedly of specific, severe symptoms, such as chest pain, abnormalities in the cardiac rhythm, dizziness, or depersonalization phenomena, rele-vant diagnostic investigations should be performed to rule out (or con-firm) the presence of the corresponding physical conditions (Table 2–12). Finally, the full organic work-up is warranted in all patients whose panic attacks occur for the first time later in life (after the age of 45) or in those cases where panic attacks have some atypical features. Examples of the lat-ter include loss of consciousness or a "clouded" state of consciousness, uri-nary incontinence, severe headache, slurred speech, and amnesia.

The relationship between panic disorder and thyroid disease in gen-eral, and hyperthyroidism in particular, is complex. Hyperthyroidism can be considered a cause of panic attacks if the etiological relationship between the two is clearly demonstrated. This is the case with patients with hyperthyroidism and panic attacks whose panic attacks subside fol-lowing treatment with antithyroid therapy and normalization of thyroid

TABLE 2–12. Sequential Three-Step Process in Organic Work-up of Panic Patients

1. Diagnostic investigations for all panic patients

    Routine physical examination

    Routine laboratory testing (complete blood count, electrolytes, calcium, glycemia)

    Thyroid function tests (levels of serum T_3, T_4, and TSH)

2. Additional diagnostic investigations for panic patients with recurrent, specific, and/or severe symptoms, such as chest pain, abnormalities in cardiac rhythm, dizziness, and depersonalization phenomena

    Electrocardiogram (ECG), cardiological examination (to check for cardiac arrhythmias)

    Echocardiogram (cardiac ultrasound), cardiological examination (to check for mitral valve prolapse)

    Vestibular function testing, neurological examination (to check for vestibular dysfunction)

    Electroencephalogram (EEG), neurological examination (to check for epilepsy)

3. Diagnostic investigations for all patients whose panic attacks occur for the first time later in life (after age 45) or whose panic attacks have atypical features

    Full organic work-up, with emphasis on those investigations that are relevant for each particular patient (and are based on the patient's symptom profile)

T_3, triiodothyronine; T_4, thyroxine; TSH, thyroid-stimulating hormone.

function. In this situation, a diagnosis of panic disorder would obviously be ruled out. In other cases, panic attacks do not abate even after the thyroid condition has been treated successfully, so that the thyroid condition (hyperthyroidism or hypothyroidism) may be thought of as playing a role in precipitating panic attacks, but not accounting entirely for their appearance. There are situations in which making a causal attribution might be so speculative that the question of whether panic attacks are better understood as a manifestation of thyroid dysfunction or as part of panic disorder is best left open and both conditions treated regardless of the precise nature of their relationship.

Sudden tachycardia (up to 150 beats/minute) is commonly reported during panic attacks. Although such tachycardias are relatively benign, they can also occur as a consequence of life-threatening cardiac arrhythmias; therefore, the possibility of such an etiology should be further investigated.

Dizziness, lightheadedness, fainting feeling, loss of balance, and "walking on waves" are frequent symptoms during panic attacks; they are especially common among patients with agoraphobia. Depending on the severity of these symptoms and presence of any other symptoms suggestive of organic etiology (e.g., vertigo, nausea), vestibular dysfunction, inner ear disease, and neurological, cerebrovascular, and cardiovascular conditions may need to be ruled out.

Panic disorder and mitral valve prolapse have several symptoms in common, including palpitations, chest pain, and manifestations of autonomic hyperarousal. The degree of association between panic disorder and mitral valve prolapse varies from one study to another, but on the basis of one meta-analysis of a large number of studies (Katerndahl, 1993), it does appear that mitral valve prolapse is more than twice as common among panic patients than it is among those without panic disorder. Data on the prevalence of panic disorder among patients with mitral valve prolapse appear far less consistent; however, the overall impression is that panic disorder is not more frequent among patients with mitral valve prolapse than in the general population. There is a consensus that despite our lack of understanding of the relationship between panic disorder and mitral valve prolapse, this link does not seem to be etiologically important and it does not have implications for treatment. That is, panic attacks in patients with mitral valve prolapse are not a consequence of mitral valve prolapse, and panic patients with mitral valve prolapse should be treated in the same way as those without mitral valve prolapse.

Certain patients with panic disorder have various and for the most part nonspecific changes on electroencephalograms (EEG). Some of these patients have more prominent symptoms of depersonalization and/or derealization and may be more likely to be irritable and aggressive during, just before, or immediately after panic attacks. It is possible that panic attacks in such cases represent a manifestation of a seizure disorder, just as it is possible that panic attacks are present with seizures, especially seizures that characterize temporal lobe (partial complex) epilepsy. In addition to an EEG, a detailed neurological examination and relevant diagnostic tests are warranted if, during panic attacks, patients experience the phenomena of "déjà vu" or "déjà vecu," marked hypersensitivity to light or sound, and other symptoms unusual for panic.

Hypoglycemia is a relatively rare cause of panic attacks; in such cases, attacks occur only in states of hunger and disappear following the administration of intravenous glucose or intake of food.

Panic attacks can occur as a consequence of intoxication with cannabis and stimulant drugs (cocaine, amphetamine, caffeine) or in the context of alcohol, benzodiazepine, or opiate withdrawal. The diagnosis of panic disorder should not be made if there is close temporal proximity between the use of a substance and the onset of panic attacks. In other words, the diagnosis of panic disorder can be made if panic attacks persist for a long time after the intoxication or a withdrawal syndrome.

Psychiatric Differential Diagnosis of Panic Disorder
Although psychiatric differential diagnosis of panic disorder may include quite a few disorders, generalized anxiety disorder and hypochondriasis are of greatest conceptual and practical relevance. These relationships will be discussed in some detail in further text. With regard to other psychiatric disorders, the crucial step in making a distinction from panic disorder is ascertaining whether the panic attacks are better understood as being part of these disorders, and not a feature of panic disorder. To establish this, patients should be carefully examined for signs and symptoms of other disorders (e.g., a psychotic illness or depression), and the nature of panic attacks needs to be clarified. Panic attacks may be exclusively situationally bound and/or situationally predisposed, as in social anxiety disorder and specific phobias, or related only to certain themes and issues (e.g., trauma-related topics and stimuli in posttraumatic stress disorder and obsessions about contamination in obsessive-compulsive disorder).

Generalized anxiety disorder can be distinguished from panic disorder on the basis of the criteria listed in Table 2–13. The separation of the previous diagnostic entity of "anxiety neurosis" into "panic disorder" and "generalized anxiety disorder" remains controversial and is not accepted by all clinicians and researchers.

In view of the often puzzling, numerous, and severe physical symptoms during recurrent panic attacks, patients with panic disorder can be so focused on their body, preoccupied with symptoms, and concerned about

TABLE 2–13. Distinguishing Between Panic Disorder and Generalized Anxiety Disorder

Criteria	Panic Disorder	Generalized Anxiety Disorder
Presence of panic attacks	Yes	No
Physical symtpoms of anxiety	More pronounced, but occurring episodically (during panic attacks)	Less pronounced, but more persistent
Profile of symptoms	Autonomic hyperactivity symptoms more typical	Symptoms of tension (both somatic and psychological) more typical
Appraisal of symptoms	Typically catastrophic	Usually noncatastrophic
Onset	Usually abrupt	Gradual
Seeking medical help	Relatively quick	Usually delayed

the possibility of having a serious medical condition that their clinical presentation may be very similar to that of the patients with hypochondriasis. However, there are ways of distinguishing between panic disorder and hypochondriasis (Table 2–14). First, patients with panic disorder are troubled by physical symptoms that occur episodically, during panic attacks, whereas physical symptoms in hypochondriacal patients are present with greater constancy. Physical symptoms in panic disorder are usually those of autonomic hyperactivity, whereas physical symptoms in hypochondriasis are more varied, and often include aches and pains. The perceived threat in panic disorder is more immediate (Salkovskis and Clark, 1993), with physical symptoms being appraised as meaning a disease with rapid progression and quick, fatal outcome (e.g., myocardial infarct); the perceived threat in hypochondriasis is more remote, and physical symptoms are appraised as suggesting a disease with a somewhat slower progression, albeit with the

TABLE 2–14. Distinguishing Between Panic Disorder and Hypochondriasis

Criteria	Panic Disorder	Hypochondriasis
Occurrence of physical symptoms	Mainly during panic attacks	More persistent
Nature of physical symptoms	Autonomic hyperactivity symptoms	Greater variety of symptoms
Nature of the perceived threat	More immediate (death from a rapidly developing disease)	More remote (death from a slowly progressing disease)
Seeking medical help	Prompt, urgent, but usually limited to panic attacks	Less urgent, but more persistent

same, fatal outcome (e.g., cancer). Because of these differences in the appraisal of danger, panic patients are more likely to seek medical help promptly when they have a panic attack, whereas patients with hypochondriasis seek such help with less urgency. Stated succinctly, panic patients are more likely to fear dying, whereas those with hypochondriasis are more likely to be afraid of death (Noyes, 1999).

Differential Diagnosis of Agoraphobia
Agoraphobia needs to be differentiated from several psychiatric conditions (Table 2–15). The most common issue in the differential diagnosis of agoraphobia is its distinction from specific phobias and social anxiety disorder. Patients with agoraphobia, specific phobias, and social anxiety disorder may fear and avoid the same or similar situations, but patients with agoraphobia are typically afraid of numerous and quite diverse situations (which are interconnected, however, by their common link to panic attacks). Reasons for fear and avoidance may be more useful in distinguishing between these phobic disorders than are the types of situations that are feared and avoided. Thus, fear and avoidance of agoraphobic situations are invariably related to panic attacks or symptoms of anxiety and panic (e.g., dizziness, urgent need to urinate). The types of specific phobias that may need to be distinguished from agoraphobia usually include situational phobias (e.g., claustrophobia, fear of flying, driving phobia) and, less often, phobia of heights. The relationship between these specific phobias and agoraphobia is presented in more detail in Chapter 5, along with the criteria for distinguishing between them. Likewise, the relationship between social anxiety disorder and agoraphobia and criteria for making a distinction between them are further discussed in Chapter 4.

As for other anxiety disorders that are relevant in the differential diagnosis of agoraphobia, obsessive-compulsive disorder needs to be consid-

TABLE 2–15. Differential Diagnosis of Agoraphobia

Other anxiety disorders

    Specific phobias, especially claustrophobia, fear of flying, driving phobia and fear of heights

    Social anxiety disorder

    Obsessive-compulsive disorder

    Posttraumatic stress disorder

    Separation anxiety disorder

Depression

Psychotic disorder

ered if there is a suggestion that patients avoid going out for fear that places outside their home are contaminated. The avoidance in posttraumatic stress disorder may be widespread and resemble the agoraphobia-associated avoidance, but all the situations avoided in posttraumatic stress disorder are directly or indirectly related to the trauma.

Separation anxiety disorder is typically seen in childhood, but it has also been described in adults. Patients with this condition are concerned about separating from attachment figures and being on their own; as a result, they avoid possible separation and loneliness, which may lead to an avoidance profile similar to the one that is seen in agoraphobia. However, patients with agoraphobia worry about catastrophes that may befall them, whereas patients with separation anxiety disorder are usually concerned that something terrible might happen to their attachment figures, which only strengthens their fears upon separating from these figures.

Staying-at-home behavior is often seen in depression. Although it may resemble agoraphobic avoidance, such behavior is not driven by fear. It is due to a pervasive loss of volition, interest, and energy, which is typical of depression. It is important to remember this distinction, because many patients with agoraphobia become depressed, and in that clinical scenario, the staying-at-home behavior may be a consequence of depression rather than a manifestation of agoraphobia.

In relatively rare situations, a psychotic illness may need to be considered in the differential diagnosis of agoraphobia. This may be the case with patients who avoid various public places and going out, because they have a delusional conviction that they are being followed or that someone might attempt to kill them.

EPIDEMIOLOGY

The highlights of the epidemiology of panic disorder are presented in Table 2–16. Panic attacks are commonly seen in various psychiatric and physical disorders, and they also appear to be common in people who have no other health problems. It is estimated that the lifetime prevalence of panic attacks in the general population is 7.3%–10% (Von Korff et al., 1985; Eaton et al., 1994), but the prevalence rates tend to be very different in various countries. Thus, almost one-tenth of the population can expect to experience a panic attack sometime during their life, but most of these individuals do not develop panic disorder and do not seek help.

Two major epidemiological studies in the United States produced different prevalence findings of panic disorder. Whereas the lifetime prevalence of panic disorder in the Epidemiologic Catchment Area study (based

TABLE 2–16. Epidemiological Data for Panic Disorder

- Lifetime prevalence in the United States: 1.7% (Epidemiologic Catchment Area study); 3.5% (National Comorbidity Survey)

- Lifetime prevalence in different countries: 1.4%–2.9% (except for Asian countries, where the lifetime prevalence rates were 0.4%–1.5%)

- One-year prevalence rate: 2.2% (National Comorbidity Survey); revised 1-year prevalence rate of clinically significant panic disorder in the United States: 1.4%

- In the general population, panic disorder without agoraphobia is more common than panic disorder with agoraphobia.

- In clinical settings, panic disorder with agoraphobia is more common than panic disorder without agoraphobia.

- Women are more often represented than men (ratio of 1.5–2.5:1), particularly in clinical settings (ratio of 2.5–3:1).

- Panic disorder with agoraphobia is 2.5 to 4 times more common in women than in men.

- Typical age of onset: third decade of life

- Mean age of onset: around age 25 years

- Bimodal distribution in age of onset: the first peak in the age group 15–24 and the second peak in the age group 45–54 years

- More prevalent among widowed, separated, and divorced individuals, among the less educated, and among urban dwellers

- High prevalence in primary-care and certain specialized medical-care settings, as well as in hospital emergency rooms, reflects characteristic patterns of help seeking

on the DSM-III criteria) was 1.7% (Regier et al., 1988; Eaton et al., 1991), the lifetime prevalence rate of panic disorder in the National Comorbidity Survey (based on the DSM-III-R criteria) was 3.5% (Eaton et al., 1994). A 1-year prevalence rate of panic disorder in the National Comorbidity Survey was 2.2% (Eaton et al., 1994). Because of an impression that the National Comorbidity Survey may have overestimated the prevalence rates of panic disorder, there have been attempts to obtain more realistic epidemiological figures. Thus, a revised 1-year prevalence rate of panic disorder in the United States among individuals over 18 years of age, taking into account the clinical significance of the condition, was estimated at 1.4% (Narrow et al., 2002).

The prevalence rates of panic disorder were generally lower in Asian countries; the lowest lifetime prevalence rate (0.4%; Hwu et al., 1989) was found in Taiwan, but then the prevalence rates of all psychiatric disorders were lower in Taiwan. The lifetime prevalence rates of panic disorder were 1.0% in Japan (Aoki et al., 1994) and 1.5% in South Korea (Lee et al., 1990a). The lifetime prevalence rates in other countries ranged between 1.4% in

Canada (Bland et al., 1988b) and 2.9% in Italy (Faravelli et al., 1989). These differences reflect different diagnostic criteria and different instruments used in different studies and, to a certain extent, cultural differences.

In the general population, panic disorder without agoraphobia seems to be more common than panic disorder with agoraphobia, as the former type is found in one-half to two-thirds of all persons with panic disorder (American Psychiatric Association, 2000). In contrast, panic disorder without agoraphobia is less often encountered in clinical samples than is panic disorder with agoraphobia. This finding suggests that individuals with panic disorder who seek help are more likely to have agoraphobia, and that panic disorder with agoraphobia is a more severe variant of the condition. As for agoraphobia, it is far more frequently encountered as part of panic disorder than as a condition unrelated to panic disorder. Indeed, agoraphobia without a history of panic disorder occurs so rarely that the validity and utility of this diagnostic category has been put into doubt (Goisman et al., 1995).

Like most other anxiety disorders, panic disorder is more frequent among women, and both the Epidemiologic Catchment Area study and the National Comorbidity Survey found that women were 2–2.5 times more likely to have panic disorder than men (Regier et al., 1988; Eaton et al., 1991, 1994). Also, the higher prevalence of panic disorder among women was consistently found in different countries. While the ratio of women to men with panic disorder in general population is in the range of 1.5–2.5:1, in clinical populations it is 2.5–3:1 (Katerndahl and Realini, 1993). This suggests that women are more likely to seek help for panic disorder, either because panic disorder is more severe in women (especially when agoraphobia co-occurs with panic disorder) or because they are generally more likely to seek help for health-related problems. Men, by contrast, may be more inclined than women to attempt to alleviate their panic attacks and anticipatory anxiety through the use of alcohol, which makes it less likely for them to appear in clinical samples of panic patients.

When panic disorder is associated with agoraphobia, 75%–80% of patients are women, with the female-to-male ratio being approximately 2.5–4:1 (Eaton et al., 1994; Yonkers et al., 1998). The preponderance of women among patients with agoraphobia is usually explained as a consequence of social and cultural factors; thus agoraphobia has been portrayed as a "caricature of the traditional female roles," with society generally reinforcing dependence and avoidance as coping mechanisms in women (Clum and Knowles, 1991). Also, an expression of fear and avoidance behavior may be more socially acceptable in women than in men (Fodor, 1974; Chambless and Mason, 1986).

In comparison with other phobic disorders, agoraphobia has a markedly different prevalence in the general population and in clinical settings. Specific phobias are more frequently encountered than agoraphobia in the general population (Kessler et al., 1994; Magee et al., 1996), but this relationship is the reverse in clinical populations, with agoraphobia there being more prevalent than specific phobias. This finding confirms that agoraphobia tends to be more disabling than specific phobias, which is the main reason for agoraphobic individuals' greater likelihood of seeking help and for agoraphobia being more represented in clinical settings.

Although panic disorder can begin at any age, its onset is rare in children and elderly. Most commonly, the onset of panic disorder is in the early to mid-20s, with the mean age of onset being around 25 years (Eaton et al., 1994). There also seems to be a bimodal distribution in the age of onset of panic disorder: the first peak was noted in the age group of 15–24 years, whereas the second peak was found in the age group of 45–54 years (Eaton et al., 1994). Thus, it is not at all rare to see the onset of panic disorder in mid-life, after the age of 40. Panic disorder with agoraphobia tends to have an earlier onset than panic disorder without agoraphobia, but both usually begin in the third decade of life.

Panic disorder is more common among the widowed, divorced, and separated than among married individuals (Lepine and Lellouch, 1994). People who live in an urban environment and have lower levels of education also appear to be at greater risk of developing panic disorder (Eaton et al., 1994).

Patients with panic disorder have a characteristic pattern of help seeking. Because of their physical symptoms, they often seek help in hospital emergency departments and primary-care settings; the current prevalence rate of panic disorder in the primary-care setting in various countries was estimated to be around 1%, but varied from 0.2% to 3.5% (Ustun and Sartorius, 1995). About 13% of patients in primary care were found to have panic disorder in another study (Katon et al., 1986). The frequency with which panic disorder is found in certain specialized medical settings is often higher—for example, the prevalence of panic disorder among cardiology clinic patients with atypical (noncardiac) chest pain was as high as 58% (Beitman et al., 1987). Other studies suggest that 16%–23% of outpatients in cardiac clinics have panic disorder (Chignon et al., 1993; Barsky et al., 1996). Patients with panic disorder are also more likely to be seen in gastroenterology, neurology, and vestibular disorders clinics. Because of the somatic nature of their symptoms and this pattern of help seeking, many cases of panic disorder are missed or misdiagnosed.

COURSE AND PROGNOSIS

The course of panic disorder is difficult to study for several reasons. Some of them are unique to panic disorder, whereas others are also applicable to long-standing conditions in general.

- First, it is difficult to find representative samples of persons with panic disorder who have not had any treatment. Studies of the course of panic disorder have almost invariably been conducted in patients who received treatment at some point in the course of panic disorder; hence, very little is known about the course of untreated panic disorder.
- Second, even after treatment has been completed, many panic patients occasionally or continuously receive additional pharmacological and/or psychological treatment, so that studying the course of panic disorder under absolutely "naturalistic" conditions (i.e., when patients receive no treatment at all) is difficult.
- Third, the course of treated panic disorder may depend on the type of treatment received, and samples of patients who received different types of treatment should not be simply added to a study to create larger samples.
- Fourth, there are no universally accepted definitions of response, improvement, remission, relapse, exacerbation, and recurrence of panic disorder. This means that criteria for characterizing the course of panic disorder are often arbitrary and differ from one study to another.
- Fifth, some patients exhibit significant improvement in one aspect of panic disorder (e.g., they may have only occasional panic attacks or no panic attacks at all), while their improvement in other aspects of panic disorder is much less impressive (e.g., they may still resort to phobic avoidance). In such cases, it is difficult to characterize overall improvement.
- Finally, regardless of how long follow-up studies last, there are some patients whose status might change during further follow-up, but how many would experience such a change remains unknown because of the need to impose a cross-sectional cut-off. Thus, patients who were panic-free and judged to be in remission at the end of a 5-year follow-up period might subsequently have a recurrence.

Keeping in mind these methodological problems and limitations, it is not surprising that results of follow-up studies of panic disorder are inconsistent. However, some conclusions about the course of panic disorder are still warranted (Table 2–17).

TABLE 2–17. Long-Term Course of Treated Panic Disorder

Characterization of Course	Percentage Estimate
Recovery	*30%–35%*
Complete or almost complete remission	
No impairment in functioning	
No need for treatment	
Chronic, with Fluctuations	*50%*
Mild and/or occasional symptoms	
Minor and/or occasional interference with functioning	
Occasional, sometimes a prolonged need for treatment	
Chronic, Without Fluctuations	*15%–20%*
Continuous and moderate to severe symptoms	
Complications of panic disorder more likely	
Continuous interference with functioning	
Continuous need for treatment	

First, panic disorder tends to be a chronic condition in the majority of patients. For example, after a 5-year follow-up of patients with panic disorder, only 12% had no symptoms at all and were not receiving any treatment (Faravelli et al., 1995). Similar findings were reported by two recently published long-term follow-up studies, conducted 11 years (Swoboda et al., 2003) and 15 years (Andersch and Hetta, 2003) after pharmacological treatment of panic disorder. At 11-year follow-up, only one-third of patients were considered to be in complete remission, although two-thirds did not have a panic attack during the year preceding the follow-up. At 15-year follow-up, 18% of patients showed complete recovery (no panic attacks and no pharmacotherapy for 10 years prior to follow-up), whereas 13% were recovered, but still taking medication. At 11-year and 15-year follow-up, the number of patients who met diagnostic criteria for panic disorder was 12.5% and 18%, respectively. At 15-year follow-up, 51% of patients reported recurrent panic attacks. As for agoraphobia, significant avoidance was found in 46% of patients at 11-year follow-up and in 20% of patients at 15-year follow-up. These findings suggest that complete and permanent recovery in panic disorder—when all the relevant criteria for such a recovery are taken into account—does not occur very often.

A second conclusion is that despite chronicity, the overall outcome of treated panic disorder is favorable. This means that most patients have relatively minor problems in one or more domains of panic disorder; these problems generally do not interfere with their functioning, interfere only mildly to moderately, or interfere only at certain times. For example, in the 11-year and 15-year follow up studies of panic disorder (Andersch and Hetta, 2003; Swoboda et al., 2003), the vast majority of patients (78%–94%) did not show impairment in functioning in the areas of work and family life.

Third, the precise proportion of panic patients with fluctuations is unknown, but rough estimates suggest that up to 50% exhibit a fluctuating course (American Psychiatric Association, 2000). The course of panic disorder in these cases is usually characterized by occasional and/or mild panic attacks, limited-symptom panic attacks, and a fluctuating, mild to moderate anticipatory anxiety and phobic avoidance. Depending on the extent of these problems and their previous treatment experience, panic patients may seek help or cope on their own. When panic disorder exhibits a fluctuating course, exacerbations can be precipitated by factors such as interpersonal conflicts, excessive consumption of caffeine, or hormonal changes during a premenstrual period. The frequency of panic attacks may decrease dramatically during pregnancy or they may completely disappear during that time (e.g., Villeponteaux et al., 1992). In the postpartum period, however, panic attacks may return with an even greater frequency and severity.

A fourth conclusion about the course of panic disorder is that in a minority of patients (15%–20% of all treated patients), various components of the disorder are continuously or almost continuously present, and patients usually remain impaired and require ongoing treatment. This group of patients is also most likely to develop complications of panic disorder, particularly depression and alcohol-related problems.

The course of agoraphobia may follow the course of panic disorder, so that with fewer and less severe panic attacks, agoraphobia also becomes less prominent, and vice versa. In other cases, there does not appear to be such a close relationship between panic attacks and agoraphobic avoidance, and agoraphobia takes a course of its own, regardless of the presence or absence of panic attacks. For example, agoraphobia may persist in patients who have not had any panic attacks for a long time.

Prognosis

Several follow-up studies (Noyes et al., 1993; Katschnig et al., 1995; O'Rourke et al., 1996; Andersch and Hetta, 2003) have identified factors that are predictive of a more chronic course and a relatively poor prognosis of panic disorder (Table 2–18). These factors include being single, earlier onset of panic disorder, longer duration of panic disorder before the

TABLE 2–18. Factors Indicating a More Chronic Course and Relatively Poor Prognosis in Panic Disorder

Being single
Earlier onset of panic disorder
Longer duration of panic disorder before onset of treatment
Greater severity of panic attacks
Greater severity of agoraphobia
Presence of a personality disorder
Co-occurrence of depression
Poor response to initial treatment

onset of treatment, greater severity of panic attacks and agoraphobia, presence of a personality disorder, co-occurrence of depression, and poor response to initial treatment. Women may be more likely than men to have recurrences of panic disorder (Yonkers et al., 1998), but this effect may be mediated through women's greater propensity to develop agoraphobia, which is itself associated with a poorer prognosis.

Complications

Panic disorder is often complicated by agoraphobia and depression and less often by alcohol-related disorders. The relationships between panic disorder on one hand and agoraphobia, depression, and alcohol-related disorders on the other are discussed in Relationship Between Panic Disorder and Other Disorders (above). The risk for depression seems to be increased if panic patients also have agoraphobia and social anxiety disorder. The long-term risk for developing alcohol-related problems and other substance abuse or dependence disorders among patients with panic disorder may also be high.

Panic disorder was found to be associated with much higher rates of suicide, suicide attempts, and suicidal ideation than those in the general population. This was intuitively surprising, as one would not expect more suicide and parasuicidal phenomena and behaviors among the patients who often have a very strong fear of death and dying. But suicide was reported as a cause of death in as many as 20% of patients with panic disorder (Coryell et al., 1982), whereas lifetime suicide attempt rates were 20% in an epidemiological study (Weissman et al., 1989; Johnson et al., 1990) and 42% in one clinical study (Lepine et al., 1993). Suicidal ideation in panic disorder was even more frequent—in 44% of an epidemiological sample (Weissman et al., 1989; Johnson et al., 1990) and in 60% of a clinical sample (Lepine et al., 1993).

The results of subsequent research (e.g., Hornig and McNally, 1995; Warshaw et al., 2000) suggest that the increased suicidality in panic disorder patients can be attributed to co-occurrence of panic disorder with other conditions—depression, alcohol-related disorders, and some personality disorders—that are known to be associated with a higher risk of suicide and parasuicidal phenomena and behaviors. An increased risk of suicidality is conferred not only by the presence of these disorders in their full-blown, diagnosable form, but also by their diagnostically subthreshold manifestations. In the absence of co-occurring psychiatric disorders, panic patients do not seem to have a higher risk of suicide and suicide attempts.

Another intriguing finding about the course of panic disorder is a higher mortality rate among patients with panic disorder, particularly among men with this condition. Men with panic disorder seem to have a higher risk for developing cardiovascular and cerebrovascular diseases and die earlier from these diseases than men without panic disorder (Coryell et al., 1982; 1986; Weissman et al., 1990; Allgulander and Lavori, 1991; Kawachi et al., 1994).

It is not clear whether the increased risk of cardiovascular and cerebrovascular morbidity and mortality is a direct or indirect consequence of panic disorder. It has been hypothesized that panic disorder may lead to ventricular arrhythmias, coronary artery disease, myocardial infarction, and/or sudden cardiac death as a result of hyperventilation (Kawachi et al., 1994), sympathetic hyperactivity and "mental stress" (Katon, 1990; Fleet et al., 2000a), or decreased vagal tone and the associated decreased heart rate variability (Kawachi et al., 1995; Fleet et al., 2000a; Gorman and Sloan, 2000). It is also possible that the presence of panic disorder confers an increased risk of heart disease because panic patients may be more likely to have hypertension (White and Baker, 1986; Davies et al., 1999) and high blood cholesterol levels (Bajwa et al., 1992). They may also be physically inactive and avoid exercise (as a consequence of the fear of the exercise-induced physical symptoms), smoke more cigarettes, and start smoking earlier (Pohl et al., 1992; Amering et al., 1999; Breslau and Klein, 1999). Finally, there may be a link with cardiovascular disease via depression, which often accompanies panic disorder and has an established association with cardiovascular disease.

Panic Disorder and Quality of Life

It is now well established that panic disorder has an adverse effect on the quality of life (e.g., Markowitz et al., 1989; Candilis et al., 1999). The impairment in one or more domains of functioning as a result of panic disorder can be quite severe. Thus, patients with panic disorder have often been found to have significant problems in marital and family functioning, in the areas of occupational and academic functioning, and also in terms of general social and interpersonal functioning. Because they often feel that no one understands them, including their own families and close friends, panic patients may gradually withdraw from such contacts and find themselves isolated. The other response to this strong sense of not being understood may be anger and hostility toward close family members, resulting in marital and family strife.

Many panic patients feel that they are unable to work or that their work performance is not satisfactory. Frequent absence from work may lead to a loss of job, and rates of unemployment among patients with panic disorder tend to be high (Leon et al., 1995). The consequences of unemployment include financial difficulties, and many panic patients receive financial assistance or disability payments (Klerman et al., 1991). Some patients drop out of school and find it difficult to participate in various social interactions and activities.

Finally, panic disorder is associated with increased health-care utilization. Panic patients have been found to seek treatment in emergency medical departments and various medical and psychiatric settings and to use primary care and specialized medical services far more often than patients with other psychiatric disorders and patients without psychiatric illness (Markowitz et al., 1989; Klerman et al., 1991; Leon et al., 1995; Katon, 1996). The combination of panic disorder patients' frequent presentation to medical facilities and relatively poor recognition of panic disorder in such settings (e.g., Fifer et al., 1994; Fleet et al., 1996) is associated with substantial costs, mainly because of expensive and often unnecessary medical diagnostic procedures used for assessment (e.g., Salvador-Carulla et al., 1995; Katon, 1996).

ETIOLOGY AND PATHOGENESIS

Etiological factors unique to panic disorder have not been discovered. It is often assumed that panic disorder is a consequence of various, more or less specific interactions between these factors, but we still do not have a complete understanding of them.

Most clinicians seem to believe that there is a certain predisposition for panic attacks and panic disorder, but there appears to be no predisposition common to all persons with panic disorder. The predisposition is usually conceptualized in terms of genetic and/or psychological vulnerability. Panic attacks then occur through various pathophysiological (e.g., hyperventilation) and/or cognitive and other psychological (e.g., catastrophic appraisal of physical sensations) mechanisms. However, reasons for triggering these mechanisms (and not others) often remain elusive. The main models that attempt to account for etiology and pathogenesis of panic disorder are presented below.

BIOLOGICAL MODELS

Table 2–19 summarizes the hypothesized pathophysiological mechanisms that may be relatively specific for panic attacks and panic disorder.

Genetic Factors

In most family studies conducted so far, the lifetime prevalence rate of panic disorder among first-degree relatives of probands with panic disorder has been 10%–17.3%, which compares to the lifetime prevalence rate of panic disorder among control subjects of 0.8%–3.5% (Crowe et al., 1983;

TABLE 2–19. Hypothesized Pathophysiological Mechanisms That May Be Relatively Specific for Panic Attacks and Panic Disorder

- An abnormally sensitive anxiety-regulating mechanism (originating in the amygdala) lowers the "threshold" for tolerating sensory information, so that ordinary sensory information activates autonomic responses (through brain-stem nuclei) and the accompanying catastrophic cognitions (through the cortex), leading to a panic attack.

- Panic attacks can be artificially induced by increasing the respiration rate (hyperventilation), inhaling carbon dioxide, or disrupting the acid–base balance.

- Acute hyperventilation leads to a panic attack via hypocapnia and alkalosis.

- A panic attack is a consequence of hypersensitivity to carbon dioxide of the brain-stem chemoreceptors, so that they react excessively to an even minor increase in concentration of carbon dioxide.

- A panic attack is a consequence of the premature and inappropriate activation of the alarm mechanism, which aims to prevent choking and ensure survival. This alarm mechanism involves hyperventilation and attempts to lower the concentration of carbon dioxide in an individual who is hypersensitive to carbon dioxide and therefore has a lower threshold for activating the alarm mechanism (theory of the false suffocation alarm).

- A panic attack is a consequence of the increased central noradrenergic activity (hypersensitivity of the presynaptic α_{-2} receptors, increased firing rate of the locus coeruleus).

- Failure of the GABA system to inhibit the locus coeruleus leads to a panic attack.

Noyes et al., 1986; Mendlewicz et al., 1993; Weissman, 1993; Fyer et al., 1995). Compared to first-degree relatives of persons without panic disorder, first-degree relatives of persons with panic disorder may be 17.7 times more at risk of developing panic disorder (Weissman, 1993). This risk is partly related to the age of onset of panic disorder: the earlier the age of onset (prior to the age of 20), the more likely it is for first-degree relatives to also have panic disorder (Goldstein et al., 1997). Thus, early-onset panic disorder may have a stronger familial or genetic component than panic disorder with a later onset in life.

Recent research suggests that there may be a genetic link between panic disorder, major depression, alcoholism, social anxiety disorder, and bipolar affective disorder. In comparison with first-degree relatives of persons without panic disorder, first-degree relatives of persons with panic disorder had higher rates of social anxiety disorder and major depression (Goldstein et al., 1994; Maier et al., 1995), whereas alcoholism was almost four times more common among male relatives (Crowe et al., 1983). Panic disorder was also more common among relatives of persons with major depression than among relatives of individuals without major depression. The occurrence of panic disorder in patients with bipolar affective disorder appears to be determined by genetic factors (Mackinnon et al., 1997).

Studies of panic disorder among twins have produced conflicting results. While some studies found a higher concordance rate for panic disorder among monozygotic twins than among dizygotic twins (Torgersen, 1983; Skre et al., 1993), there was no such difference in at least one twin study (Andrews et al., 1990). In addition, the concordance rate for panic disorder in monozygotic twins was 31% (Torgersen, 1983), suggesting that nongenetic factors play an important role in the development of the condition. The risk of inheriting panic disorder, calculated on the basis of a female twin study, was estimated at 30%–40% (Kendler et al., 1993); as a way of comparison, this estimate is considerably lower than the corresponding figures for schizophrenia and bipolar affective disorder.

The mode of inheriting panic disorder is not known, but genetic linkage studies indicate that a single-gene transmission is unlikely. Genetic predisposition for panic disorder may be nonspecific, because a general tendency to respond with anxiety is perhaps more likely to be inherited (Torgersen, 1983; Andrews et al., 1990). A higher prevalence of panic disorder in certain families and among first-degree relatives of persons with panic disorder still does not constitute evidence that panic disorder is a genetically based condition, because the relative contribution of shared environmental factors remains unknown.

Neuroanatomical Model of Panic Disorder

In an attempt to tie panic disorder to specific brain structures, it was initially proposed (Gorman et al., 1989) that panic attacks originate in brain-stem structures, specifically locus coeruleus and raphe nuclei. The limbic system was believed to play the main role in the development of anticipatory anxiety, whereas prefrontal cortex was thought to be responsible for panic-related avoidance. This model has recently been revised (Gorman et al., 2000), and it now incorporates some contributions from psychological theories of panic disorder.

In its current version (Gorman et al., 2000), the model proposes that persons with panic disorder inherit and/or develop early in life an abnormally sensitive mechanism that regulates anxiety. The brain structure that is crucial for the functioning of this mechanism is now believed to be the central nucleus of the amygdala, which is well connected with the prefrontal cortex, hippocampus, thalamus, hypothalamus, periaqueductal gray matter, locus coeruleus, and other parts of the brain stem. According to this model, the overly sensitive anxiety-regulating mechanism lowers the threshold for tolerating sensory information, so that ordinary sensory information activates autonomic responses (through brain-stem nuclei) and the accompanying catastrophic cognitions (through the cortex). The model also suggests that medications that reduce intensity and/or frequency of panic attacks do so by decreasing the activity of the amygdala (and thereby affect the activity of the hypothalamus and brain stem); cognitive-behavior therapy and other efficacious psychotherapies, by contrast, affect higher brain structures connected with the amygdala, especially the hippocampus and prefrontal cortex.

Induction of Panic Attacks

Biological studies of panic disorder have often relied on the provocation of panic attacks by means of an intravenous infusion or inhalation of various substances. The purpose of these studies was to shed more light on possible mechanisms involved in the precipitation of panic attacks. The main problem with these studies, however, has been the uncertainty as to whether their findings might be generalized to naturally occurring panic attacks.

The most important finding of panic induction studies was that panic attacks were induced much more often in individuals with panic disorder than in those without panic disorder. For example, panic attacks were induced by sodium lactate infusions in 67% of individuals with panic disorder, 7%–22% of those with other psychiatric disorders, and 13% of persons without any psychiatric disorder (Liebowitz et al., 1985; Cowley and Arana, 1990). This finding has been a subject to two different interpretations. First, the occurrence of panic attacks was regarded as a direct consequence of the pathophysiological changes produced by "panicogenic" substances: second, it was proposed that cognitive factors (e.g., fear of physical symptoms, catastrophic appraisal of physical symptoms) accounted for the occurrence of panic attacks, as physical symptoms are induced in the vast majority of individuals, whereas only some go on to develop a panic attack.

Various substances have been used in panic induction studies. Some of them, such as carbon dioxide, sodium lactate, and sodium bicarbonate, change the acid–base balance and affect levels of carbon dioxide and respiration rate, leading to panic. This mechanism may be a consequence of hypersensitivity to carbon dioxide and/or may involve hyperventilation (both described below). Other substances (e.g., yohimbin, fenfluramine, m-chlorophenylpiperazine, flumazenil, and cholecystokinin) induce panic attacks by acting on the norepinephrine, serotonin, or gamma-aminobutyric acid (GABA) neurotransmitter systems and the corresponding receptors.

Role of Hyperventilation

Acute hyperventilation is a pathophysiological mechanism that causes many symptoms of panic. However, hyperventilation is not always sufficient, nor is it necessary for panic attack to occur, as panic attacks in many individuals are neither preceded by nor associated with hyperventilation.

The pathophysiological changes in acute hyperventilation occur as a result of the deficit of carbon dioxide; when carbon dioxide is lost through overbreathing it is not compensated for by its production through metabolism. The consequently decreased blood level of carbon dioxide (hypocapnia) and alkalosis lead to symptoms typical of panic attacks. Hypocapnia causes cerebral vasoconstriction and decreased delivery of oxygen to the brain tissue, which is clinically manifested through such symptoms as lightheadedness, dizziness, fainting feeling, blurred vision, and even depersonalization, derealization, disorientation, confusion, and agitation. Alkalosis leads to hypocalcemia, and this in turn causes numbness or tingling sensations. The clinical consequences of further pathophysiological changes are tachycardia, palpitations, chest pain or tightness in the chest, and shortness of breath.

In chronic hyperventilation, all the pathophysiological changes are compensated for, except for hypocapnia. Therefore, persons who habitually hyperventilate may develop symptoms of acute hyperventilation with minimal increase in their breathing rate.

Other Respiratory Dysfunction in Panic Disorder

Inhalation of 5%–35% carbon dioxide is much more likely to induce panic attacks in patients with panic disorder than in persons who have never experienced panic attacks (Gorman et al., 1984). The pathophysiological mechanism involves respiratory acidosis, hypercapnia, and hypercalcemia, which cause dyspnea, choking feeling, and panic. This state may trigger hyperventilation to compensate for the respiratory and metabolic changes, but hyperventilation only leads to further symptoms of panic (Gorman et al., 1988). These observations and findings have served as the foundation for the hypothesis that panic attacks are a consequence of the hypersensitivity to carbon dioxide of brain-stem chemoreceptors (Gorman and Papp, 1990; Papp et al., 1993). Because of this hypersensitivity, chemoreceptors react excessively to an even minor increase in the concentration of carbon dioxide, leading to symptoms of dyspnea and choking feeling followed by hyperventilation, all of which lead to panic.

D. Klein (1993) has proposed a theory of the "false suffocation alarm" as an explanation for panic attacks. According to this theory, panic attack is a consequence of the premature and inappropriate activation of the alarm mechanism, which aims to prevent choking and ensure survival. This alarm mechanism involves hyperventilation—and an attempt to lower the concentration of carbon dioxide in an individual who is hypersensitive to carbon dioxide and therefore has a lower threshold for activating the alarm mechanism. The reaction is triggered especially in those situations that signal a possibility of lack of oxygen and the consequent suffocation (for example, being in a small, enclosed space). Klein (1993) has listed several clinical findings in support of his theory and its specificity for panic disorder. Among them, the most significant seem to be the following: (1) dyspnea is a frequent symptom during panic attacks, but it is not a manifestation of "normal" anxiety or fear, and (2) panic disorder is the most common anxiety disorder among people with respiratory diseases. The "false suffocation alarm" theory has been tested and re-examined, and the results have been mixed, with only partial support for the main tenets of the theory.

Dysfunction of Neurotransmitter Systems

As already noted, there is no neurotransmitter abnormality that is specific for panic disorder. As in generalized anxiety disorder, which most resembles panic disorder in terms of neurotransmitter abnormalities, it appears that the norepinephrine, serotonin, and GABA systems are involved, in proportions and combinations that vary from one person to another.

Norepinephrine
Early studies of the pathophysiology of panic disorder focused on the role of the locus coeruleus, which is located in the pons and contains about one-half of all noradrenergic neurons in the central nervous system. The locus coeruleus appears to play a key role in coordinating the functioning of the sympathic nervous system, as it is well connected with the hippocampus, amygdala, limbic system, and cerebral cortex (particularly the frontal lobe). Through the descending pathways that originate in the locus coeruleus, it also affects peripheral sympathetic activity.

Two lines of evidence suggest that there may be increased central noradrenergic activity in panic disorder. One is the finding from animal studies that stimulation of the locus coeruleus leads to anxiety reactions that are very similar to panic attacks in humans (Redmond, 1979). The other is that several medications efficacious in panic disorder (e.g., tricyclic antidepressants and benzodiazepines) decrease the firing rate of the locus coeruleus. However, the locus coeruleus may have a more broad role and may play a part in general arousal responses as well as in responses to novel stimuli (Aston-Jones et al., 1984). Also, not all medications that decrease the firing rate of the locus coeruleus (e.g., propranolol, morphine) are efficacious in the treatment of panic disorder.

In patients with panic disorder, panic attacks can be induced by yohimbin, an α-2 adrenergic antagonist that increases the activity of the locus coeruleus and noradrenergic function (Charney et al., 1984). Likewise, symptoms of panic and anxiety can be alleviated by clonidine, an α-2 adrenergic agonist that inhibits the locus coeruleus. The latter finding has led to a hypothesis that panic disorder may be characterized more specifically by hypersensitivity of presynaptic α-2 receptors (Charney and Heninger, 1986) and the consequently increased noradrenergic stimulation. Such presynaptic hypersensitivity may be counteracted by imipramine, which would help explain, at least in part, the efficacy of imipramine in the treatment of panic disorder. However, the postulated central noradrenergic dysregulation in panic disorder seems more complex than originally thought.

Serotonin
The administration of fenfluramine (which enhances the release of serotonin) and *m*-chlorophenylpiperazine (which is an agonist at some serotonin receptors and antagonist at other serotonin receptors) to patients with panic disorder tends to induce anxiety and panic attacks. Numerous studies suggest a role of the serotonin system in the etiology and pathogenesis

of panic disorder, but it is a matter of considerable speculation as to the exact mechanisms through which this occurs. Thus, it is not clear whether the function of serotonin in panic disorder is decreased or increased. It has been hypothesized that serotonin 1_A receptor dysfunction may be relatively specific for panic disorder (Lesch et al., 1992), but this has not been confirmed. In view of these uncertainties, it is not surprising that the exact mechanism through which selective serotonin reuptake inhibitors work in panic disorder remains unclear and that different hypotheses have been put forward in an attempt to explain this.

Gamma-aminobutyric Acid

The GABA system has been implicated in the anxiety disorders in general. Administration of antagonists at the benzodiazepine-$GABA_A$ receptors (e.g., flumazenil) induces panic attacks in patients with panic disorder (Nutt et al., 1990), whereas administration of agonists (e.g., benzodiazepines) alleviates anxiety and panic, although not reliably so. It is largely on the basis of these findings that alterations at the level of the benzodiazepine-$GABA_A$ receptors have been hypothesized in panic disorder.

Since GABA normally inhibits functioning of the locus coeruleus, thereby decreasing anxiety and preventing panic attacks, the main idea in this hypothesis is that the GABA system fails to inhibit the locus coeruleus. This may occur as a consequence of various primary abnormalities and mechanisms. For example, individuals with panic disorder may have fewer benzodiazepine-$GABA_A$ receptors, a possibility suggested by the finding of decreased benzodiazepine receptor binding in imaging studies (Malizia et al., 1998; Bremner et al., 2000). Another possibility is that levels of GABA are decreased in patients with panic disorder (Goddard et al., 2001b). The sensitivity of benzodiazepine-GABA receptors may be decreased in panic disorder (Roy-Byrne et al., 1990) or, more generally, altered (Nutt et al., 1990). Finally, there may be a deficiency in endogenous anxiolytic substances or an excess of endogenous, anxiogenic/panicogenic substances, which act via benzodiazepine-GABA receptors.

Neuroimaging Studies

The results of magnetic resonance imaging (MRI) and position emission tomography (PET) studies in panic disorder have not been consistent. We do know, however, that cerebral structural abnormalities and changes in metabolism and blood flow in patients with panic disorder tend to be found more often in temporal lobes; some of these changes are unilateral, whereas others are bilateral. A full understanding of these findings is still lacking, and it is not clear whether such changes play some role in the pathogenesis of panic disorder or whether they are merely an epiphenomenon of panic disorder.

Psychological Models

Cognitive Approaches

All cognitive theories of panic disorder (Table 2–20) share a view that, in a way similar to other anxiety disorders, panic disorder is characterized by the exaggerated appraisal of threat and danger. It is the *nature* of this threat that distinguishes panic disorder from other anxiety disorders. Whereas the threat in conditions like phobias and posttraumatic stress disorder is mainly external, the perceived threat in panic disorder is of an internal nature. That is, the threat in panic disorder is perceived to originate within one's body, which accounts for panic patients' hypervigilance about their physical sensations and bodily functions. As a result, patients may be more prone to misinterpret certain physical events and/or may be more afraid of physical anxiety symptoms. This may represent an ongoing, relatively specific cognitive vulnerability for panic disorder; alternatively, such hypervigilance about one's body and physical sensations and symptoms may be a consequence of panic disorder.

Catastrophic Misinterpretation of Benign Physical Sensations and Symptoms

The most influential cognitive model of panic disorder was postulated by Clark (1986, 1988). Its main idea is that panic attack is a consequence of catastrophic misinterpretation of benign physical sensations and symptoms.

Table 2–20. Cognitive Aspects of Panic Disorder

Common to All Anxiety Disorders
Exaggerated perception and appraisal of threat and danger
Relatively Specific for Panic Disorder
Threat is perceived as originating within one's body
Hypervigilance about physical sensations and symptoms and bodily functions
Greater likelihood of misinterpreting physical sensations and symptoms as a sign of impending catastrophe
Beliefs about dangerousness of anxiety and its (physical) symptoms, leading to fear of anxiety and its (physical) symptoms
Greater need for control over physical sensations and symptoms and bodily functions

In other words, physical sensations and/or symptoms do not lead to a panic attack unless they have been misinterpreted in a catastrophic fashion. According to this model, physical sensations and symptoms are experienced as dangerous because they are appraised as portending a catastrophic outcome, such as death or a life-threatening physical condition, or, less often, loss of control or loss of sanity.

Physical sensations and symptoms, such as symptoms of autonomic hyperactivity, initially occur as a physiological component of anxiety and are subsequently subjected to misinterpretation. For example, palpitations are typically misinterpreted as meaning that the person is having a heart attack or is about to die; this misinterpretation then intensifies anxiety and leads to further arousal and more physical symptoms. These symptoms are in turn further misinterpreted in a catastrophic manner, which creates a vicious cycle and a panic attack. Sensations and symptoms most likely to be misinterpreted are usually those that occur suddenly, that have not been experienced before, and for which the person does not have a ready explanation.

The proneness to misinterpret physical sensations and symptoms catastrophically may be a consequence of interacting with parents who are preoccupied with health, symptoms, and bodily functions; as such, this proneness may be present long before the very first panic attack. It may also be reinforced by the attention and care that the person received after the first panic attack. If the tendency to make such catastrophic misinterpretations persists after the first panic attack, the person will be very likely to become apprehensive about future panic attacks, and thus develop panic disorder.

According to Clark's theory, panic disorder is maintained by one or both of the following mechanisms:

1. Persistent hypervigilance about physical sensations and symptoms makes the person even more sensitive to them and lowers the threshold at which sensations and symptoms are experienced. As a result, there are more "opportunities" to misinterpret sensations and symptoms catastrophically.
2. Avoidance of all physical activities (e.g., sport, exercise, physical recreation) that could induce physical sensations and symptoms that the person might misinterpret prevents the person from finding out that these sensations and symptoms are not dangerous.

The catastrophic-misinterpretation model of panic disorder has received substantial support, although it has not been able to give a convincing account of all instances of panic attacks (e.g., nocturnal panic attacks). It also appears that panic attacks are not always preceded by cat-astrophic misinterpretation of physical sensations and symptoms (Rach-man et al., 1988; Wolpe and Rowan, 1988), so that such an appraisal is not always necessary for panic attacks to develop. However, catastrophic appraisal of physical sensations and symptoms may be necessary for panic attacks to occur when physical symptoms of anxiety and panic have been induced by hyperventilation or other panic induction techniques. Like-wise, the occurrence of panic attacks under these circumstances can be pre-vented if symptoms are not misinterpreted. The latter has been used for therapeutic purposes, and the model has been successful as the basis for cognitive therapy, which has proved to be efficacious in the treatment of panic disorder.

Beliefs About the Dangerousness of Anxiety
Another important cognitive model of panic disorder was derived from the concept of anxiety sensitivity (Reiss and McNally, 1985). This concept denotes beliefs that anxiety and its symptoms have dangerous conse-quences, with these consequences being physical (e.g., a serious disease, death), psychological (e.g., loss of sanity), and/or social (e.g., humiliation). According to this model, anxiety sensitivity is akin to a stable personality dimension and represents a specific risk factor for developing panic disor-der (Taylor, 1995). In other words, strong beliefs that anxiety symptoms are dangerous are present before the first panic attack and predict the development of panic disorder. However, the relationship of these beliefs with some of the other anxiety disorders has also been demonstrated (Reiss et al., 1986; Taylor et al., 1992), and it appears that high anxiety sen-sitivity confers a more general vulnerability to develop anxiety disorders, not just panic disorder. Also, high levels of anxiety sensitivity do not sug-gest that the person will inevitably develop panic disorder or any one of the anxiety disorders.

The relationship between anxiety sensitivity and trait anxiety has been a subject of some debate. These constructs may emphasize different aspects of the personality-based experience of anxiety (Taylor, 1995), or there may be a hierarchical relationship between them, so that anxiety sen-sitivity is seen as a dimension of trait anxiety (Lilienfeld et al., 1993). Anxi-ety sensitivity appears to have a genetic component (Stein et al., 1999b), but it may also be caused by parental reinforcement of the child's sick role (Watt et al., 1998) and/or parental threatening, hostile, and rejecting behaviors (Scher and Stein, 2003).

Regardless of the exact nature of anxiety sensitivity, the concept has been of great interest and value in the study of the psychopathology of panic disorder. Thus, the phenomenon of anticipatory anxiety, as conceptualized in current models and definitions of panic disorder, has much overlap with the concept of anxiety sensitivity; for example, high levels of anticipatory anxiety are unlikely in the absence of high levels of anxiety sensitivity. If this is the case, the link between anxiety sensitivity and panic disorder may be better understood through a relationship between anxiety sensitivity and anticipatory anxiety than through a relationship between anxiety sensitivity and panic attacks.

Panic Attacks as False Alarms

Barlow (1988) has proposed a model of panic disorder that includes components from biological, basic emotion, learning (behavioral), and cognitive theories. His theory first makes a distinction between fear and anxiety (Table 2–21). Fear is one of the "basic emotions" with a distinct physiological pattern (autonomic hyperarousal), which represents an acute, short-lasting response to the perceived, immediate danger ("true alarm"). Anxiety is a longer-lasting "state of mood," which lacks a distinct physiological pattern and is more cognitive in nature, being characterized by apprehension about harm and danger in the future. Within this framework, panic attack is conceptualized as fear but, more precisely, as a "false alarm," because real danger is not present. Thus, except for the presence or absence of real danger, there is no difference between panic attacks and fear in terms of biological (autonomic hyperarousal), cognitive (appraisal of threat as immediate), and behavioral ("fight-or-flight") responses.

Barlow (1988) has suggested that there has to be both a biological and psychological vulnerability for the first panic attack to develop. Biological vulnerability refers to a susceptibility to be easily aroused, especially in response to stress; psychological vulnerability, which results from adverse childhood events and interactions with parents, pertains to the lack of

TABLE 2–21.Distinctions Between Fear and Anxiety and Between Panic Attacks and Anticipatory Anxiety[a]

Characteristics	Fear and Panic Attacks	Anxiety and Anticipatory Anxiety
Appraisal of threat	Clear and immediate	Somewhat vague and more distant (in the future)
Physiological response	Autonomic hyperarousal	Less clear, often absent
Behavioral response	"Fight or flight"	No clear and immediate behavioral response
Onset, course, and duration	Abrupt onset, acute, short-lasting	Gradual onset, chronic, long-lasting

[a]Distinctions according to Barlow (1988).

security and a strong sense that one has little or no control over one's life. Barlow's theory accounts for two further developments after the initial panic attack. The first one is the occurrence of the specific type of anxiety or anxious apprehension that pertains to a possibility of having another panic attack. Panic attacks are then usually perceived as even more unpleasant, uncontrollable, and even dangerous, so that these particular appraisals of panic contribute to the maintenance of panic disorder.

In the second development, following the first panic attack, a link is established between the experience of the "false alarm" on one hand and physical symptoms and the accompanying "negative" cognitions on the other—this is a process referred to as "interoceptive conditioning." As a result of this process, the occurrence of physical symptoms or certain associated thoughts may trigger panic attacks; these conditioned panic attacks have been called "learned alarms."

Through the false-alarm model of panic disorder, an important attempt has been made to integrate knowledge about panic and anxiety from different perspectives. Certain components of the model remain somewhat controversial—for example, the distinction between panic (fear) and anxiety—but overall, the model has been widely accepted and used as a foundation for a specific and efficacious type of cognitive-behavioral therapy, panic control treatment.

Other Cognitive Factors

Another phenomenon that may be important in the development of panic disorder is a loss of the sense of control. Patients often describe panic attacks as a "complete loss of control." If this is the case, can a restoration of this sense of control, even if it is an illusion, prevent panic attacks? This strategy has been tested in a study (Sanderson et al., 1989) in which panic attacks were induced by carbon dioxide inhalations. Subjects who were led to believe that they had some control over the situation by changing the concentration of carbon dioxide during inhalations, and thereby decreasing the likelihood of having panic attacks, had significantly fewer panic attacks than those who did not have this illusion of control. This study shows that, at least in some individuals, loss of the sense of control is associated with panic attacks. But this loss may precede panic attacks, just as it may be a consequence of panic disorder.

Expectations of panic attacks in general, and expectations of the attacks in certain situations in particular, have been associated with the development of agoraphobia (see Table 2–10). Furthermore, the more a person expects a panic attack to occur, the more likely it is for panic to actually occur (Margraf et al., 1986). This is so because the vigilance and arousal accompanying such expectations make it easier for physical symptoms to appear; a catastrophic appraisal of such symptoms then leads to a panic attack.

Psychodynamic Approaches

Modern psychodynamic accounts of panic disorder (Table 2–22) all share a view that panic attacks are not quite spontaneous (unexpected); rather, panic attacks are usually preceded by events that have a unique, unconscious meaning for the person. This meaning then triggers a panic attack by automatically activating relevant neurophysiological mechanisms.

What are the unconscious meanings and mechanisms that could trigger a panic attack? According to the integrative model formulated by Shear and colleagues (1993), panic attacks are triggered by the frightening thoughts and fantasies related to the fear of separation and abandonment by the mighty parental figures and others onto whom such feelings have been transferred. This particular fear is a consequence of the interaction between the innately anxious, inhibited child and the overcontrolling, critical parents and the consequent conflict between dependence and independence. Other manifestations of this unresolved conflict are the following, alternating or simultaneously present, phenomena: excessive reliance on others, fear of interpersonal intimacy, and/or a failure to attain a satisfying measure of independence. As a result of such dynamics, panic patients often harbor negative, angry, and hostile feelings toward their parents and other persons who are important in their lives, but at the same time are extremely afraid of such feelings and use various defense mechanisms to avoid these feelings. Thus, the main problem that panic patients

TABLE 2–22. Psychodynamic "Themes" in Panic Disorder

- Panic attacks are triggered by events that have a unique, unconscious meaning for the person.
- Fears of separation and abandonment
- Unresolved conflict between dependence and independence

  Excessive reliance on others

  Fear of interpersonal intimacy

  Failure to attain a satisfying measure of independence
- Ambivalent attitudes toward significant others
- Finding a bearable "interpersonal distance," so that significant others are neither too close (controlling) nor too far (impossible to rely on)

face is to find a bearable "interpersonal distance," so that significant, "mighty" others are neither too close nor too far.

While the mainstream psychodynamic approach to panic disorder emphasizes underlying intrapsychic conflicts, self psychology proposes a "deficit model." According to this approach, panic disorder is conceptualized as a result of structural defect, with consequent deficiencies in the control of anxiety (Kohut, 1971; 1977). This defect is attributed to the parents' inability to empathize with the child, so that the child cannot feel secure. A fragile and incohesive self then develops and, as such, it is prone to fragmentation, which is the essence of the experience of panic (Diamond, 1985, 1987).

Childhood Separation Anxiety and School Phobia or Refusal

Childhood separation anxiety and the associated problem of school phobia or school refusal have a unique place in considerations about the etiology of panic disorder and agoraphobia: this phenomenon has served an explanatory role for understanding panic disorder and agoraphobia from biological, evolutionary, and psychological perspectives. Separation anxiety has been conceptualized as a biologically determined, automatic response to separation from the mother or the mothering figure (Klein, 1981). This response is seen as a form of the child's effective protest and serves the purpose of "assuring" that the mother will return as quickly as possible. Ultimately, separation anxiety is important for survival of the individual and humankind as well. According to this model, a panic attack is a consequence of the inborn lowered threshold at which separation anxiety is activated. In other words, hypersensitivity to separation is at the root of a panic attack; the attack occurs even when separation is merely being thought about or anticipated.

The findings that separation anxiety is more prominent among girls (Zitrin and Ross, 1988; Silove et al., 1993) and that it has a genetic basis only in females (Silove et al., 1995) have also been interpreted in terms of the theory of evolution. That is, strong separation anxiety in women (but not in men) was seen as adaptive and helping the survival of the species, because it "forced" women to stay with their children and thereby protect the children and care for them (Silove et al., 1995). If this is the case, then agoraphobia could be understood as a result of the conflict between these traditional, survival-driven feminine roles and expectations by contemporary Western society that women take on various social roles, be independent, and compete with men. This account of agoraphobia might also help explain why men are so underrepresented among individuals with agoraphobia.

Separation anxiety plays a pivotal role in Bowlby's (1973) attachment theory. According to this theory, separation anxiety is the "prototype" of any and every anxiety; it can be neutralized only through a secure attachment to the mother (or the mothering figure). If the mother fails to provide security to the child, an "insecure attachment" develops, while the separation anxiety persists. Therefore, agoraphobia will ensue in a child, who as a result of insecure attachment, feels that reliance on parents (and thus on others in general) is not possible but at the same time is afraid of separating from them.

The link between separation anxiety in childhood and panic disorder or agoraphobia in adults has been confirmed by studies showing that patients with panic disorder are more likely to have a history of childhood separation anxiety and school phobia (Gittelman and Klein, 1984). Also, patients with agoraphobia were more likely to have experienced prolonged separation from their mothers in childhood and were more likely to report separation or divorce of their parents and parents' deaths during childhood (Faravelli et al., 1985).

However, other research has not confirmed that there is a specific link between childhood separation anxiety and separation experiences on the one hand and panic disorder or agoraphobia on the other. That is, childhood separation anxiety and separation experiences have been found just as frequently in patients with generalized anxiety disorder, social anxiety disorder, specific phobias, obsessive-compulsive disorder, depression, and eating disorders. Therefore, childhood separation anxiety may be one of the nonspecific risk factors for developing not only panic disorder and agoraphobia but also a range of other psychiatric conditions in adulthood.

Behavioral Inhibition in Childhood

Childhood behavioral inhibition is another etiological explanatory construct often used by theorists, clinicians, and researchers of various orientations. It refers to the inborn dimension of temperament, characterized by caution, inhibition, withdrawal, and physiological hyperarousal on exposure to novel stimuli and situations. When this behavior is consistently present and particularly pronounced, it prevents exploration of the surrounding world, use of cognitive potentials, and self-assertion. Childhood behavioral inhibition was found to be a nonspecific risk factor for developing several anxiety disorders, including panic disorder, agoraphobia, and social anxiety disorder (Rosenbaum et al., 1988). Indeed, because the link between behavioral inhibition and social anxiety disorder seems stronger and perhaps somewhat more specific, the corresponding theory is presented in greater detail in Chapter 4.

Role of Other Developmental Factors and External Influences

Patients with panic disorder are more likely to report the occurrence of various unpleasant and/or traumatic events during their childhood, including physical and sexual abuse. They also tend to report difficulties in relationships with family members and a "family climate" characterized by strife (Raskin et al., 1982). Patients with panic disorder are more likely to perceive their parents as being overprotective, controlling, too critical, and too strict, lacking in warmth and care, and being less interested in their children (Arrindell et al., 1983; Leon and Leon, 1990; Faravelli et al., 1991; Silove et al., 1991).

There are two fundamental problems with research of this kind. One is the retrospective nature of this methodological approach, which has a strong propensity to be biased. The other is a lack of specificity of the research findings: traumatic experiences in childhood, unfavorable family constellation, and negative perception of parents have all been found in patients with very different forms of psychopathology.

Life Events Research

In the year preceding the onset of panic disorder, more negative life events were found among patients with panic disorder than among control group subjects. Among these life events, particularly common were separation or divorce and serious illness or death (especially sudden death) of a close family member or friend. The underlying meaning and significance of these events may be in their leading to abandonment or portending danger, in addition to such events often being experienced as loss of control (Roy-Byrne et al., 1986; Faravelli and Pallanti, 1989).

The onset of panic disorder is preceded not only by clearly unpleasant or painful events but also by such events as getting married or having a child. This suggests that some patients who develop panic disorder may be particularly sensitive to any changes in their lives (Lteif and Mavissakalian, 1995). These findings have led to a hypothesis that the nature of life events preceding panic disorder is not as important as the negative interpretation of these events (Rapee et al., 1990b); in turn, such an interpretation may be determined by various contextual factors (e.g., current health problems, perceived lack of support), personality-related factors (e.g., neuroticism), and/or childhood factors (e.g., loss of parents during childhood).

It can be speculated that life events that suddenly demonstrate the extent of a person's vulnerability and lack of control permanently activate biological alarm mechanisms. Once set in motion, these mechanisms continue to operate and thus maintain panic attacks, long after the occurrence of the unpleasant or traumatic precipitating event.

Psychological Accounts of Agoraphobia

The straightforward explanation of agoraphobia is that it is a consequence of recurrent panic attacks and anticipatory anxiety. As a result of conditioning, patients learn to fear those places and situations where they have had unpleasant, frightening panic attacks and symptoms (and where they now expect to have another attack). The avoidance of such places and situations reinforces agoraphobia, because avoidance minimizes the possibility of having panic attacks, panic symptoms, and, more generally, anxiety and discomfort. The avoided situations are believed to be dangerous because of their link with panic attacks and panic symptoms: these are situations from which patients might have difficulty escaping in case of a panic attack or in which they might feel embarrassed and there would be no one to help in case of a panic attack. The avoidance behavior prevents disconfirmation of beliefs about such situations and about panic attacks and symptoms.

In other accounts of agoraphobia, panic attacks are not postulated as being so crucial in the development of agoraphobia. Instead, the avoidance behavior might have meanings and purposes other then just minimizing the possibility of having a panic attack. The psychodynamic model of agoraphobia is a prime example of such an approach.

The classical psychoanalytic explanation (Fenichel, 1945; Miller, 1953) is that agoraphobia serves the purpose of "protecting" women from unconscious, forbidden sexual drives that suggest promiscuous tendencies. By developing agoraphobia and ultimately by becoming homebound, such women no longer have an "opportunity" to be unfaithful to their partners, who are often depicted as controlling and jealous. In this scenario, agoraphobia may also serve the purpose of "saving the marriage" (or saving the relationship, in a wider sense), and this is the "secondary gain" from having agoraphobia. But partners of agoraphobic patients may also "benefit" from agoraphobia, as it allows partners to have better control over the agoraphobia sufferers. This is consistent with the observations (e.g., Hafner, 1977) that husbands of agoraphobic patients are often reluctant to change the agoraphobic status quo, that they may sabotage the treatment of patients, and that they actually get worse (become more jealous or develop sexual dysfunction) as patients get better.

The hypothesis that agoraphobia has a "marriage-saving" function has not been confirmed: studies generally show that marital functioning improves, rather than deteriorates, in the course of behavioral treatment of

agoraphobia, and that treatment does not affect patients' partners in a negative way (Lange and van Dyck, 1992; Emmelkamp and Gerlsma, 1994).
Moreover, studies could not confirm that marriages of most patients with
agoraphobia differed significantly from the marriages of persons without
agoraphobia (Buglass et al., 1977; Arrindell and Emmelkamp, 1986;
McLeod, 1994). There is a subset of patients with agoraphobia, however,
who are in a dysfunctional marital relationship such as that outlined above
that is very prominent and precedes the onset of agoraphobia. This may
play some role in the etiology of agoraphobia. A recent review (Marcaurelle
et al., 2003) has concluded that the issue of the role of marital dysfunction in
the development of panic disorder with agoraphobia remains open.

Patients with agoraphobia who have significant marital problems
often exhibit a paralyzing ambivalence about what to do. They often want
to leave their partners, or separate from or divorce them, but are equally
afraid of doing so; weighing the reasons for and against separation or
divorce may be all-encompassing and exhausting. Such ambivalence may
reflect an underlying conflict between autonomy and attachment (or independence and dependence), which is presumed to be an important etiological factor in agoraphobia (Frances and Dunn, 1975).

More broadly, agoraphobia is often portrayed as a prototype or even a
caricature of dependence and dependent behavior. However, patients
with agoraphobia do not necessarily feel "comfortable" about such dependence and may be quite resentful and hostile toward the persons on whom
they have become dependent.

Finally, there has been some speculation about childhood "precur-
sors" of agoraphobia. Observations and research findings (Goldstein and
Chambless, 1978) suggest that agoraphobic patients come from families in
which mothers had a dominant and controlling position, and in which
independent behavior and open expression of feelings and needs were dis-
couraged or even punished. Children growing up in such families adopt a
style of avoiding to deal with problems and leave it to others to take
responsibility and "do things" for them, because they do not feel capable of
acting responsibly and functioning on their own. Although there may be a
link between these features in childhood and behaviors typical of agoraphobia in adulthood, again, the specificity of this link is questionable.

TREATMENT

In view of the chronic course of panic disorder in most cases, short-term
treatment is usually not sufficient. Even when patients improve significantly after several weeks or months of treatment, as they often do, some

treatment measures need to be continuously administered because of the possibility of relapse and complications.

When patients with panic disorder first present for treatment, they are typically distressed by panic attacks and frightened of their consequences. Therefore, they are likely to urgently seek some plausible explanation for their symptoms and reassurance that the feared catastrophe will not happen—and quick relief from at least some of their symptoms. All this can be achieved through relatively simple measures, such as psychoeducation and provision of support, in addition to administration of medications, if appropriate. The subsequent course of therapeutic action is a matter of negotiation between patients and their therapists, and this occurs ideally after patients have been well informed about further treatment and available treatment options. In this process, it is important to identify patients' expectations from treatment and explore any discrepancies between these expectations and treatment realities.

Regardless of the treatment modality used, short-term (1–3 months) goals of treatment of panic disorder generally include a significant decrease in the frequency and intensity, or even disappearance of, panic attacks, and a decrease in the intensity of anticipatory anxiety and panic-related avoidance. Although maintenance of the previously achieved treatment gains and further symptomatic improvement are important treatment goals in the long-term (more than 1–3 months) treatment of panic disorder, the focus of treatment shifts largely to improving quality of life, minimizing impairment and likelihood of relapses and complications, and decreasing vulnerability to panic disorder (Starcevic, 1998). Long-term treatment of panic disorder takes different forms, such as maintenance pharmacotherapy, weekly sessions of psychotherapy, occasional "booster" sessions of cognitive-behavioral therapy (CBT), or any combination of these treatment modalities.

PHARMACOLOGICAL TREATMENT

Indications for Pharmacotherapy and Goals of Pharmacological Treatment

Medications are usually used in the treatment of panic disorder when the condition is of moderate to severe intensity, when patients are in such distress that a quick relief is needed, and/or when panic disorder co-occurs with another psychiatric disorder, especially depression.

To the extent that panic disorder is characterized by the preponderance of unexpected panic attacks *at the time of commencing treatment*, it appears that pharmacotherapy, or at least antidepressants, will be useful, because antidepressants have been found to have a specific, suppressing effect on unexpected panic attacks, without significant effects on other components of panic disorder (Uhlenhuth et al., 2000, 2002). In other words, panic disorder without agoraphobia may be more likely to respond to treatment with antidepressants alone, whereas antidepressants may not be sufficient in the treatment of panic disorder with agoraphobia.

The main short-term goals of pharmacological treatment of panic disorder are a decrease in the intensity and frequency of panic attacks and decrease in general symptoms of anxiety. The aim of pharmacotherapy should also be disappearance and suppression, blocking, or prevention of panic attacks. As already noted, pharmacological treatment is less efficacious in alleviating anticipatory anxiety and panic-related avoidance, but when this does occur, it is usually a consequence of the primary effect on (unexpected) panic attacks. The main long-term goals of pharmacological treatment are prevention of complications of panic disorder and improvement in quality of life.

Choice of Medication

Three groups of medications are approximately equally efficacious in the treatment of panic disorder: selective serotonin reuptake inhibitors (SSRIs), tricyclic antidepressants (TCAs), and high-potency benzodiazepines (alprazolam, clonazepam). Of the SSRIs, the evidence of efficacy exists for paroxetine (Oehrberg et al., 1995; Lecrubier et al., 1997; Ballenger et al., 1998), sertraline (Londborg et al., 1998; Pohl et al., 1998; Pollack et al., 1998), fluvoxamine (den Boer et al., 1987; Black et al., 1993; Hoehn-Saric et al., 1993b), citalopram (Wade et al., 1997), and fluoxetine (Michelson et al., 1998). Escitalopram, the active isomer of citalopram, has recently been found to be efficacious in the treatment of panic disorder (Stahl et al., 2003).

Of the TCAs, imipramine (Cross-National Collaborative Panic Study, 1992) and clomipramine (Cassano et al., 1988; Johnston et al., 1988; Fahy et al., 1992; Modigh et al., 1992; Gentil et al., 1993) were found to be efficacious in panic disorder. When clomipramine was compared with imipramine (Cassano et al., 1988; Modigh et al., 1992; Gentil et al., 1993), it was found to be somewhat more efficacious, with an earlier onset of efficacy.

Although various benzodiazepines have been used in the treatment of panic disorder, the convincing evidence of their efficacy exists for alprazolam (Ballenger et al., 1988; Cross-National Collaborative Panic Study, 1992) and clonazepam (Tesar et al., 1991).

It is important to note that the placebo response rates in pharmacological studies of panic disorder are often quite high: up to 51% in some

TABLE 2–23. Factors to be Taken into Consideration When Choosing a Medication for Treatment of Panic Disorder

Factors	Likely Choice
Side-effect profile and general tolerability	Favors SSRIs and benzodiazepines over TCAs
Presence of co-occurring conditions, especially depression	Favors SSRIs and TCAs over benzodiazepines
History of alcohol or other substance abuse or dependence	Favors SSRIs and TCAs over benzodiazepines
Speed of antipanic response	Favors benzodiazepines over SSRIs and TCAs
Toxicity or lethality in overdose	Favors SSRIs and benzodiazepines over TCAs

SSRIs, selective serotonin reuptake inhibitors; TCAs, tricyclic antidepressants.

studies (Pohl et al., 1998). Apart from raising concerns about the methodology and interpretation of results of various drug trials, this finding suggests that nonspecific treatment factors (such as expectations from the treatment that patients may have and the therapeutic relationship with the physician) may play an important role in the treatment of panic disorder.

Because there are no differences in efficacy between the three groups of medications, the choice of medication depends on the factors listed in Table 2–23. The relative importance of each of these factors in every patient with panic disorder then determines which medication is used.

Although SSRIs and TCAs are now considered first- and second-line choice of treatment, respectively (Table 2–24), both SSRIs and TCAs can initially be administered together with a benzodiazepine, or treatment can be initiated with a benzodiazepine only. This decision is likely to depend on the combination of factors listed in Table 2–23.

A recent report (Bruce et al., 2003) suggests that making decisions about pharmacological treatment of panic disorder is fairly complex, without these

TABLE 2–24. Choice of Medication in Treatment of Panic Disorder

Rank	Medication
First-line	a. SSRIs (especially paroxetine, sertraline, fluvoxamine, and citalopram)
	b. SSRI + high-potency BDZ (alprazolam, clonazepam)
Second-line	a. TCAs (clomipramine, imipramine)
	b. TCA + high-potency BDZ (alprazolam, clonazepam)
Third-line	High-potency BDZs only
Fourth-line	Classical, irreversible MAOIs (phenelzine), venlafaxine, or reboxetine

BDZ, benzodiazepine, MAOI, monoamine oxidase inhibitor; SSRI, selective serotonin reuptake inhibitor; TCA, tricyclic antidepressant.

decisions necessarily being based on current treatment guidelines. This report indicates that benzodiazepines may still be the most commonly used form of pharmacotherapy for panic disorder in the United States and that a majority of patients taking SSRIs also use benzodiazepines at the same time. The two most likely reasons for the apparent preference of benzodiazepines over SSRIs are their rapid onset of action and better tolerability (Bruce et al., 2003). An earlier study (Schweizer et al., 1993) has already indicated that, in comparison with patients treated with imipramine, panic patients treated with alprazolam were less likely to drop out of treatment and more likely to experience substantial relief from panic attacks.

Selective Serotonin Reuptake Inhibitors and Tricyclic Antidepressants in Treatment of Panic Disorder

There are several reasons for the current status of SSRIs as the first-line pharmacological treatment for panic disorder (see Table 2–23). Their side effects are generally better tolerated than the side effects of TCAs, and they are safer in overdose than TCAs (an important consideration for many patients with panic disorder who develop depression and become suicidal). They are also not associated with dependence to the extent that benzodiazepines are, and SSRIs are often efficacious in pharmacological treatment of many disorders that tend to co-occur with panic disorder (e.g., generalized anxiety disorder, social anxiety disorder, depression). Perhaps the greatest disadvantage of the SSRIs is the fact that their full antipanic efficacy appears only after they have been administered continuously for 4–6 weeks. This delayed efficacy may be even more pronounced with TCAs, where antipanic effect often appears after 8–12 weeks of treatment.

Comparisons between clomipramine and SSRIs (den Boer et al., 1987; Lecrubier and Judge, 1997; Lecrubier et al., 1997; Wade et al., 1997) did not show significant differences in efficacy, but SSRIs tended to be better tolerated. A recent meta-analysis (Bakker et al., 2002b) has confirmed that there are no differences in efficacy between TCAs and SSRIs, but the number of dropouts was significantly higher among panic patients treated with TCAs. However, another review of the comparative efficacy and tolerability of SSRIs and TCAs (Otto et al., 2001) found no differences, adding to the growing impression that good tolerability of SSRIs might have been exaggerated.

Indeed, side effects of SSRIs can be troublesome to some patients with panic disorder, with the discontinuation of SSRIs in at least one study (Cowley et al., 1997) being attributed to their side effects in a substantial proportion of patients. The problems with SSRI side effects are particularly prominent at the beginning of treatment. Because the occurrence of side effects is unpredictable, patients should be well informed about them before commencing treatment. Most common among these side effects are nausea, vomiting, diarrhea, other gastrointestinal disturbances, agitation, headache, and insomnia. If they are severe, some patients describe them in terms of "worst ever experience." Most patients have these side effects only initially and should be encouraged to continue taking SSRIs. To prevent insomnia, patients should generally take SSRIs in the morning. Alternatively, a hypnotic medication can be taken on an as-needed (prn) basis if patients have already developed insomnia.

The occurrence of side effects of TCAs is more predictable than that of SSRIs; for example, most patients taking a TCA will have dry mouth. The main issue is whether patients can tolerate the side effects of TCAs (which most commonly include anticholinergic symptoms, such as dry mouth, blurred vision, constipation, and urinary hesitancy, plus sedation, weight gain, postural hypotension, tachycardia, sexual dysfunction, and lowering of the seizure threshold). Some of these side effects are dose-dependent (e.g., sedation) and may disappear with a reduction in dose, whereas others occur regardless of dosage. In view of their side-effect profile and specific organ toxicity, TCAs are contraindicated in patients with cardiac arrhythmias, enlarged prostate, glaucoma, and epilepsy.

If SSRIs or TCAs are commenced at their usual antidepressant dosage, agitation, restlessness, and increased anxiety ("jitteriness syndrome") are particularly common. This phenomenon seems to be relatively specific for panic disorder. Therefore, it is important to start an SSRI at one-quarter to one-half of its initial antidepressant dose. In practice, this means that paroxetine should be commenced at 5–10 mg/day, sertraline at 12.5–25 mg/day, citalopram at 5–10 mg/day, fluvoxamine at 25 mg/day, and fluoxetine at 2.5–5 mg/day. When using a TCA, the starting dose should be 10 mg/day of imipramine or clomipramine. These initial doses should be increased as quickly as the tolerability of the medication allows. For an SSRI or a TCA to reach its therapeutic dosage, several weeks may need to elapse; the rate of increasing the dose should be tailored to each individual patient. This phase of treatment is often critical, as patients do not yet experience the benefits of pharmacotherapy while possibly having prominent side effects. It is not surprising, then, that dropout rates are highest during this period.

The other commonly used strategy to counteract initial agitation and increase in anxiety with SSRIs or TCAs is to coadminister alprazolam or clonazepam. This combination is also useful for quick alleviation of distress and panic symptoms and for producing an earlier response, as confirmed by the results of studies in which clonazepam was coadministered with sertraline (Goddard et al., 2001a) and paroxetine (Pollack et al., 2003). The combined treatment with an SSRI or a TCA and alprazolam or clonazepam can last for 6–12 weeks—a period during which the dosage of an SSRI or a TCA is gradually increased to a therapeutic range, while a benzodiazepine is subsequently discontinued. Alternatively, combined antidepressant–benzodiazepine treatment can be continued for prolonged periods of time, depending on the circumstances of individual patients.

The usual medication doses for panic disorder are shown in Table 2–25. A target dose among SSRIs has been established only for paroxetine: 40 mg/day (Ballenger et al., 1998). However, if the patient responds fully to a daily dose of 20 or 30 mg paroxetine, there is no need to further increase the dose. Sertraline was found to be efficacious in decreasing panic attacks at all three doses (50 mg/day, 100 mg/day, 200 mg/day) that were used (Londborg et al., 1998). Citalopram and fluoxetine may be more efficacious in doses of 20–30 mg/day and 20 mg/day, respectively, than in lower doses (Wade et al., 1997; Lepola et al., 1998; Michelson et al., 1998). If there is no satisfactory response to a dose of fluoxetine of 20 mg/day, patients may benefit from a higher dose (Michelson et al., 2001). Also, citalopram may have a somewhat slower onset of action (Wade et al., 1997).

A higher dose of imipramine (e.g., 200 mg/day) was associated with greater likelihood of response and more treatment gains (Mavissakalian

TABLE 2–25. Medication Dosages Efficacious in Panic Disorder

Medication	Dose Range
Selective Serotonin Reuptake Inhibitors	
Paroxetine	40–60 mg/day
Sertraline	100–200 mg/day
Fluvoxamine	150–300 mg/day
Citalopram	20–40 mg/day
Fluoxetine	20–30 mg/day
Tricyclic Antidepressants	
Clomipramine	75–250 mg/day
Imipramine	150–300 mg/day
Benzodiazepines	
Alprazolam	2–6 mg/day
Clonazepam	1–4 mg/day

and Perel, 1989; 1995). Therefore, the dose of imipramine should be pushed relatively quickly to at least 150 mg/day, unless patients experience intolerable side effects.

Benzodiazepines in Treatment of Panic Disorder

Some patients are so troubled by their symptoms and the overall experience of panic that they urgently seek alleviation of anxiety and panic. Because of the quick onset of anxiolytic and antipanic action, benzodiazepines are particularly advantageous in the treatment of such patients, as patients can experience significant relief, with a complete disappearance of panic attacks within days or 1 to 2 weeks. In addition, benzodiazepines are generally well tolerated, have fewer side effects, and, if taken alone, are safe in overdose. The main disadvantages of benzodiazepines include therapeutic drug dependence and lack of efficacy in depression and some of the co-occurring anxiety disorders (e.g., obsessive-compulsive disorder).

The most important and most common side effect of benzodiazepines is sedation, which patients typically experience through drowsiness and/or difficulty keeping their attention focused. If sedation is accompanied by problems with motor coordination, driving skills or skills needed for other complex activities may be impaired. Sedation and the accompanying impairment in motor coordination are potentiated by the use of alcohol, and patients should be warned of the potential consequences of sedation and should be advised not to use alcohol along with benzodiazepines. Sedation is dose-dependent and tolerance to sedation develops fairly quickly, so that higher doses of benzodiazepines are required to produce the same initial degree of sedation. In clinical practice, this means that sedation usually occurs at the very beginning of treatment or immediately after a dose of a benzodiazepine has been increased; there is usually no need to decrease the dose because of sedation. However, if sedation does persist, the dose may be decreased.

Another relatively common side effect of benzodiazepines is a certain memory impairment. It occurs most commonly in the form of anterograde amnesia and is usually not clinically significant. Some patients exhibit "paradoxical reactions" to benzodiazepines; they are called this because of the resulting irritability and disinhibited and even aggressive behavior, instead of the expected effects of anxiolysis and sense of calm.

Alprazolam and clonazepam are the most commonly used benzodiazepines in the treatment of panic disorder. The initial dose of alprazolam is usually 1 mg/day, and the initial dose of clonazepam is 0.5 mg/day. The dose is then gradually increased, according to response and side effects (e.g., sedation). Clonazepam may have an advantage over alprazolam in that it has a longer duration of action and is therefore less likely to be associated with discontinuation problems. In addition, because of these properties, it is easier to administer clonazepam—usually twice a day—whereas the total daily dosage of alprazolam needs to be divided into three to four doses. For clonazepam it appears that doses of 1 mg/day and above are more efficacious than a dose of 0.5 mg/day; the dose of 1–2 mg/day is also better tolerated (Rosenbaum et al., 1997). Alprazolam has been subsequently manufactured in an extended-release form, allowing administration twice a day.

The optimal length of treatment of panic disorder with benzodiazepines is not known. There is general agreement that because of dependence issues (see below), benzodiazepines should be used for as brief a time as possible; this usually translates to 6–12 weeks of treatment. It appears, however, that quite a few patients require long-term treatment with benzodiazepines, which may extend over several months or even years. When benzodiazepines are used as maintenance treatment, patients usually do not show a tendency to escalate the dosage nor to develop tolerance to their anxiolytic effects (Nagy et al., 1989; Schweizer et al., 1993).

Long-Term Pharmacological Treatment

How long should panic patients be treated with medications? Because panic disorder tends to have a chronic course, pharmacological treatment should be continued for at least 6–12 months after the patient has attained remission and the panic attacks have either disappeared completely or their frequency and severity have decreased significantly. In practice, patients often take medications for longer periods of time. After 1 year, a physician needs to review whether pharmacotherapy is to continue. In doing so, the physician should bear in mind that there is a high risk of relapse upon cessation of medication, unless the patient has learned strategies for coping with panic symptoms and anxiety. A decision to stop medication should be made jointly by the physician and patient after the patient has been well informed of the risks involved in medication cessation.

Relapse seems to occur even in the course of continuing and/or adequate long-term pharmacotherapy, with as many as 46% of patients reporting a relapse after they had achieved remission (Simon et al., 2002). Relapse figures upon discontinuation of medication vary, with about 37% of panic patients relapsing within 6 months after cessation of antidepressants (Mavissakalian and Perel, 2002), and 67% relapsing over the course of 3 years (Toni et al., 2000). An even greater number of panic patients may relapse after the cessation of benzodiazepines (Noyes et al., 1991).

What can be done to minimize the risk of relapse after discontinuing pharmacotherapy? There is some evidence that administration of anti-panic medication for longer periods of time is associated with a lower relapse rate: fewer patients who took imipramine for 18 months relapsed in comparison with patients who took imipramine for 6 months (Mavis-sakalian and Perel, 1992). However, a more recent study (Mavissakalian and Perel, 2002) could not confirm that a relapse rate was associated with the duration of imipramine treatment. The other strategy to minimize the risk of relapse is to add psychological interventions, most notably CBT, to the ongoing pharmacotherapy (see Combined Treatments, below).

In the course of long-term treatment with SSRIs, most patients either do not gain weight or gain weight only minimally. This is another advantage of SSRIs over TCAs. The most troublesome long-term side effects of SSRIs are various problems with sexual functioning. The SSRI-associated sexual dysfunction usually takes the form of ejaculatory disturbances (delayed or absent ejaculation) in men and anorgasmia in women. Less commonly, patients taking SSRIs have erectile problems and decreased sexual desire.

Clinical experience and follow-up studies of panic patients suggest that a certain number of patients develop depression in the course of long-term pharmacotherapy. While it is not clear whether this phenomenon is related to the type of medication that patients are taking, its clinical implications are obviously important and patients need to be closely monitored for any symptoms and signs of depression.

In long-term pharmacological treatment of panic disorder, medications do not seem to exhibit a decrease in efficacy (Uhlenhuth et al., 1988; Lecrubier and Judge, 1997; Lepola et al., 1998; Michelson et al., 1999). Therefore, the dose of medication during long-term treatment does not need to be increased, and it is likely to be the same as the one that initially produced remission of panic disorder.

Although SSRIs are often not considered to be dependence-producing medications, discontinuation symptoms have been observed and well described in many patients who stopped taking SSRIs abruptly. These symptoms are usually headache, dizziness, sweating, nausea, exhaustion, muscle pain, and flu-like symptoms, but various other symptoms may appear as well. Discontinuation symptoms are more likely to be seen after abrupt cessation of SSRIs with a short half-life (e.g., paroxetine) than after abrupt cessation of SSRIs with a longer half-life (e.g., fluoxetine). It is good clinical practice to decrease the dose of SSRIs gradually, before their complete cessation. Depending on the dosage and type of SSRI used, this process usually takes between 1–2 weeks and 2–3 months.

Specific Issues in the Course of Long-term Treatment
with Benzodiazepines

The main issue during long-term treatment with benzodiazepines is therapeutic dependence on these medications, often labeled as "addiction." Although therapeutic drug dependence and dependence on alcohol and certain illicit drugs ("addiction") are both characterized by the occurrence of withdrawal symptoms upon abrupt cessation of the drug, there are important differences between the two. Unlike addiction, therapeutic dependence on benzodiazepines is *not* associated with tolerance (increasing the dosage to produce the same initial anxiolytic effect or the initial dosage producing a decreased effect), craving for the medication, and adverse health and/or social consequences, such as an all-encompassing preoccupation with benzodiazepines.

There is no evidence that patients with panic disorder are more likely to develop benzodiazepine abuse or dependence in the absence of current or past alcohol or other substance abuse or dependence (e.g., Andersch and Hetta, 2003). Therefore, it is erroneous to assume automatically that benzodiazepines are "addictive" and on that basis deprive panic patients of the drug's potential benefits. However, benzodiazepines should generally not be prescribed to panic patients with current or past substance use problems. Caution is also warranted when administering benzodiazepines to patients who have a family history of substance abuse or dependence and personality features (e.g., dependent) that might make it more difficult for them to stop taking benzodiazepines.

Benzodiazepine withdrawal symptoms are more likely to occur if the patient has been taking a benzodiazepine with a shorter half-life (e.g., alprazolam), if its dose has been higher (e.g., more than 2 mg of alprazolam per day), and if a benzodiazepine has been taken continuously over a longer period of time (generally more than 1–2 months). Withdrawal symptoms may resemble a recurrence of anxiety disorder. Symptoms such as increased anxiety, tension, restlessness, agitation, insomnia, and panic attacks are quite common, especially a short time after a benzodiazepine has been ceased. Severe withdrawal symptoms usually occur later: tachycardia, hypertension, profuse sweating, nausea, vomiting, tremor, muscle pain, unstable gait, transient hallucinations, and, rarely, grand mal seizures. The prevention of a severe withdrawal syndrome entails its early recognition on the basis of the relatively specific symptoms (hypersensitivity to light, sound, smell or taste, various perceptual disturbances, distorted body image, tinnitus, tingling sensations, depersonalization, derealization) along with its early treatment.

After a sudden cessation of benzodiazepines, the withdrawal syndrome is not the only potential consequence. Patients may experience a "rebound," which refers to the worsening of initial symptoms of an anxiety disorder. The symptoms of rebound often overlap with manifestations of benzodiazepine withdrawal syndrome, and it is important to attempt to distinguish between the two because their course and treatment implications are different. While the course of the withdrawal syndrome is transient (duration no longer than 10–20 days) and calls mainly for the treatment of the withdrawal itself, rebound essentially means a recurrence of the original disorder, for which a long-term treatment strategy is necessary.

The best way to prevent benzodiazepine withdrawal syndrome is to taper benzodiazepines very gradually and carefully before their discontinuation. In addition, CBT can be helpful in the process of tapering benzodiazepines in patients with panic disorder (Otto et al., 1993; Spiegel et al., 1994). In the course of decreasing the dosage, it is crucial to address patients' specific fears of the withdrawal symptoms, as these fears often determine the outcome of the taper. Although the rate of taper depends primarily on the duration of treatment with a benzodiazepine and its dosage, the rate should be adjusted according to the characteristics of the individual patient. The rate of taper should always be negotiated with the patient, without any pressure or hurry. It is more important that patients avoid withdrawal symptoms (which can occur even with a relatively slow taper) and feel comfortable as they go through a tapering process than it is to complete this process within a set, predetermined period. Thus, there are large variations in the duration of taper, and it is not unusual for this to last 6 months or longer. In principle, a decrease in the total daily dosage by 0.25–0.5 mg alprazolam per week or 0.125–0.25 mg clonazepam per week is adequate to minimize the risk of withdrawal symptoms.

Pharmacotherapy of Treatment-Resistant Panic Disorder

An adequate trial of pharmacotherapy for panic disorder consists of 6–8 weeks of treatment with a first-, second-, or third-line medication given in a maximum dose that the patient can tolerate. All too often, patients are labeled "treatment-resistant," even though they have not taken a medication long enough or in an adequate dosage. Still, about 20%–30% of panic patients do not respond to pharmacotherapy. If there has been no response at all to an SSRI, a TCA, or a high-potency benzodiazepine, treatment with a medication from another first, second-, or third-line group can be tried (Table 2–26).

Another option in case of lack of response to pharmacotherapy with a first-, second-, or third-line medication is a classical, irreversible monoamine oxidase inhibitor (MAOI) (Table 2–26). There is some evidence

Table 2–26. Pharmacological Options for Treatment-Resistant Panic Disorder

Partial Response to First-, Second-, or Third-Line Pharmacotherapy

Augmentation strategies

    SSRI + pindolol

    SSRI + TCA

    SSRI (or TCA or BDZ) + gabapentin

Lack of Response to First-, Second-, or Third-Line Pharmacotherapy

Monotherapy with another SSRI, a TCA, or a high-potency BDZ

Monotherapy with a classical, irreversible MAOI (phenelzine)

Monotherapy with

    Venlafaxine

    Reboxetine

    Mirtazapine

    Nefazodone

    Valproate

BDZ, benzodiazepine; MAOI, monoamine oxidase inhibitor; SSRI, selective serotonin reuptake inhibitor; TCA, tricyclic antidepressant.

(Sheehan et al., 1980) that phenelzine (45–90 mg/day) may be efficacious in treating panic patients. Several other medications (venlafaxine, reboxetine, mirtazapine, nefazodone, and valproate) can also be used as alternatives (Table 2–26), but sufficient evidence of their efficacy in panic disorder is currently lacking. It is likely that more data on the efficacy of these medications in the treatment of panic disorder will emerge in the near future; for example, a recent randomized, controlled trial (Versiani et al., 2002) has demonstrated efficacy of reboxetine, a selective norepinephrine reuptake inhibitor. There has also been some indication (e.g., Pollack et al., 1996) that venlafaxine might be an efficacious alternative to SSRIs. The potential advantages of nefazodone over SSRIs in the treatment of panic disorder include a low likelihood of causing the "jitteriness syndrome" and of sexual side effects.

If there has been a partial response to pharmacotherapy with a first-, second-, or third-line medication, augmentation strategies can be considered (Table 2–26). For example, an SSRI can be augmented with pindolol, a strategy that has received some empirical support (Hirschmann et al., 2000). An SSRI can also be combined with imipramine or clomipramine (Tiffon et al., 1994), but plasma levels of imipramine or clomipramine may become quite high and patients need to be closely monitored for any signs of TCA toxicity. Finally, gabapentin can be added to first-, second-, or third-line medication for panic disorder.

PSYCHOLOGICAL TREATMENT

Cognitive Therapy

Cognitive therapy of panic disorder is based on the cognitive theory of panic disorder and, more specifically, on the assumption that panic attacks are a consequence of catastrophic misinterpretation of benign physical sensations and symptoms. Hence, the immediate goal of cognitive therapy of panic disorder is to normalize interpretations of physical sensations and symptoms. Furthermore, cognitive therapy is undertaken with the goals of decreasing or eliminating the fear of anxiety symptoms and the fear of panic attacks. In order to achieve this, cognitive therapy has to "dismantle" the underlying beliefs about the dangerousness of anxiety and panic. The emphasis in cognitive therapy is *not* on the control and total disappearance of anxiety, panic, and its symptoms; rather, the goal is for panic patients to be able to appraise anxiety and panic in a nonthreatening and realistic manner, and thereby cope with anxiety and panic more effectively. Cognitive therapy of panic disorder proceeds through several steps (Table 2–27) that are described below.

Identification of Specific Panic- and Anxiety-Relevant Catastrophic Cognitions or Automatic Thoughts

The first step is to identify catastrophic cognitions or automatic thoughts that patients have about specific anxiety symptoms and panic. This is done by directly asking patients what they think would happen as a result of the

TABLE 2–27. Process of Cognitive Therapy of Panic Disorder

---

1. Identification of catastrophic cognitions or automatic thoughts that patients have about specific anxiety symptoms and panic

2. Challenging the identified catastrophic cognitions

   Looking for evidence that specific catastrophic cognitions are (in)correct

   Proposing alternative, normalizing explanations for the relevant physical sensations and symptoms

   Weighing "pros" and "cons" for catastrophic cognitions

3. Using "behavioral experiments" to have a more convincing evidence that the alternative explanation is correct

4. Replacing catastrophic cognitions with normalizing, rational and more logical interpretations

---

symptoms. The appraisals of symptoms may be easy to access, as in the case of patients who spontaneously say that they believe they are going to lose control and faint when they feel dizzy. In other cases, it is more difficult to grasp the underlying appraisal of the symptoms, and patients need to be "led" from one question to another to access it. Thus, in the case of patients who feel dizzy, it may be that they consider this symptom dangerous because of the belief that dizziness leads to fainting and falling; consequently, they anticipate that they will humiliate themselves, sustain a serious injury, or even die.

Challenging Identified Catastrophic Cognitions

The next step in cognitive therapy (Table 2–27) is to challenge the previously identified catastrophic cognitions. This step involves several procedures.

Looking for evidence that specific catastrophic cognitions are (in)correct. The first procedure is looking for evidence that specific catastrophic cognitions are (in)correct. For example, patients can be asked questions such as "How do you know that you will lose control when you feel dizzy?" or "What makes you believe that you will die when you are dizzy?". Whatever reasons patients come up with, they ultimately suggest to patients that their beliefs are not well founded.

Proposing alternative, normalizing explanations. The next procedure is offering alternative explanations for the relevant physical sensations and symptoms, and discussing them with patients. Implementation of this technique is crucial, as it introduces a normalizing interpretation of the symptom(s) and of the overall panic experience, and "invites" patients to consider this instead of clinging to their usual catastrophic appraisal. The successful use of this technique depends on patients' understanding (previously achieved through psychoeducation) of the basic physiological processes involved in the anxiety response. For example, it can be suggested to patients that dizziness is often a consequence of the pathophysiological chain of events that occur during hyperventilation; in turn, hyperventilation and panic are explained as having no serious short-term or long-term consequences, regardless of how unpleasant they may be.

Weighing pros and cons for catastrophic cognitions. After patients have been presented with alternative explanation(s) for their symptoms, their task is to weigh pros and cons of their particular beliefs. For example, patients who believe that they will faint and collapse when they feel dizzy may try to support this belief by asserting that because of their usually low blood pressure, they will faint and collapse. This line of reasoning should be contrasted with information, provided by the therapist, that blood pressure usually rises during panic attacks, which makes it rather unlikely for patients to faint and collapse, despite feeling dizzy or lightheaded. The weighing of pros and cons may take some time, as patients often need to rehearse this part of the process of challenging their catastrophic beliefs. Ultimately, they will be able to replace these beliefs with normalizing, rational, and more logical interpretations.

Behavioral Experiments
Sometimes it is not sufficient for patients to go through the process of challenging their cognitions—they may seek more convincing evidence that the alternative explanation is correct. In such cases, using "behavioral experiments" (Clark and Beck, 1988) may be particularly useful. This technique consists of the deliberate induction of one or more symptoms of anxiety that patients are particularly afraid of; after patients have induced this symptom, they try to modify their previous catastrophic appraisal of it on the basis of the alternative explanations presented to them. For example, for patients who are especially afraid of dizziness and have a catastrophic belief that they will faint and collapse as a result of dizziness, the behavioral experiment consists of asking them to hyperventilate for a few minutes. Hyperventilation produces dizziness among other symptoms, and patients find out that while dizziness is unpleasant, it does not lead to fainting and collapsing. For many patients, such a direct demonstration that the feared symptom (e.g., dizziness) does not lead to a catastrophe (e.g., fainting, collapsing) is quite convincing and leads to a change in their catastrophic beliefs about specific symptoms.

Replacing Catastrophic Cognitions with Normalizing, Rational, and More Logical Interpretations
As already suggested, replacement of catastrophic cognitions with normalizing appraisals of sensations, symptoms, and panic occurs throughout the treatment, and not as any particular stage of cognitive therapy. It can be conceived of as both the mechanism of cognitive change and one of the treatment goals.

Other Aspects of Cognitive Therapy
Another aspect of cognitive therapy of panic disorder is the work on dysfunctional expectations of panic attacks. Because many panic patients erroneously believe that expectations of attacks are firmly associated with the actual occurrence of attacks, it is important for them to realize that manipulating their expectations cannot reliably make the occurrence of panic

attacks more or less likely. In other words, instead of focusing on the expectation of panic attacks, patients are encouraged to learn strategies for coping with anxiety and panic. Once they have learned to cope with them more effectively, it will be less relevant whether panic attacks are expected or not expected, and indeed, whether panic attacks occur or do not occur.

In the course of cognitive therapy, general anxiety-related cognitive distortions are addressed, so that panic patients become better equipped to recognize them and change these dysfunctional patterns of thinking. This pertains to the "all-or-nothing," dichotomized, and/or rigid style of thinking; underestimation of one's own abilities; and exaggerated perception of threat and danger. Through Socratic dialogue and challenge of entrenched notions, assumptions, interpretations, and beliefs, it is demonstrated to patients that such cognitive style and distortions only contribute to the maintenance of anxiety in general and panic disorder in particular.

The use of cognitive therapy techniques is not simple and requires a considerable degree of patients' psychological-mindedness and sophistication. First, it may be difficult for some patients to accept the idea that the goal of treatment is not necessarily elimination of symptoms, but learning how to cope with symptoms and anxiety. Other patients may have difficulty accepting alternative, rational explanations for their symptoms and for panic attacks, as if having adopted a stance that "reason and logic cannot cure." The reason for this may be in the general lack of common sense and logic in the "neurotic paradox:" regardless of how many times patients have experienced certain symptoms and panic attacks with no catastrophe occurring, they may believe that the catastrophe is still looming and continue to expect the worst outcomes from the attacks, while also believing that the catastrophe has not occurred yet because they were "lucky" or because they used avoidance or escape to avert it. Some of these beliefs may need to be addressed for the treatment to proceed successfully.

The role played by "safety behaviors" (e.g., avoidance) and "safety devices" (e.g., medications that are carried around at all times) in maintaining panic disorder is considered crucial in cognitive therapy. This needs to be clarified to patients, and they should be encouraged to first identify all instances in which they are using safety behaviors and safety devices, and then abandon them. Safety behaviors pertain to all the behaviors that are designed to prevent the feared catastrophe; most commonly, this is avoidance, even if subtle, of various situations and/or activities (e.g., exercising) in which patients might be likely to experience the feared sensations and symptoms. If patients persistently cling to their safety behaviors and/or safety devices, they may reinforce an erroneous belief that, owing to their use, they have been able to prevent catastrophic outcomes.

Probably the most difficult component of the cognitive therapy package is participation in behavioral experiments. Many panic patients are understandably concerned about the technique in which the feared symptoms are being deliberately induced. Therefore, the rationale for conducting behavioral experiments and the corresponding procedures need to be carefully explained to patients.

Efficacy of Cognitive Therapy and Its Limitations
Cognitive therapy has proved to be an efficacious treatment modality in panic disorder, with 90% of patients being panic-free upon completion of treatment, and 70% remaining panic-free at 1-year follow-up (Clark et al., 1994b). More specifically, cognitive therapy was found to result in diminished beliefs in catastrophic misinterpretations of bodily sensations and symptoms during panic attacks; this outcome correlated with both decreased severity and frequency of panic attacks (Bakker et al., 2002a). Studies of the efficacy of cognitive therapy in panic disorder should rely more on specific and relevant outcome measures, such as fear of panic symptoms and appraisal of their consequences, because these reflect the goals of cognitive therapy more adequately than general outcome measures such as the severity and frequency of panic attacks.

Because of the demanding nature and somewhat radical goals of treatment, cognitive therapy in its unmodified form may be suitable for some panic patients only. Modifications include use of symptom control or symptom alleviation techniques (whether psychological or pharmacological), which may make it easier to administer cognitive therapy. Whereas "pure" cognitive therapy has been considered more useful in the treatment of panic attacks, but not in the treatment of agoraphobia, behavior therapy techniques (exposure) have been deemed more efficacious in the treatment of agoraphobia than in treatment of panic attacks (van den Hout et al., 1994). The logical implication is that cognitive and behavioral techniques should be combined in the presence of both panic attacks and agoraphobia.

Panic Control Treatment

Panic control treatment (Barlow, 1988; Barlow et al., 1989) is a commonly used form of CBT for panic disorder, with greater emphasis on behavioral components of treatment. It is based mainly on the model of panic attacks as "false alarms" and the concepts of interoceptive conditioning and "learned alarms." As its name implies, and in contrast to the goals of treatment in cognitive therapy, the main goal of panic control treatment is a better control of symptoms of anxiety and panic.

The main technique of panic control treatment is "interoceptive exposure," which is similar to behavioral experiments used in cognitive therapy. However, the rationale for using these techniques and the way in which they are administered are different. In interoceptive exposure (Table 2–28), the emphasis is on exposure to the deliberately induced symptoms, along with techniques for controlling symptoms (e.g., relaxation and controlled, slow breathing) and reattribution of symptoms to innocuous causes (i.e., normalization of patients' interpretations). The purpose of interoceptive exposure is to enable patients to have a greater sense of control over their symptoms, anxiety, and panic. In addition, the behavioral model on which interoceptive exposure is based holds that alleviation of anxiety occurs through habituation to the symptoms and eventual extinction of the conditioned anxiety response.

In behavioral experiments, the emphasis is on demonstrating to patients that deliberately induced, feared symptoms do not lead to the expected catastrophes, so that the subsequent alleviation of anxiety occurs through cognitive change. Also, symptom control techniques are not used in behavioral experiments and in "pure" cognitive therapy; they are actually regarded by some cognitive therapists as just another "safety mechanism" that interferes with cognitive change. That is, cognitive therapists argue that there is no need for patients to control symptoms, because they are learning through cognitive therapy that they have no reason to fear symptoms.

Various symptoms can be induced, depending on what particular patients find most distressing. Exposure to these symptoms is gradual, and in accordance with the hierarchical principles embedded in general exposure-based therapies (see Exposure-Based Therapy for Agoraphobia below). Interoceptive exposure may be contraindicated in patients with asthma, other respiratory diseases, or heart disease, because the symptoms (e.g., shortness of breath, chest pain, accelerated heart rate) induced during interoceptive exposure are then practically indistinguishable from symptoms of the primary medical condition. In addition, there is a possibility of interoceptive exposure exacerbating respiratory or heart disease.

After several sessions of interoceptive exposure, in which symptoms are induced through an "artificial" procedure (usually hyperventilation),

TABLE 2–28. Components of Interoceptive Exposure

1. Exposure to deliberately induced symptoms

2. Use of symptom-controlling techniques (e.g., relaxation, controlled, slow breathing)

3. Reattribution of symptoms to innocuous causes (normalizing patients' interpretations) following the process of challenging catastrophic symptom appraisals

patients should expose themselves to the "naturally occurring" physical symptoms. That means that patients should resume physical activities that they have been avoiding for fear of provoking these physical symptoms. The panic control treatment is conducted over 12–15 sessions, with a frequency of one session per week. There are various modifications to this regimen, and the treatment has also been used in a group format (Telch et al., 1993).

Panic control treatment has been found to be efficacious in panic disorder. In studies of this treatment, between 79% and 87% of patients were symptom-free at the end of treatment (Barlow et al., 1989; Klosko et al., 1990), whereas 83% were panic-free at 6-month follow-up (Telch et al., 1993) and more than 80% were panic-free at 2-year follow-up (Craske et al., 1991).

Panic Symptom Control Techniques

The most common techniques used for alleviation of symptoms of anxiety and panic are controlled, slow breathing (breathing retraining) and relaxation.

Controlled, Slow Breathing (Breathing Retraining)
In view of the role of hyperventilation in the pathophysiology of at least some panic attacks, the use of the controlled, slow breathing can avert hyperventilation or restore the normal breathing pattern in patients who are already hyperventilating. Insofar as the panic symptoms are caused by hyperventilation, restoration of the normal breathing pattern can alleviate or even eliminate these symptoms.

Controlled, slow breathing relies on three components: primary use of the diaphragm (instead of the chest) for breathing, normal-sized breaths (rather than deep breaths), and pacing of the breathing rhythm so that the respiratory rate decreases to approximately 10 cycles/minute. The latter means that the patient needs to learn to breathe in cycles that consist of 3 seconds of inhaling and 3 seconds of exhaling.

The technique of controlled, slow breathing is relatively easy to learn. It has to be practiced on a daily basis, however, before patients feel confident to use it in a variety of situations, including those in which they expect to have a panic attack or after the occurrence of initial panic symptoms.

Relaxation
Various relaxation techniques have been used for a long time in the treatment of various anxiety states, most notably generalized anxiety disorder (see Chapter 3). A modified progressive muscle relaxation technique,

called "applied relaxation" (Öst, 1987a; 1988), has been used in treatment of panic disorder. Its goal is to quickly produce a relaxed state, so that this state will neutralize autonomic arousal and provide patients with some sense of control. As with controlled, slow breathing, applied relaxation should be practiced regularly and used when the first manifestations of autonomic arousal occur and upon exposure to situations in which anxiety symptoms are anticipated. Applied relaxation as the only treatment modality in panic disorder has not proved to be particularly efficacious, however (Barlow et al., 1989).

Exposure-Based Therapy for Agoraphobia

The behavioral technique of exposure is the key component in the treatment of agoraphobia. Even if the formal exposure-based therapy is not used, at least some basic principles of exposure should be incorporated into every treatment approach to agoraphobia.

Gradual exposure in vivo is by far the most common type of exposure therapy for agoraphobia (Table 2–29). Its use entails a construction of phobic hierarchies on the basis of a behavioral analysis, with initial exposure to situations that elicit the least amount of anxiety (and that are least avoided). Patients need to remain in agoraphobic situations during exposure until the level of anxiety has started to subside; patients should also make every effort not to escape from the situations. They should work simultaneously on two to three agoraphobic situations at any stage of the treatment.

The exposure is to be conducted by patients (self-directed exposure) after they have been adequately informed through psychoeducation about the purpose of treatment and its technical aspects. The main role of the therapist is to plan exposure together with patients and to review the progress that they are making in the course of treatment. Patients should be encouraged to take the greatest possible responsibility for conducting the treatment, as that increases their sense of ownership of the treatment results.

TABLE 2–29. Aspects of Gradual Exposure in vivo for Use in Agoraphobia

- Self-directed exposure is the cornerstone of treatment
- Gradual exposure to the hierarchically constructed agoraphobic situations
- Exposure to two to three agoraphobic situations at any stage of the treatment
- Therapist-assisted exposure in the beginning of treatment for some patients with very severe forms of agoraphobia (e.g., those who are homebound)
- Partner-assisted exposure at certain stages of treatment
- Regular, continuous exposure (several hours every day) is preferable
- Shorter duration of exposure and "exposure-free" days should be avoided

The therapist should not accompany patients during exposure, except in the initial stages of treatment of some patients with very severe forms of agoraphobia (i.e., those who are homebound and are extremely disabled by agoraphobia). The patients' partners, family members, or friends may accompany them occasionally, during exposure to particularly difficult situations.

Patients should conduct exposure every day for at least 1 hour. It is preferable that exposure sessions last several hours and that patients not skip a day or two in the course of treatment. To facilitate monitoring and review of treatment, it is of paramount importance that patients keep a good record of their exposure exercises, which includes the following components: (1) type of situation to which they expose themselves; (2) degree of fear or discomfort experienced in these situations; (3) symptoms that occur during the exposure; and (4) duration of each exposure session. The exposure to a particular situation is completed after the degree of the recorded fear or discomfort has been reduced to manageable or negligible levels, and physical symptoms experienced in this situation have ceased to be disabling.

Patients can use various techniques to reduce their anxiety during exposure: relaxation, controlled, slow breathing, paradoxical interventions (e.g., imagining the "worst possible scenario" during exposure), and cognitive therapy techniques. The use of medications in the course of exposure-based treatment, particularly benzodiazepines, is controversial; this issue is discussed in more detail in Combined Treatments (below).

The typical length of treatment of agoraphobia with exposure in vivo is between 8 and 12 weeks. The usual frequency of therapist sessions is once to twice a week, with self-directed exposure proceeding between these sessions. More recently, there have been trends to reduce both the number of therapist sessions and the overall duration of treatment.

It may be difficult for some patients to initiate or complete exposure in vivo, and refusal or dropout rates may be as high as 40%. Some of the problems that occur before and during exposure that affect the compliance with treatment and its outcome include fluctuating levels of motivation, lack of trust in the therapist, disbelief that exposure might be efficacious, a too quick progression through the hierarchy of phobic situations (with consequently unmanageable, high levels of anxiety induced by exposure), failure to remain in the situation long enough for habituation to take place, discontinuous exposure sessions, and excessive use of companions, safety devices (e.g., medications), or safety behaviors during exposure (e.g., taking a seat only at the end of a theater row, which would allow easy escape in case of panic).

Exposure in vivo has been clearly efficacious in the treatment of agoraphobia. In numerous studies (McPherson et al., 1980; Munby and

Johnston, 1980; Jansson and Öst, 1982; Burns et al., 1986; Jacobson et al., 1988; Trull et al., 1988; Fava et al., 1995), between 60% and 75% of patients were symptom-free or exhibited only minimal avoidance at the end of treatment. Moreover, this improvement has a tendency to be maintained over prolonged periods of time (Munby and Johnston, 1980; Burns et al., 1986; Jansson et al., 1986; Margraf et al., 1993; Marks et al., 1993; Fava et al., 1995); in one study (Fava et al., 1995), 67% of patients who remitted after exposure-based treatment remained in remission at 7-year follow-up.

Some minor avoidance may persist after exposure-based treatment has been completed; although patients are usually not distressed by such avoidance, especially when their level of functioning has returned to normal, it is still possible for these patients to resort to full-scale agoraphobic avoidance at some point in the future. This does not happen very often, but when it does happen, it is usually in response to a stressor. If the fear of certain symptoms (e.g., dizziness) persists and drives patients to continue with avoidance, despite gains previously made during exposure, this fear needs to be specifically addressed. That can be done through cognitive therapy techniques or interoceptive exposure.

The variants of exposure-based treatments for agoraphobia include a combination of exposure in vivo and imaginal exposure (for those situations where in vivo exposure is not practical) and massed or ungraded exposure ("flooding") for those patients who are able to tolerate high levels of anxiety upon immediate exposure to the most anxiety-eliciting situations. Good results have also been reported for self-help–based or computer-assisted exposure therapy, with very little or no therapist involvement. However, in the more complex and severe cases of agoraphobia, more therapist involvement and time are needed.

Several mechanisms of change and improvement in the course of exposure have been postulated. These include habituation (decrease in anxiety upon repeated exposure to phobic stimuli), extinction (decrease in anxiety because it is not reinforced by further phobic avoidance), gradual loss of catastrophic appraisals and beliefs related to the phobic situations, and improved perception of self-efficacy.

Supportive Psychotherapy

There appear to be few, if any, issues that are specific for supportive psychotherapy of panic disorder. This treatment approach seems to be used often, but because of its nonspecific nature, it is usually considered an auxiliary rather than a main modality for bringing about relevant therapeutic changes. Hence, this background role of supportive psychotherapy tends to be underestimated.

In view of some general characteristics of patients with panic disorder and dominant themes in their lives, supportive psychotherapy aims to overcome patients' mistrust, foster their sense of security, and facilitate their reliance on others. This is also done with a further aim of building strong therapeutic alliance and securing patients' active participations in other, more specific treatment modalities. Panic patients who are struggling with ambivalence and indecisiveness often ask for advice or reassurance, and sometimes attempt to engage the therapist in making decisions for them. The therapist may have to walk a very fine line between providing patients with reasonable support, encouragement, and reassurance and discouraging their excessive dependence.

Marital or Couple Therapy

Marital or couple therapy may be indicated when pathological interactions between patients and their partners seem to play a pivotal role. This is more likely to be encountered in panic patients with agoraphobia; as already noted, a dysfunctional relationship between the partners may contribute to the persistence of agoraphobia, and in such cases, marital or couple therapy may be both appropriate and useful. However, marital or couple therapy is not a substitute for other, more specific psychological treatment approaches, such as cognitive, behavioral, and cognitive-behavioral therapies.

Marital or couple therapy is usually not the initial treatment for panic disorder. Many patients do improve in their functioning with partners after they have undergone a course of the more specific psychological therapy. Therefore, a decision to use marital or couple therapy is likely to be based on the persistence of significant problems in the marital or partner relationship after treatments such as exposure in vivo have been used to reduce panic-related avoidance. Less often, CBT may not be efficacious because the agoraphobic patients' partners sabotage treatment or the interference of pathological partner relationships with CBT is too strong.

Patients' partners need to be highly motivated for marital or couple therapy to be useful. This may or may not entail partners' realization that they share some responsibility with patients for the development and maintenance of the disorder. Marital or couple therapy can itself rely on behavioral and cognitive techniques or be based on other theoretical models. Perhaps the most important component of this type of treatment is fostering of open communication between the partners. This involves direct expression of feelings and needs, as well as expectations that partners may have of each other, but have not been able to articulate before. Their understanding of these issues and willingness to deal constructively with areas of conflict are crucial for overall improvement in their relationship and, consequently, for improvement in some of the clinical manifestations of panic disorder.

Psychodynamic Psychotherapy and Psychoanalysis

Psychodynamic therapy and psychoanalysis are generally used if general indications for these forms of psychotherapy are present. These include the patient's ability to make meaningful connections between various experiences, phenomena, symptoms, and external events, along with the willingness to understand these connections and relationships in relevant context ("introspectiveness"), ability to withstand unpleasant emotions and frustrations, delay gratification, resist impulsive urges and form reasonably mature interpersonal relationships, motivation for change and psychological growth, and willingness to invest time and energy into a treatment process.

Of all the anxiety disorders, panic disorder has received the most attention from psychodynamically oriented psychotherapists in recent times. A specific form of treatment, termed "panic-focused psychodynamic psychotherapy," has been developed (Milrod et al., 1997). This is a modified type of psychodynamic psychotherapy; in addition to goals common to other psychodynamic psychotherapies, its goals are specific for panic disorder and pertain to alleviation or disappearance of the main components of panic disorder. With such goals, it is not surprising that psychodynamic psychotherapy has been used in conjunction with pharmacotherapy—whether simultaneously or following a sufficient decrease in symptoms by means of pharmacotherapy. Moreover, one randomized, controlled study (Wiborg and Dahl, 1996) has demonstrated that treatment of panic disorder with manualized, brief dynamic psychotherapy and clomipramine resulted in a significantly lower rate of relapse than that after treatment with clomipramine alone. This finding is important because it suggests that psychodynamic psychotherapy may decrease panic patients' vulnerability to relapse.

In the course of psychodynamic psychotherapy of panic disorder, the relatively specific issues that are worked through are fears of separation and abandonment, fear of one's own anger and aggressive feelings, and conflictual and ambivalent feelings about attachment and dependency (with the alternating, varying degrees of interpersonal mistrust and idealizing tendencies). The treatment aim is gaining insight into the unconscious conflicts surrounding these issues and into their origin; in other words, dynamic (developmental) understanding of these conflicts and their relevance in the here-and-now situation is sought, along with their resolution through transference and interpretation.

COMBINED TREATMENTS

Combining efficacious pharmacological and psychological treatments for panic disorder is an important issue for clinical practice, albeit one that has divided the profession. The issue of combined treatments will be reviewed in some detail in this section. The reader should bear in mind that many of the problems identified in the context of panic disorder also apply to other anxiety disorders.

Whenever two treatment procedures are combined, the fundamental question pertains to the benefit of such a combination. In other words, does a combination of pharmacotherapy and CBT in panic disorder achieve better results than either treatment alone? It is this question that has generated the most controversy.

The Case Against Combining Pharmacotherapy and Cognitive-Behavioral Therapy

Many CBT therapists regard a combination of CBT and pharmacotherapy as unnecessary. In support of their view are studies suggesting that combined treatment confers no benefit over and above CBT alone (or some components of CBT, such as exposure therapy) in both short-term (Marks et al., 1983; Wardle et al., 1994) and long-term treatment of panic disorder, especially after discontinuation of medications (e.g., Mavissakalian and Michelson, 1986a; Marks et al., 1993; Otto et al., 1996; Barlow et al., 2000). According to this view, combined treatments might even be detrimental.

What makes the combined treatments potentially detrimental? There are several reasons for such an outcome, and they all represent a variation on the theme, "no pain, no gain." In other words, this view postulates that treatment progress entails better coping with anxiety and panic, which can be achieved only if patients confront anxiety-provoking situations and panic symptoms without the mitigating or facilitating effects of the concomitantly administered medication. Also, exposure to physical symptoms of anxiety and panic while patients are taking medications is not adequate, because intensity of the symptoms has been decreased by medications (Westra and Stewart, 1998). More specifically, the following arguments have been raised:

1. By decreasing anxiety, medications promote passivity and reduce motivation for participation in CBT.
2. During the concomitant administration of pharmacotherapy and CBT, patients may be more likely to attribute progress to medications than to learning new skills through CBT and personal mastery (e.g., Marks

et al., 1993; Basoglu et al., 1994); this makes it difficult for patients to develop a sense of ownership of their treatment gains.

3. Medications interfere with the acquisition of new skills through CBT, because of the "state-dependent" learning of these skills. That is, the skills learned while patients are taking a medication cannot be effectively used in various situations outside treatment or when patients are not taking the medication.

4. Medications serve as safety devices when taken in the course of CBT; as such, medications perpetuate the erroneous notion that physical symptoms are dangerous and should be best dealt with by suppression.

Although there is no conclusive evidence that any of these assumptions are correct, they have been influential in promoting a view that combining medications and CBT is detrimental, in addition to being useless.

The Case for Combining Pharmacotherapy and Cognitive-Behavioral Therapy

The combining of pharmacotherapy and CBT, or components of CBT, is frequent in the course of treating panic disorder. It is apparently preferred by patients (Craske, 1996), perceived by patients as the most efficacious form of treatment (Ballenger and Lydiard, 1997), and endorsed by international experts in the field (Uhlenhuth et al., 1999) and treatment guidelines for panic disorder (e.g., American Psychiatric Association, 1998). Medications are also used when the primary treatment modality is CBT, but it appears that this use is not reported at all or its potential benefits are downplayed. For example, one study (Fava et al., 1995) that reported good results of exposure therapy in the treatment of panic disorder with agoraphobia made only cursory mention that patients were permitted to use benzodiazepines and that one-fourth of the patients were taking these medications at the conclusion of the study.

One meta-analysis of the treatment of panic disorder (van Balkom et al., 1997) found combination treatment to be more efficacious than either pharmacotherapy or CBT alone. Also, combined treatment was more efficacious than CBT alone immediately after the completion of treatment (de Beurs et al., 1995; Oehrberg et al., 1995; Barlow et al., 2000), but this advantage was not found later, after the medication had been discontinued, when combined treatment actually fared worse than CBT alone (Barlow et al., 2000). Therefore, it has been proposed that combined treatments may offer a short-term advantage but a long-term disadvantage. Combined treatment was associated with a lower likelihood of relapse when compared to pharmacotherapy alone (Biondi and Picardi, 2003).

It has been suggested that antidepressants (imipramine) improve motivation and thereby make it more likely for patients to engage in CBT for agoraphobia, especially self-directed exposure between sessions (Telch et al., 1985). Other studies (Zitrin et al., 1980; Mavissakalian and Michelson, 1986b) have also found a beneficial effect of imipramine on exposure therapy for agoraphobia. At the very minimum, pharmacotherapy may not have an adverse effect on the long-term outcome of CBT (e.g., Oei et al., 1997).

In summary, research has produced conflicting data about the benefits of combined treatment. Nevertheless, the combination of pharmacotherapy and CBT is not only frequent in clinical practice but also seems to be a preferred treatment modality, despite the problems with its use. Perhaps this discrepancy between research findings and the reality of clinical practice is due to studies neglecting to address the fundamental issues of when and how to combine treatments to maximize, not minimize, the benefits of such a combination.

What Are the Indications for the Combined Treatment Approach?

A lack of clarity about when to use combined treatment has contributed to the ongoing controversy and confusion about its value. It appears that combined pharmacotherapy and CBT might be useful in the following situations and for the following purposes:

1. When there is greater severity of panic disorder, which includes a more severe agoraphobia (Spiegel and Bruce, 1997; American Psychiatric Association, 1998; Starcevic et al., 2004)
2. When it is difficult to conduct CBT because of the high level of anxiety and frequent or severe panic attacks (Spiegel and Bruce, 1997)
3. When the likelihood of relapse, particularly after the cessation of pharmacotherapy, needs to be minimized (Biondi and Picardi, 2003)
4. When there is insufficient response to either pharmacotherapy or CBT (American Psychiatric Association, 1998)
5. When psychiatric conditions and/or psychiatric complications of panic disorder (e.g., depression) co-occur (Starcevic et al., 2004)

How Should Pharmacotherapy and Cognitive-Behavioral Therapy Be Combined?

In terms of sequence, there are basically three ways in which pharmacotherapy and CBT can be combined.

First, CBT may be added to the initially used pharmacotherapy. This seems to be the most common way of combining treatments in clinical practice: many patients are first treated with a medication, and by the time they present to a facility in which CBT is offered, they are likely to be using pharmacotherapy (e.g., Wardle, 1990). Indeed, when the clinician encounters a panic patient in specialized settings such as anxiety disorders clinics, the patient is likely to have been taking, and may still be taking, a medication; more often than not, this medication is a benzodiazepine. In this situation, CBT may be added with the goal of expanding a response to pharmacotherapy and increasing the likelihood that gains of pharmacotherapy will last longer.

Second, pharmacotherapy may be added to the initially used CBT. This may occur when patients are too distressed to participate in CBT because of the severity of anxiety and/or panic disorder. The other reason for adding pharmacotherapy to CBT is the presence of psychiatric conditions (e.g., depression) or complications of panic disorder that may respond to pharmacotherapy.

Finally, both CBT and pharmacotherapy may be commenced at approximately the same time. This does not seem to occur very often, as most clinicians prefer one or the other treatment approach initially, and then add the other treatment modality if the initial one does not produce an adequate response or if they want to augment the response to the initially administered treatment.

Regardless of the sequence in which CBT and pharmacotherapy are administered, it is crucial not to combine them "mechanically" (e.g., Biondi and Picardi, 2003), but in a manner that makes clinical sense. This means that the clinician should take care to avoid favoring one type of treatment, while suggesting indirectly that he or she does not value the other treatment as much. The combined treatment is less likely to be efficacious if the clinician lacks a positive attitude toward it. In addition, it is very important that patients understand the rationale for using combined treatments. It is important to check whether patients feel confused about the conflicting messages that they might have been receiving about the value of different treatments and the different underlying models of etiology.

There has been some debate as to which type of medication might be more suitable in combination with CBT for treating panic disorder. Benzodiazepines tend to be regarded more negatively in this context than antidepressants, and are usually considered to interfere more with CBT because of their quick onset of action, patients' tendency to attribute treatment gains to them, and the state-dependent learning with which they are readily associated. Although some studies (e.g., Echeburua et al., 1993; Marks et al., 1993; Wardle et al., 1994; Otto et al., 1996) did not find a combination of benzodiazepines and situational exposure useful, other studies indicated that the benefit of such a combination might depend on the sequence of administering these treatments (Spiegel and Bruce, 1997) and on whether benzodiazepines are administered regularly or on an as-needed (prn) basis (Westra et al., 2002). In particular, as-needed use of benzodiazepines in conjunction with CBT was associated with a negative outcome of CBT, whereas regular use of benzodiazepines did not interfere significantly with CBT (Westra et al., 2002).

The relative advantages and disadvantages of combining benzodiazepines or antidepressants with CBT have not been studied systematically, and there is as yet no evidence to support the notion that antidepressants are to be preferred over benzodiazepines for the purpose of combining pharmacotherapy with CBT. This means that the practicing clinician should be guided by general considerations when making a decision to use specific medications for panic disorder. This decision should not depend on whether combined treatment is contemplated.

3
Generalized Anxiety Disorder

Generalized anxiety disorder (GAD) is characterized by chronic pathological worry and other manifestations of nonphobic anxiety, which are accompanied by various symptoms of tension. Physical symptoms of anxiety are usually less prominent in GAD than in panic disorder, and behaviors that are often seen in other anxiety disorders, such as avoidance, are conspicuously absent. Unlike all other anxiety disorders, GAD is more likely to co-occur with a primary condition for which help has been sought—usually another anxiety disorder or depression—than to be the main reason for which the person seeks professional help.

CLINICAL FEATURES

Generalized anxiety disorder has been described as the "basic" anxiety disorder (Barlow, 1988). This implies that many of its features characterize all anxiety disorders and it is not surprising that it has been difficult to single out clinical features and other characteristics that might be specific for GAD. Bearing this in mind, GAD can be conceptualized as a heterogeneous condition, that encompasses in various proportions the following "clusters" of clinical features: (1) pathological worry and other cognitive aspects of chronic anxiety, (2) symptoms of tension, and (3) various physical symptoms, many of which reflect autonomic hyperactivity.

Pathological Worry and Other Cognitive Aspects of Chronic Anxiety

Generalized anxiety disorder has been redefined as a condition in which pathological worry is the most conspicuous feature. Pathological worry has been subject of much interest and research over the last 10–15 years, and following DSM-IV-TR, it is now conceptualized as being excessive, uncontrollable, present almost constantly, and relating to several "topics" or "domains" (Table 3–1). In addition, pathological worry often pertains to events and circumstances that are located in the remote future, and this may be one of the distinguishing features of GAD-specific worry (Dugas et al., 1998a).

Patients with GAD worry about matters that may seem minor or unrealistic, but they also worry about problems such as poor health of loved ones, a conflictual marital relationship, and poor performance at work or in school. Regardless of whether patients worry about minor or major matters, what they worry about almost always pertains to something in the future, and the future is usually perceived negatively. That is, GAD patients look forward to the future with much apprehension, as they might get sick, lose a job, or have no money, their children might have an accident, etc. Although the events that they worry about may happen, they overestimate the probability that these events will happen. The worry themes are not unusual or odd in themselves, as many people without GAD do worry about similar things. Therefore, for the conceptualization of pathological worry, it is more important *how* persons worry rather than *what* they worry about.

TABLE 3–1. Characteristics of Pathological Worry

1. Excessive in intensity
2. Constant or almost constant (present more often than not; most of the day, nearly every day)
3. Chronic
4. Ruminative and uncontrollable; although it is self-initiated, it has an intrusive quality (e.g., the person states that he or she is unable to stop worrying)
5. Relates to several "topics" or "domains" (e.g., the person worries about health, finances, and work at the same time)
6. Often pertains to remote future circumstances (Dugas et al., 1998a)

Patients with GAD usually worry about more issues or matters than "normal" worriers. Also, the worry in GAD is constant or almost constant, and it seems to patients that they have been troubled by their tendency to worry for a very long time ("I have always been a worrier" is a typical statement made by GAD patients). Patients often realize that they worry excessively, but at the same time feel that they cannot do anything to prevent or resist worry or to stop worrying. As a result, they are preoccupied with their worries so much that they find it difficult to distract themselves and to focus on something else.

The thought processes of patients with GAD are often characterized by the escalating pattern of "what if . . ." style of questioning, whereby one imagined catastrophe leads to another. For example, a patient with health-related worries expressed the corresponding concerns in the following sequence: "What if they find that I have cancer? What if I have to undergo surgery? Will I be allergic to the anesthetic? What if my children have to watch me dying? How will they manage financially after my death?"

Many patients with GAD have trouble tolerating any ambiguity and uncertainty (Ladouceur et al., 1997). They tend to interpret ambiguous situations as implying some hidden danger, so that they have even more reasons to worry. The sense of uncertainty undermines their confidence and makes patients more vigilant; patients are then also more likely to have trouble making decisions.

Sometimes patients with GAD have difficulty identifying what they worry about or are vague about it. For example, they may have nonspecific concerns about some existential and philosophical issues (such as the meaning and purpose of life and death) or state that they are anxious "about everything." They may also report what has been referred to as "free-floating anxiety"—a pervasive anxious feeling, without a clear focus of anxiety.

Symptoms of Tension

In addition to worry that is excessive, constant, and uncontrollable, patients with GAD are troubled by tension that can be experienced in many different ways (Table 3–2). Thus, patients often state that they are constantly nervous, keyed up, on edge, unable to relax, restless, "cranky," "ready to explode," unable to tolerate anything, and the like. Another aspect of tension is difficulty in concentrating and, even more so, being unable to quickly shift the focus of attention from one subject to another. Finally, as a result of the ongoing, excessive perception of threat, GAD patients tend to be hypervigilant: they are constantly "on alert," expecting something

TABLE 3–2. Manifestations of Tension in Generalized Anxiety Disorder

Psychological Aspects of Tension

Nervousness

Feeling keyed up, on edge, unable to relax

Inner restlessness

Irritability: feeling "cranky" or "ready to explode," getting easily annoyed or angry, having decreased tolerance of frustration

Difficulty concentrating

Hypervigilance: feeling constantly "on alert," expecting something bad to happen, getting startled easily

Physical (Somatic) Aspects of Tension

Muscle tightness or stiffness (muscle tension): stiff neck, back pain, shoulder pain, tension headache

Muscle spasms

Tic-like movements, jerks

Fine tremor

Difficulty in swallowing ("psychogenic dysphagia")—fear of choking on food

Consequences of Tension

Sleep disturbance: trouble falling asleep, "broken sleep," unrefreshing sleep

Agitation

Fatigue, exhaustion

---

bad to happen, and get startled easily by ordinary and innocuous stimuli, such as a knock on the door or the telephone ringing.

A very common physical aspect of tension is muscle tightness or stiffness (or muscle tension), which often leads to pain. As a result, GAD patients often complain of a stiff neck, back pain, or shoulder pain. Tension headache is another typical feature of GAD, with the headache usually being located in the back or frontal regions or described as "aching all over." Patients may also complain of muscle spasms, tic-like movements, jerks, and fine tremor. These symptoms may be particularly prominent in eyelids and other facial muscles. Another manifestation of tension is difficulty in swallowing, sometimes referred to as "psychogenic dysphagia"; this may lead to the fear of choking on food.

In addition, many patients have disturbed sleep as a consequence of tension; they usually have trouble falling asleep, but many have "broken sleep" or wake up feeling that their sleep has not been refreshing. Another consequence of tension is feeling tired or even exhausted.

Other Physical Symptoms

Generalized anxiety disorder is also characterized by various other physical symptoms, which may dominate the clinical presentation. Although the emphasis in current conceptualization of GAD is on pathological worry and tension, some patients with GAD present mainly with physical symptoms. In such cases, patients are more likely to seek help in general medical or primary care settings. There is nothing about these symptoms that is specific for GAD, as they often appear in other anxiety disorders, particularly panic disorder. Unlike panic disorder, in which physical symptoms are usually severe but appear episodically during panic attacks, physical symptoms in GAD are usually less intense but more enduring.

Some of the physical symptoms reflect autonomic hyperarousal: tachycardia, palpitations, sweating, and tremor. Not infrequently, GAD patients complain of gastrointestinal symptoms, such as nausea, upset stomach, and diarrhea. Other symptoms seen among GAD patients include dizziness, lightheadedness, hot and cold flushes, numbness, and tingling sensations. Breathing difficulties, tightness in the chest, and chest pain are sometimes severe and lead patients with GAD to seek help in cardiology clinics, not unlike panic patients (Logue et al., 1993).

Physical symptoms may be the main vehicle through which GAD patients express distress; the means of expressing distress are usually determined by various personal and cultural factors. Unexplained physical symptoms, which result from the process of somatization, are not rare among patients with GAD.

Relationship Between Generalized Anxiety Disorder and Other Disorders

The relationship between GAD and other disorders is unique in that GAD almost "needs" other disorders to be present in order for it to be noticed. That is, GAD is usually diagnosed as a condition co-occurring with another disorder, and less often as the only disorder for which help is being sought. This has led some investigators and clinicians to doubt the validity of GAD as an independent psychopathological and diagnostic entity. When GAD is a chronologically primary condition, it is possible that it represents a risk factor or predisposition for the development of some conditions with which it commonly co-occurs.

Most patients with GAD have at least one other psychiatric disorder; the figures vary, but as many as 89% of GAD patients in the primary care setting have been found to have additional psychiatric conditions (Olfson et al., 1997). In contrast to other anxiety disorders, in which the rates of co-occurrence of other disorders are often much higher in clinical than in general populations, GAD has similar rates of co-occurrance in both populations. Psychiatric conditions that most frequently co-occur with GAD are major depressive disorder (up to 46% of patients currently and up to 64% over lifetime), social anxiety disorder (59% over lifetime), specific phobias (55% over lifetime), dysthymic disorder (8% currently and up to 39.5% over lifetime), and panic disorder (27% over lifetime) (Brawman-Mintzer et al., 1993; Wittchen et al., 1994; Brawman-Mintzer and Lydiard, 1996). Of these conditions, the most important relationship is the one with depressive disorders (major depressive disorder and dysthymic disorder).

Generalized anxiety disorder also has some association (up to 15% of patients) with alcohol abuse and dependence (Brawman-Mintzer and Lydiard, 1996). Alcohol-related problems are less prominent, however, in patients with "pure" GAD than in those with some other anxiety disorders, especially social anxiety disorder, posttraumatic stress disorder, and panic disorder. The onset of GAD may occur in people who have been abusing alcohol, e.g., following alcohol withdrawal. Some symptoms of alcohol withdrawal or withdrawal from other substances may be difficult to distinguish from autonomic hyperactivity and tension symptoms seen in patients with GAD. Alcoholism may also appear some time after the onset of GAD, as part of the patients' self-medicating strategy of coping with anxiety; however, this is less common than with patients suffering from social anxiety disorder.

Personality disorders may be present in a substantial number of GAD patients, with the most common types of personality disturbance being dependent and avoidant personality disorders (Mavissakalian et al., 1993).

Generalized Anxiety Disorder and Depression

The relationship between GAD and depression is important for several reasons (Table 3–3). First, symptoms of chronic anxiety and depression often overlap, and the differentiation between GAD and depression may sometimes be very difficult. In fact, some of the key symptoms of GAD and the corresponding diagnostic criteria are the same as those in depression; this pertains to sleep disturbance, concentration difficulties, and fatigue or exhaustion. Even pathological worry, now considered a defining feature of GAD, was found to characterize major depressive disorder (Starcevic, 1995). The symptoms that can most reliably distinguish depression from

TABLE 3–3. Aspects of the Relationship Between Generalized Anxiety Disorder and
Depression and Clinical Implications

Aspects	Clinical Implications
Overlap between symptoms of GAD and depression	Difficulties in distinguishing between GAD and depression
Depression is the most frequent complication of GAD and the most common reason for GAD patients to seek help.	When GAD patients present for help, symptoms and signs of depression need to be investigated.
High likelihood that a substantial proportion of GAD patients will develop depression	Depression may be prevented by administration of antidepressants and/or by vigorous psychological treatment of GAD.

chronic anxiety and GAD are loss of interest and anhedonia (Clark et al.,
1994a; Mineka et al., 1998); symptoms that are most likely to suggest that an
anxiety disorder (mainly panic disorder, but possibly also GAD) is the main
condition are those of autonomic hyperactivity and arousal (Clark and Watson, 1991).

Depression is the most frequent complication of GAD and the most
likely reason for GAD patients to seek help. Therefore, by the time GAD
patients see a physician or other therapist, a possibility of the co-occurring
depression should always be kept in mind. The high probability that GAD
patients will develop depression has important treatment implications:
depression may perhaps be prevented by the administration of antidepressants and/or by vigorous psychological treatment of GAD. If depression has already developed, the use of antidepressant medication is the
logical treatment strategy. Although a more typical sequence is for depression to appear some time after the onset of GAD, both disorders may occur
at approximately the same time, and in some patients GAD may be
chronologically secondary to depression.

Generalized Anxiety Disorder and Social Anxiety Disorder

Generalized anxiety disorder and social anxiety disorder often co-occur in
clinical practice, with rates of social anxiety disorder in clinically primary
GAD ranging between 23% and 59% (Sanderson et al., 1990; Brawman-
Mintzer et al., 1993). Social anxiety disorder and GAD have some features
in common, including early and gradual onset. Both disorders may have a
similar origin, but the perceived threat in GAD spreads to various issues
and areas, whereas the perceived threat in social anxiety disorder remains

in the realm of social and interpersonal interactions and situations. Thus, GAD is a wider psychopathological concept, which often encompasses features of social anxiety disorder. It is not surprising, then, that even in the absence of a diagnosis of social anxiety disorder, concerns about performance and negative evaluation are frequently the focus of worries of GAD patients, and sometimes these concerns dominate the clinical presentation of GAD.

Generalized anxiety disorder and the generalized type of social anxiety disorder also have in common the pervasiveness of clinical features and their frequent conceptualization as a form of personality disturbance rather than a mental state (DSM Axis I) disorder.

ASSESSMENT

Diagnostic Issues

The assessment of GAD has been hampered by the frequently changing conceptualization and diagnostic criteria. Generalized anxiety disorder has gone from a residual diagnostic category in DSM-III (to be used only if diagnostic criteria for other anxiety disorders and depression have not been met) to a condition characterized by both physical and psychological symptoms in DSM-III-R and disorder whose defining feature is pathological worry in DSM-IV and DSM-IV-TR. It is not clear how GAD will be defined in DSM-V, as there is some dissatisfaction with its DSM-IV/DSM-IV-TR conceptualization. The lack of continuity in terms of how GAD has been conceptualized over time is a significant problem, because it is uncertain whether different versions of DSM-defined GAD refer to the same condition.

In addition, there are significant differences between the DSM-IV-TR and ICD-10 definitions of GAD and between the corresponding diagnostic criteria (Table 3–4). As a result, although the DSM- and ICD-defined GAD overlap, they are not identical disorders.

Generalized anxiety disorder is perhaps the most controversial diagnostic category in the group of anxiety disorders, and there have been repeated calls for reexamination of its diagnostic criteria, its status as an independent nosological entity, and its construct validity (e.g., Breier et al., 1985; Bienvenu et al., 1998; Starcevic and Bogojevic, 1999). In a way, this is somewhat paradoxical for a condition considered to be the "basic" anxiety disorder. The most compelling reason for this state of affairs is the fact that GAD co-occurs so frequently with other psychiatric disorders that it is rarely seen in relative isolation from them. As a result, GAD is more likely

TABLE 3–4. Differences in Conceptualization of Generalized Anxiety Disorder in DSM-IV-TR and ICD-10

Criteria	DSM-IV-TR	ICD-10
Nosological status	Independent diagnostic category	Residual diagnostic category; criteria for diagnosing other anxiety disorders and depression must not be met
Pathological worry	Must be present for diagnosis to be made	Not necessary for diagnosis
Symptoms of autonomic hyperactivity and other physical symptoms	Not necessary for diagnosis	Must be present for diagnosis to be made
Duration of symptoms	At least 6 months	Several months

to be a secondary condition than a disorder for which patients seek help, and many clinicians do not regard it as particularly relevant for clinical practice. Recent data suggest that in the community, the rates of co-occurrence of other disorders with GAD are not significantly higher than the corresponding rates for other anxiety disorders; however, this does not seem to have changed clinicians' perception of GAD as a disorder with dubious clinical validity.

Assessment Instruments

The most commonly used instrument for assessment of the degree of pathological worry (which is not necessarily related to GAD) is the Penn State Worry Questionnaire (Meyer et al., 1990). This is a brief, easy-to-administer, self-report measure, that is also useful for monitoring changes in the degree of pathological worry during treatment.

The Hamilton Anxiety Rating Scale (Hamilton, 1959) is one of the most frequently used instruments for measuring the degree of general anxiety, which cuts across several types of anxiety disorders. This clinician-administered instrument has been used as a gold standard in pharmacotherapy trials of GAD. The scale assesses both the psychological and somatic symptoms of anxiety, but it does not specifically address worry; symptoms of autonomic arousal are emphasized, which are now considered less important for GAD. The Hamilton Anxiety Rating Scale can be useful for treatment monitoring purposes if administered along with the Penn State Worry Questionnaire.

As an alternative to the Hamilton Anxiety Rating Scale, a self-report Beck Anxiety Inventory (Beck et al., 1988) can be used because its administration is simpler. The Beck Anxiety Inventory emphasizes somatic symptoms of anxiety, which are not specific for GAD.

In an attempt to develop a brief, yet comprehensive measure of the severity of GAD, Sheehan and co-workers have recently proposed the Worry-Anxiety-Tension Scale (Sheehan et al., 2000). This self-report instrument measures separately the degree of all three main components of GAD: pathological worry, general anxiety, and tension. Although the instrument is somewhat simplistic, it represents a step in the right direction, as it generates a total score for the severity of GAD and separate scores for the severity of its main components.

Differential Diagnosis

Generalized anxiety disorder needs to be distinguished from normal worries and various physical and psychiatric conditions, as well as substance-induced disorders (Table 3–5). Generalized anxiety disorder may be the anxiety disorder that most resembles "normal" anxiety. Criteria for distinguishing between normal worries and GAD have been spelled out in Clinical

TABLE 3–5. Differential Diagnosis of Generalized Anxiety Disorder

1. Normal worries
2. Physical conditions (e.g., hyperthyroidism)
3. Substance-related conditions
   Intoxication with psychostimulants (e.g., amphetamine)
   Caffeinism
   Alcohol withdrawal syndrome
   Benzodiazepine withdrawal syndrome
4. Psychiatric disorders
   Mood disorders (major depressive disorder, dysthymic disorder)
   Mixed anxiety and depressive disorder
   Panic disorder
   Obsessive-compulsive disorder
   Hypochondriasis
   Specific phobias
   Posttraumatic stress disorder
   Adjustment disorders
   Personality disorders (avoidant, dependent)

Features (above). Normal worries are not accompanied by the degree of tension, multiple manifestations of tension, and/or physical symptoms of anxiety seen in GAD. Likewise, there is no interference with functioning and no impairment in people with normal worries and normal anxiety.

Medical Differential Diagnosis
As for physical conditions, symptoms of GAD may appear in the course of hyperthyroidism and, less often, as part of asthma, chronic lung disease, various heart conditions, hypertension, diabetes mellitus, and certain neurological, metabolic, and other endocrinological diseases. A diagnosis of GAD is not warranted if it is clear that GAD-like features are secondary to any physical condition, particularly if successful treatment of the physical condition brings about a disappearance of the symptoms of GAD. If the features of GAD persist despite improvement in physical condition, it is not likely that these features are attributable to the physical condition and a diagnosis of GAD is probably justified.

Generalized anxiety disorder is relatively frequently seen in patients with irritable bowel syndrome, but the etiological significance of this association, if any, is not well understood.

Medical work-up of patients with GAD should include routine laboratory analyses with thyroid function tests. Depending on the age of the patient, symptoms, and specific circumstances, the work-up may also include a cardiological examination with electrocardiogram. A thorough medical work-up is particularly important in elderly patients with GAD and a GAD-like picture, because of the increased probability of an association with various medical conditions.

Substance-Related Disorders and Generalized Anxiety Disorder
Generalized anxiety disorder needs to be differentiated from intoxication with stimulant substances, such as amphetamine. In clinical practice, the most common stimulant-related disorder is intoxication with caffeine; it is important to distinguish between GAD and caffeine intoxication, as the two may have similar clinical features. However, unlike GAD, caffeine intoxication is likely to be accompanied by characteristic somatic symptoms such as frequent urination, upset stomach and other gastrointestinal problems, tachycardia or other heart rhythm disturbances, and blushing. Because of this phenomenological overlap, all patients with GAD-like clinical presentation should routinely be asked about their consumption of coffee and caffeinated beverages.

Sometimes GAD may also need to be distinguished from alcohol or benzodiazepine withdrawal syndromes.

Psychiatric Differential Diagnosis

In the psychiatric differential diagnosis, the first task is to distinguish GAD from a depressive disorder (both major depressive disorder and dysthymia) because of the significant overlap between their typical symptoms. Also, both GAD and depression are characterized by a predominantly dysphoric mood or "negative affect" (Clark and Watson, 1991). The relationship between GAD and depression and criteria for distinguishing between the two are presented in greater detail in Relationship Between Generalized Anxiety Disorder and Other Disorders (above); aspects of this relationship are presented in Table 3–3.

Mixed anxiety and depressive disorder is a controversial diagnosis, which exists in ICD-10 but not in the DSM system (except as a provisional diagnosis that requires further study). It can be used if neither the diagnosis of a specific anxiety disorder, including GAD, nor the diagnosis of a depressive disorder can be made. In other words, mixed anxiety and depressive disorder can be conceptualized as a residual diagnosis for patients with diagnostically "subthreshold" manifestations of GAD and depression. It appears that a number of patients for whom this diagnosis may be appropriate is not small, particularly in primary care settings.

As for other anxiety disorders, it is interesting to note that the concept of worry has a place analogous to that of panic attacks. That is, just as panic attacks occur in various disorders and are not typical only of panic disorder, pathological worry is not confined only to GAD and is found in other psychiatric conditions, and other anxiety disorders in particular. What differentiates pathological worry in GAD from pathological worry in other anxiety disorders are its focus and pervasiveness. The focus of worry in other anxiety disorders is more circumscribed: patients with panic disorder are excessively concerned about future panic attacks and their consequences, whereas those with social anxiety disorder worry about being judged too harshly by others. Not only do patients with GAD worry about matters and issues from different domains, they may also worry about worrying—a phenomenon referred to as "meta-worry" (Wells, 1994).

Criteria for differentiating between GAD and panic disorder are listed in Table 2–13.

Obsessive-compulsive disorder sometimes needs to be considered in the differential diagnosis of GAD, because of the similarities between obsessions and pathological worry that characterize these conditions; both of these phenomena are experienced as uncontrollable and repetitive. In addition, obsessions involving doubting and centered on the need to check may seem similar to pathological worry, as many of these obsessions and pathological worries pertain to a hypothetical danger in the future. In most cases, however, GAD and pathological worry can be differentiated from obsessive-compulsive disorder and obsessions (see Table 3–6 and Chapter 6).

Patients with GAD who worry excessively about health and disease usually do not suspect that they already have a serious physical disease, as in hypochondriasis. Likewise, patients with GAD do not exhibit typical hypochondriacal behaviors, such as seeking reassurance from various doctors and subjecting themselves to numerous, unnecessary medical investigations.

Patients with GAD differ from patients with some types of specific phobias, particularly phobia of choking and disease phobia, in terms of having a more broad type of anxiety. Their fears lack a phobic quality and they do not exhibit the phobia-related avoidance behavior.

Generalized anxiety disorder differs from posttraumatic stress disorder and adjustment disorders in that it is not necessarily preceded by and is not etiologically associated with a trauma or a stressful event.

Finally, GAD may resemble some personality disorders, especially avoidant and dependent personality disorders, because of its chronic course and early onset in many of its sufferers. While the personality disorders from DSM Cluster C are often characterized by long-standing manifestations of anxiety, the pattern of pathological worry, various symptoms of tension, and other somatic symptoms is usually absent, unless these personality disorders are accompanied by GAD. Unlike GAD, the avoidant and dependent personality disorders are characterized by marked patterns of social avoidance and excessive dependency, respectively.

TABLE 3–6. Distinguishing Between Generalized Anxiety Disorder and Obsessive-Compulsive Disorder

Criteria	Pathological Worry in GAD	Obsessions in OCD
Quality of the experience	Not alien, "crazy," or inappropriate	Ego-dystonic, alien, "crazy," or inappropriate
Intrusiveness	Less pronounced	More pronounced
Content	Real-life problems (health, work, school, relationships, finances)	Referring to something abhorrent or shameful (e.g., contamination, aggressive or sexual urges) and/or implying one's personal involvement or responsibility
Relationship with images	Usually not present	Often very strong
Need to neutralize	Usually not present	Usually very strong

GAD, generalized anxiety disorder; OCD, obsessive-compulsive disorder.

Epidemiology

Highlights of the epidemiology of GAD are shown in Table 3–7. Epidemiological data on GAD vary significantly because of the frequently changing diagnostic criteria from DSM-III to DSM-IV-TR, differences in the conceptualization of GAD and the corresponding diagnostic criteria between the DSM and ICD classifications, and differences between instruments used in the epidemiological studies.

In the U.S. National Comorbidity Survey, which used the DSM-III-R criteria, lifetime prevalence of GAD was 5.1% (Wittchen et al., 1994). When the ICD-10 criteria for GAD were used, lifetime prevalence was estimated at 8.9% (Wittchen et al., 1994). Depending on the diagnostic criteria used and the country in which epidemiological studies were conducted, lifetime prevalence ranged from 1.9% to 10.5% (Uhlenhuth et al., 1983; Faravelli et al., 1989; Hwu et al., 1989; Lee et al., 1990a, 1990b; Wacker et al., 1992).

The lifetime prevalence of GAD without any co-occurring conditions was found to be much lower—only 0.5% (Wittchen et al., 1994). This finding suggests that GAD rarely occurs alone, not only in clinical population

---

TABLE 3–7. Epidemiological Data for Generalized Anxiety Disorder

- Lifetime prevalence in the United States: 5.1% (DSM-III-R criteria)
- Lifetime prevalence in various countries, according to various diagnostic criteria: 1.9%–10.5%
- Rarely occurs alone: 66.3% had at least one additional current disorder (most commonly depression, social anxiety disorder, and panic disorder); 90.4% had at least one additional disorder co-occurring with GAD during their lifetime (with depression and panic disorder being most common)
- Most common anxiety disorder among children and the elderly
- Relatively high prevalence in all age groups
- One of the most common psychiatric disorders in primary care
- Often diagnosed as a condition co-occurring with another disorder (e.g., depression) for which help was originally sought
- About two-thirds of GAD sufferers are women
- More common in urban populations and among separated, divorced, widowed, and unemployed persons, homemakers, and people with lower income
- Typical age of onset: 15–25 years; onset occurs in childhood and adolescence in a sizeable proportion
- Characteristic help-seeking patterns: most persons with GAD do not seek help at all; there is a long period between onset and the time of seeking help; help is usually sought in primary care for a condition that complicates the course of GAD (e.g., depression)

but in epidemiological samples as well. As many as 66.3% of persons with GAD in the community had at least one additional current disorder, most commonly depression, social anxiety disorder, and panic disorder; the life-time rate of psychiatric disorders co-occurring with GAD was 90.4%, with depression and panic disorder being the most common co-occurring disorders (Wittchen et al., 1994).

Generalized anxiety disorder has been reported to be either the most common anxiety disorder among the elderly (with a 1-year prevalence rate of 7.1%; Uhlenhuth et al., 1983) or the third most common anxiety disorder in this age group, following specific phobias and agoraphobia (Blazer et al., 1991a). Likewise, GAD and its nosological precursor in children, overanxious disorder, were consistently found to be very frequent (3.6%–5.9%) in children (Bowen et al., 1990; McGee et al., 1990). In comparison with other anxiety disorders, this high prevalence of GAD in all age groups, from childhood to old age, is rather unique.

It is estimated that about one-half of persons with GAD seek help from primary care physicians (Wittchen et al., 1994). Thus, GAD is one of the most common psychiatric disorders encountered in primary care, with the prevalence of 7.9% being second only to that of depression (Goldberg and Lecrubier, 1995). A recent study (Wittchen et al., 2002) has found that GAD is the most frequent anxiety disorder in primary medical care. Moreover, GAD sufferers also tend to see various medical specialists, most commonly gastroenterologists (Kennedy and Schwab, 1997); however, they seem to attend specialized medical clinics generally less often than persons who have panic disorder.

Generalized anxiety disorder occurs about twice more often among women than among men (Blazer et al., 1991b; Wittchen et al., 1994), and is encountered more often among separated, divorced, widowed, and unemployed persons and homemakers (Wittchen et al., 1994). It may be more frequent in urban populations and among people with lower income.

It is often difficult to determine the precise onset of GAD, because it usually develops gradually and many patients say that they have "always" worried and have "always" been anxious, nervous, or tense. Still, it is estimated that the onset of GAD occurs most commonly between the age 15 and 25, although in a sizeable number, first manifestations of GAD appear in childhood and early adolescence. In contrast to the gradual and insidious onset of GAD in adolescence and in the third decade, its onset later in life may be more acute, and is often associated with a stressful event (Hoehn-Saric et al., 1993a).

It is estimated that only one-third of persons with GAD seek help in the year of onset of GAD (Olfson et al., 1998), whereas those who seek help later delay doing so for an average of about 10 years. Even then, help is usually sought for a condition that complicates the course of GAD, such as depression. In view of the frequency with which other psychiatric disorders co-occur with GAD, it is not surprising that GAD is often overshadowed by disorders that receive therapeutic attention; in such cases, the presence of GAD may also be overlooked.

In contrast to the usual early onset of GAD, the average age at which persons with GAD seek professional help is 39 years. This lengthy delay before help and treatment are sought is similar to the corresponding delay in social anxiety disorder and specific phobias. By contrast, the onset of panic disorder usually occurs at a later age than GAD, but persons with panic disorder do not wait very long before seeking help; therefore, in clinical settings, patients with panic disorder are often younger than those with GAD.

COURSE AND PROGNOSIS

Generalized anxiety disorder is a chronic condition. While its clinical features tend to persist, the course of GAD is often characterized by the waxing and waning of its symptoms and by symptoms becoming more severe at times of stress.

It is difficult to conduct follow-up studies of "pure" GAD, because it so often co-occurs with other disorders. Still, a 5-year follow-up study of treated GAD patients (Woodman et al., 1999) revealed that only 18% of patients were in remission, while more than 50% continued to have symptoms, with impairment in various areas of functioning. Other studies paint a similar picture of the course of GAD. Noyes et al. (1987b) found that only one-fourth of GAD patients have "remissions," defined as 3-month periods without any symptoms. In another study (Mancuso et al., 1993), one-half of patients continued to have symptoms of GAD 16 months after the completion of treatment.

As already noted, GAD is often complicated by depression, and less often by panic disorder and alcohol-related problems. If depression develops, patients' overall condition tends to be more severe, their functioning more impaired, treatment more difficult, and prognosis worse. The development of depression in the course of GAD also increases the suicide risk.

Factors suggesting poor prognosis of GAD are its long duration before it is treated; presence of chronic physical conditions, other psychiatric disorders, and personality disorders; disturbed marital or other family relationships; and poor adjustment to the environment in which patients live.

Generalized anxiety disorder is associated with substantial impairment in occupational and social functioning and adverse effects on quality of life. In particular, GAD has been associated with decreased work productivity (Greenberg et al., 1999; Kessler et al., 1999a; Wittchen et al., 2000a). High proportions of GAD patients are unemployed and/or receive welfare or disability financial packages (Massion et al., 1993). While the degree of impairment and disability are higher when GAD is accompanied by depression, GAD has been associated with considerable impairment even in its pure form (Wittchen et al., 2000a). Patients with GAD tend to perceive themselves as being in poor health and are more likely to use health-care services (e.g., Kessler et al., 1999a; Maier et al., 2000; Wittchen et al., 2002).

ETIOLOGY AND PATHOGENESIS

There are generally two broad ways of conceptualizing the etiology and pathogenesis of GAD. Like other anxiety disorders, GAD may be conceived of as a condition that develops in the background of a specific and nonspecific predisposition, following certain precipitating events; within this framework, factors that maintain GAD can also be identified. Unique to GAD, however, among all the anxiety disorders except for generalized social anxiety disorder, is the fact that GAD has also been conceptualized as being akin to a personality disorder. When GAD is conceptualized as primarily a disturbance at the level of personality, a different etiological model—one in which a distinction between the predisposing and precipitating factors is largely irrelevant—needs to be elaborated.

In this section, contributions to the current understanding of etiology and pathogenesis of GAD will be reviewed from the major theoretical perspectives. A hypothesis that GAD is primarily a personality disorder will also be presented.

BIOLOGICAL MODELS

Genetic Factors

There is some indication that GAD may have a genetic component. This is suggested by the finding (Noyes et al., 1987b) that GAD occurs several times more frequently among first-degree relatives of individuals with GAD (19.5%) than among first-degree relatives of normal controls (3.5%). Also, the heritability of GAD among female twins was estimated at 30% (Kendler et al., 1992a). However, other findings do not support the notion that GAD is a genetically based disorder (e.g., Torgersen, 1983), and there is a possibility that higher rates of GAD in some families reflect the influence of the shared environment more than that of hereditary factors.

Other studies have examined the genetic relationship between GAD and depression. One proposal is that genes involved in GAD and major depressive disorder might be linked, so that GAD might be inherited only if a gene for depression is also inherited (Skre et al., 1993). A genetic link between GAD and depression has been postulated in women, with genetic predisposition for GAD and depression presumed to be the same. According to this model, the development of GAD or depression then depends on environmental and developmental factors and life events (Kendler et al., 1992b; Kendler, 1996).

Pathophysiological Mechanisms and Neuroanatomy

Neurotransmitter Systems

Several neurotransmitter systems have been implicated in the etiology and pathogenesis of GAD: norepinephrine, serotonin, gamma-aminobutyric acid (GABA), and cholecystokinin. Studies of some of these four systems have been undertaken largely as a result of the efficacy of medications that act via the corresponding transmitters. Thus, the efficacy of buspirone (and later, the efficacy of selective serotonin reuptake inhibitors) in the treatment of GAD was largely responsible for investigations of the etiological and pathogenetic role of serotonin; similarly, the efficacy of benzodiazepines was instrumental in promoting studies of the GABA system. A finding that there are abnormalities in the norepinephrine system in GAD provided some explanation for the efficacy in GAD of medications such as imipramine.

The results of these studies have not been consistent and did not point to any one neurotransmitter system as being more significant for GAD than others. These results also do not allow a conclusion that there are abnormalities in the neurotransmitter systems specific for GAD. In addition, it is not clear whether neurotransmitter abnormalities precede the onset of GAD or whether they are a consequence of GAD. Some of the neurotransmitter abnormalities presumed to be involved in GAD are presented in Table 3–8.

Neuroimaging Studies

There have been few imaging studies of GAD, and, as with imaging studies of most other anxiety disorders, results have been inconsistent and do not allow any firm conclusions to be made about the neuroanatomy and

Table 3–8. Some Potential Neurotransmitter Abnormalities in Generalized Anxiety Disorder

Neurotransmitter Systems	Potential Abnormalities
Norepinephrine	Hyperactivity (e.g., Sevy et al., 1989; Kelly and Cooper, 1998)
Serotonin	Hyperactivity or underactivity (role of serotonin neurotransmitter abnormalities unclear, with potential abnormalities in GAD speculated on the basis of corresponding abnormalities in other anxiety disorders)
GABA	Altered (decreased) function of GABA-$_A$ receptors, which interact with benzodiazepines (e.g., Tiihonen et al., 1997)
	Excessive release of norepinephrine, serotonin, and/or cholecystokinin via GABA

GABA, gamma-aminobutyric acid.

pathophysiology of GAD. There is some brain imaging–based evidence, though, that dysfunction of the amygdala might be involved in the pathogenesis of GAD (DeBellis et al., 2000), but this finding does not appear specific for GAD. Another imaging study (Wu et al., 1991) has suggested that the large areas of the brain—the occipital, temporal, and frontal lobes, as well as the cerebellum and basal ganglia—might be implicated in the etiology and pathogenesis of GAD.

Other Neurobiological Aspects
Several studies of patients with GAD suggest that there may be changes in the functioning of the hypothalamic–pituitary–adrenal axis, which plays a major role in response to stress. Results of these studies have been inconsistent, but there may be chronically increased cortisol levels in GAD, suggesting an exaggerated response to stress (Avery et al., 1985; Tiller et al., 1988).

Generalized anxiety disorder may be characterized more by the activation of central nervous system (and more precisely, cortical hyperactivity) than by autonomic nervous system hyperactivity. However, autonomic hyperarousal is not rare in GAD, and autonomic dysfunction in GAD may only be more subtle. A general autonomic inflexibility may be relatively specific for GAD; this is suggested by the findings of a weakened response to stress, prolonged recovery from stress (e.g., slower return to baseline of skin conductance after stress), and slower habituation to novel stimuli and stress (Hoehn-Saric et al., 1989; Brawman-Mintzer and Lydiard, 1997). Patients with GAD may also have a lowered vagal (parasympathetic) tone (Thayer et al., 1996).

Panic induction studies have shown that panic attacks can be induced in a much smaller percentage of patients with GAD than in those with panic disorder (e.g., Cowley et al., 1988; Holt and Andrews, 1989; Verburg et al., 1995; Perna et al., 1999). This finding supports the notion that GAD differs significantly from panic disorder.

PSYCHOLOGICAL MODELS

Cognitive Approaches

The reconceptualization of GAD as a condition primarily characterized by cognitive activity, worrying, was largely a result of the growing number of cognitive models of GAD. This reconceptualization has in turn led to the formulation of additional cognitive accounts of pathological worry and GAD. These models better account for the ways in which pathological worry and GAD are reinforced and maintained than for the causes of pathological worry and GAD. Nevertheless, the models are valuable for their contribution to a better understanding of the processes involved in pathological worry and GAD. Table 3–9 lists the main aspects of cognitive models in GAD.

The cognitive abnormalities in GAD have several consequences: patients often have great difficulty in distinguishing between threatening and nonthreatening situations and cues; they feel less capable of detecting threat and of understanding where the danger is coming from; and they nonetheless feel very strongly that there is much danger out there and that they should do something about it (e.g., protect themselves). As a result, patients are puzzled about the nature of their worry (what it is that they "really" worry about and/or why), which only increases their apprehensiveness and a sense of dread.

Psychodynamic Approaches

No psychodynamic model has been specifically developed for GAD, and a psychodynamic approach to GAD is based on psychoanalytic theories of anxiety in general. Psychodynamic formulations of anxiety (Freud, 1926/1959; Karasu, 1994) are still relevant for clinical practice in that they can help clinicians better understand the underlying issues and the nature and meaning of anxiety in their patients. Modern psychodynamic approaches make a distinction between two types of anxiety ("automatic" and "signal") that may be present in GAD. Their origins are then traced to specific

TABLE 3–9. Cognitive Models of Generalized Anxiety Disorder

Model	Main Components of Model
Worry as cognitive avoidance	• Worry is predominantly a thought activity, in contrast to imaginal activity (mental imagery) (Borkovec and Inz, 1990) • Emotions expressed through a thought activity (worry), in contrast to emotions expressed through imaginal activity, are not associated with sympathetic nervous system hyperactivity (Vrana et al., 1986). • Since worry inhibits autonomic arousal, it serves the purpose of avoiding somatic symptoms that accompany strong emotional states ("cognitive avoidance"); worry is maintained by the avoidance of both unpleasant emotions and the accompanying autonomic arousal (Borkovec et al., 1991, 1998).
Beliefs about benefits of worry	• Worry is maintained by beliefs that it is necessary to worry to avoid danger, prevent harm, prepare oneself for a bad outcome, and/or promote better coping (Rapee, 1991; Freeston et al., 1994). • These beliefs are maintained by nonoccurrence of the events that one worries about (Borkovec et al., 1998; Dugas et al., 1998b).
Intolerance of uncertainty as the central cognitive feature of GAD	• Intolerance of uncertainty perpetuates worry by exacerbating the "what if . . ." thinking style (Ladouceur et al., 1997; Dugas et al., 1998b).
Biased information-processing, related to exaggerated perception of threat	• Attention is focused on a wide variety of threatening cues and on detecting threat in numerous situations (MacLeod et al., 1986). • A wide variety of ambiguous stimuli and information are interpreted as threatening (Mogg et al., 1994). • Memory for all threat-related information is better (biased) (Butler and Mathews, 1983; Mathews et al., 1989).
Low self-efficacy, poor problem orientation	• GAD is associated with the belief that one is unable to exercise control over events (Kent and Gibbons, 1987); there may be lack of confidence in one's ability to cope with problems (Ladouceur et al., 1998) and/or core beliefs of self-doubt are present (Davey and Levy, 1998).

developmental issues (Table 3–10). Although it is difficult to separate them precisely along diagnostic lines, it appears that automatic anxiety is more characteristic of panic disorder, whereas signal anxiety is more typically encountered in GAD.

TABLE 3–10. Psychodynamic Conceptualization of Anxiety in Generalized Anxiety Disorder

	Automatic Anxiety	*Signal Anxiety*
Key features	1. Predominance of physical symptoms of anxiety 2. Anxiety experienced as highly disruptive	Predominance of anxious anticipation, worry, and/or "free-floating" anxiety
Explanatory model	Failure of the mothering figure to provide protection, sense of security, and love in the pre-Oedipal phase results in the inability to tolerate or endure anxiety and in the experience of anxiety in its "raw" (predominantly physical) form.	1. Anxiety serves as a "signal" to the ego to strengthen its defenses against sexual or aggressive drives. 2. Anxiety indicates the presence of unconscious, unresolved intrapsychic conflicts. 3. The origin of anxiety is in Oedipal phase.
Manifestations of anxiety	1. Fear of annihilation 2. Fear of losing one's identity through a merger with another person 3. Fear of separation 4. Fear of losing love	1. Fear of castration (fear of injury to one's physical integrity) 2. Fear of superego (fear of conscientiousness, punishment)

Role of Developmental and Childhood Factors

Patients with GAD tend to report various traumatic experiences in childhood, e.g., separation from parents, death of parents, and physical and sexual abuse. While this link does not appear to be specific for GAD (e.g., Raskin et al., 1982), other studies suggest that there may be a relatively specific relationship between GAD and these traumatic childhood experiences (e.g., Hubbard et al., 1995; Windle et al., 1995). Patients with GAD often view their parents as overprotective, controlling, and rejecting, and their families of origin as dysfunctional (e.g., Rapee, 1997), but this is very similar to how many panic patients perceive their parents and primary families (see Chapter 2). Hence, the notion that there are specific developmental antecedents to GAD cannot be supported.

Life Events Research

Life events research in GAD has suggested that the onset of GAD may be preceded by stressful or traumatic experiences more often than expected (e.g., Nisita et al., 1990). This appears to be the case more with persons in whom GAD occurs in the third decade of life or later. More typically, the onset of GAD is gradual, and stressful events are more likely to precipitate exacerbations in the course of GAD than the very onset of GAD.

The link between relatively minor stress and exacerbation of GAD symptoms (Brantley et al., 1999) may suggest that patients with GAD have generally low tolerance for stress and that they easily decompensate in response to even minor stressors.

Generalized Anxiety Disorder as a Personality-Level Disturbance

There is a long tradition of considering some types of anxiety, particularly chronic anxiety, more "characterological" in nature, hence the concepts of "trait anxiety" (versus "state anxiety") and "anxious personality disorder" (as it most recently appeared in the ICD-10). This is analogous to the states of chronic depression often being referred to as "characterological depression" and "depressive personality."

Several characteristics of GAD make it look like a personality disorder. First, in many cases, GAD starts very early, in childhood or adolescence. Second, the onset of GAD is usually gradual, with more than 80% of persons with GAD not being able to recall its precise onset (Rapee, 1985). Third, the course of GAD is usually chronic, its manifestations are persistent, and its pattern is pervasive. Fourth, the anxiety in GAD has a strong characterological "flavor" in that all aspects of personality seem to be affected by it. Is GAD then a personality disorder?

The fact that the onset of GAD may also occur later in life, after personality development has for the most part been completed, suggests that there are perhaps two types of conditions subsumed under the current concept of GAD (Table 3–11). As proposed by Brown et al. (1994), there may be a type of GAD with an early and gradual onset, which does resemble a personality disorder; this type may be more frequent, and appears to be associated with behavioral inhibition, childhood anxiety disorders, and/or childhood fears. The late-onset type of GAD is less frequent, has a more acute onset in the third decade of life or later (usually after some stressful event), and resembles an anxiety disorder. In comparison with an early-onset type, the late-onset type of GAD may have a less chronic course

TABLE 3–11. The Two Types of Generalized Anxiety Disorder

Criteria for Differentiation	Personality Disorder Type	Anxiety Disorder Type
Age of onset	Childhood or adolescence	Third decade and later
Mode of onset	Gradual	Relatively acute
Stressful event(s) preceding the onset	No	Yes
Course	More chronic	Less chronic
Association with behavioral inhibition, anxiety disorders in childhood, and/or childhood fears	Yes	No
Association with depression, other psychiatric conditions, and personality disorders	Yes	No
Frequency of occurrence	More frequent	Less frequent

and may be less likely to be associated with depression, other psychiatric conditions, and personality disorders.

If at least one type of GAD may be better conceptualized as a personality disorder, its etiology and pathogenesis still remain to be elucidated. Because of the close relationship between GAD and certain personality dimensions that are believed to be largely inherited (e.g., neuroticism, negative affectivity, and harm avoidance), it is possible that GAD is at the extreme end of these dimensions. If so, GAD may not necessarily be a distinct personality disorder, but rather a temperament-based, nonspecific vulnerability or predisposition for the development of a range of anxiety and mood disorders (e.g., Nisita et al., 1990; Brown, 1997; Akiskal, 1998).

There are certain aspects of the relationship between GAD and personality disorders which suggest that GAD may be related to personality disturbance. In comparison with panic disorder, GAD was more often found to be associated with more severe character pathology, including antisocial traits, mistrust, suspiciousness, hostility, and irritability, as well as paranoid, schizotypal, obsessive-compulsive, and passive-aggressive personality disorders (Blashfield et al., 1994). Also, it has been hypothesized that severe character pathology might be a risk factor for developing GAD, rather than being a risk factor for developing panic disorder (Nisita et al., 1990). Other personality traits and personality disorders found among patients with GAD, such as lack of self-confidence, feelings of insecurity, hypervigilance, heightened sensitivity, and dependent and avoidant personality disorders, may be nonspecifically associated with other anxiety disorders and depression as well.

Treatment

As with other anxiety disorders, early treatment of GAD is more likely to be efficacious than treatment that starts later in the course of GAD. Many persons with GAD often tolerate their anxiety and distress for many years, believing that it is in their "nature" to worry and that there is little that can be done to change that. As a result, they often seek help and treatment only when the disorder has become more severe and/or when they have developed complications. Therefore, by the time GAD patients present for treatment, they are likely to need a long-term treatment strategy that would also address any co-occurring psychiatric conditions. This strategy may entail use of combined pharmacological and psychological treatment.

Pharmacological Treatment

The goal of pharmacological treatment in GAD is a significant decrease in general anxiety. This does not seem to be a difficult goal to achieve, and there have been numerous substances, from alcohol to current investigational anxiolytics, that are able to alleviate anxiety. However, alleviating general anxiety is only one aspect of the treatment of GAD, and it is apparently not possible for medications to target all the components of this condition. For example, in comparison with specific psychological treatments, medications seem less able to alleviate pathological worry.

Many GAD patients take anxiolytic medications, usually benzodiazepines, on an as-needed (prn) basis. When they start visiting their primary care physicians more often or feel that they need to see a mental health professional, it usually means that they have greater difficulty tolerating their chronic anxiety, worries, and tension or that they have developed a complication of GAD (e.g., depression). It is often at that point that GAD patients are offered regular pharmacological treatment.

There are several relatively specific considerations in the pharmacological treatment of GAD (Table 3–12). As suggested in Table 3–12, it should not come as a surprise that antidepressants have largely replaced benzodiazepines as medications of choice in the treatment of GAD. Still, this is somewhat paradoxical, because benzodiazepines used to be considered a gold standard for pharmacological treatment of GAD. In fact, panic disorder and GAD were initially distinguished from each other on the basis of the former responding to an antidepressant, imipramine, and the latter responding to benzodiazepines. What has changed?

The modern concept of GAD is quite different from the concept of its historical precursor, anxiety neurosis: GAD is now recognized as a chronic

TABLE 3–12. Pharmacological Treatment Considerations for Generalized Anxiety Disorder

Issues and Factors	Clinical Implications
• In clinical setting, GAD is usually accompanied by another condition, most commonly depression; GAD patients are also more likely to develop depression	• Optimal medication for use in GAD is the one that is also likely to be efficacious in treatment of depression—an antidepressant.
• Benzodiazepines may be more efficacious for somatic anxiety symptoms, and autonomic hyperarousal in particular (Rickels et al., 1982; Hoehn-Saric et al., 1988; Rocca et al., 1997), which are not particularly prominent in GAD, whereas buspirone and antidepressants may be more efficacious for cognitive anxiety symptoms (e.g., worry), which are more characteristic of GAD.	• Antidepressants and buspirone may offer specific advantages over benzodiazepines in treatment of GAD.

condition, with symptoms of a more cognitive than somatic nature. Also, in clinical practice GAD is more likely to be encountered with another disorder, such as depression. All this makes antidepressants a more suitable pharmacological option than benzodiazepines. There is some suggestion (e.g., Kahn et al., 1986; Rickels et al., 1993) that in long-term treatment of GAD, antidepressants may be more efficacious than benzodiazepines. Table 3–13 lists current recommendations for pharmacotherapy of GAD.

As with other anxiety disorders, medication is usually initiated in the smallest dose; the dose is then gradually increased until optimum response is achieved. Most clinicians consider sufficient a dose on which the patient has achieved remission. That is, they do not increase the dose further if the patient no longer exhibits clinically significant symptoms of GAD.

TABLE 3–13. Choice of Medication in Treatment of Generalized Anxiety Disorder

Rank	Medication
First-line	a. Venlafaxine extended release or SSRIs (especially paroxetine) b. Venlafaxine extended release or SSRI + BDZ (short-term)
Second-line	a. TCAs (imipramine) or trazodone b. TCA + BDZ (short-term)
Third-line	Buspirone
Fourth-line	Hydroxyzine

BDZ, Benzodiazepine; SSRI, selective serotonin reuptake inhibitor; TCA, tricyclic antidepressant.

Antidepressants

Venlafaxine, selective serotonin reuptake inhibitors (SSRIs), tricyclic antidepressants (TCAs), and trazodone have all demonstrated efficacy in the treatment of GAD, but venlafaxine and SSRIs are considered the treatment of choice, mainly because of their better tolerability.

Venlafaxine is a serotonin and norepinephrine reuptake inhibitor. Several studies (Davidson et al., 1999; Gelenberg et al., 2000; Rickels et al., 2000) have established the efficacy of venlafaxine in the treatment of GAD. The efficacy of long-term (6-month) treatment with venlafaxine has also been demonstrated (Gelenberg et al., 2000; Allgulander et al., 2001). Venlafaxine is used in its extended-release form in GAD, and is administered once a day, in the morning. Venlafaxine has been found to be efficacious across the range of low to moderate doses (75–225 mg/day), with the starting dose of 75 mg/day. In low to moderate doses, venlafaxine has a side-effect profile similar to that of SSRIs (see Chapter 2). Like SSRIs, it is associated with sexual side effects, and should not be discontinued abruptly because of possible discontinuation symptoms. Less common side effects that may be seen in the course of treatment with venlafaxine include dry mouth, constipation, dizziness, sedation, and sweating. At higher doses (300 mg/day and above), which are not particularly likely to be used in "pure" GAD, venlafaxine is sometimes associated with an increase in blood pressure.

Among the SSRIs, the greatest evidence of efficacy exists for paroxetine (Rocca et al., 1997; Pollack et al., 2001; Rickels et al., 2003). It appears that the dose of 20 mg/day is adequate for most GAD patients, but some patients may need a higher dose, e.g., 40 mg/day (Rickels et al., 2003). Paroxetine was also found to be efficacious over a 32-week treatment of GAD (Stocchi et al., 2003).

Imipramine (Hoehn-Saric et al., 1988; Rickels et al., 1993) and trazodone (Rickels et al., 1993) have also been efficacious in the treatment of GAD. Depending on the symptoms of particular patients, a comparative advantage or disadvantage of these medications over SSRIs and venlafaxine is their sedative effect. This effect may be very useful for GAD patients who are troubled by insomnia and restlessness, whereas other patients may have difficulty tolerating trazodone because of sedation. Imipramine may not be tolerated because of the side effects typically associated with the use of TCAs (see Chapter 2). Other antidepressants (e.g., mirtazapine, nefazodone) may also be used in the treatment of GAD, but at present there are no data on their efficacy.

All antidepressants start showing efficacy in GAD after at least 2–4 weeks of continuous treatment. Longer periods of treatment with antidepressants (e.g., at least 6 weeks) are sometimes needed for them to show efficacy.

Table 3–14 shows the usual dosages of antidepressants and other medications used in treatment of GAD.

Benzodiazepines

Although benzodiazepines are no longer the pharmacological treatment of choice, they continue to play a role in the treatment of GAD. They are useful for treating insomnia, symptoms of tension (especially muscle tension), and symptoms of autonomic hyperactivity. Benzodiazepines can be combined with antidepressants, and because of the speed with which they exhibit their effects, they can accelerate pharmacological response and alleviate distress. In such a combination, benzodiazepines should preferably be used on a short-term basis, for several (6–10) weeks. A benzodiazepine can then be ceased very gradually, while the treatment with an antidepressant continues.

Benzodiazepines can be used as the only pharmacotherapy for GAD, but in the long term, this does not appear to be the optimal pharmacological strategy. Apart from issues of dependence, the main reason for this is a

TABLE 3–14. Medication Dosages Efficacious for Treatment of Generalized Anxiety Disorder

Medication	Dose Range
Antidepressants	
Venlafaxine extended release	75–225 mg/day
Paroxetine	20–50 mg/day
Sertraline	50–150 mg/day
Imipramine	100–150 mg/day
Trazodone	50–300 mg/day
Benzodiazepines	
Diazepam	5–30 mg/day
Oxazepam	30–90 mg/day
Lorazepam	2–6 mg/day
Clorazepate	15–60 mg/day
Buspirone	15–60 mg/day
Hydroxyzine	50–400 mg/day

fairly high likelihood that patients with GAD will develop depression over time. Also, benzodiazepines are sometimes implicated in actually causing depression over long-term treatment. If patients do need benzodiazepines over prolonged periods of time, benzodiazepines with a longer half-life (e.g., diazepam) are more suitable, because it is easier to administer them and they are less likely to be associated with significant discontinuation problems (see Chapter 2). When benzodiazepines need to be ceased after prolonged use, they should be carefully tapered to avoid withdrawal symptoms, as outlined in Chapter 2. In the absence of current and past drug and alcohol abuse or dependence, GAD patients are just as unlikely as patients with panic disorder to escalate the dose of a benzodiazepine or to abuse it.

Benzodiazepines can be taken on an as-needed (prn) basis, for example, in relatively mild cases of GAD or after treatment with an antidepressant has resulted in sustained remission and regular pharmacotherapy has been ceased.

The usual doses of commonly prescribed benzodiazepines in the treatment of GAD are shown in Table 3–14.

Buspirone

Buspirone is another pharmacotherapy option for GAD. Its advantages and disadvantages are listed in Table 3–15. Buspirone is a nonbenzodiazepine, azapirone anxiolytic, which acts as a partial agonist on serotonin 1_A receptors. There has been some controversy about the benefit of buspirone in GAD patients previously treated with benzodiazepines. The initial assertion that buspirone is less efficacious in patients who were previously exposed to benzodiazepines (Schweizer et al., 1986) appears to

TABLE 3–15. Advantages and Disadvantages of Buspirone

Advantages	Disadvantages
Does not cause sedation	Onset of therapeutic action after 2–3 weeks of administration
Not associated with dependence	Not efficacious in treatment of depression
Efficacious in treatment of cognitive anxiety symptoms	Sometimes poorly tolerated because of side effects: nausea, headache, dizziness, agitation, insomnia
	Administered twice or three times a day
	May be less efficacious in patients recently treated with benzodiazepines
	Often perceived as generally less efficacious

be correct only to a certain extent: buspirone may be efficacious if the pre-viously administered benzodiazepines were discontinued very gradually (Delle Chiaie et al., 1995). Also, the efficacy of buspirone is not affected if a benzodiazepine has not been taken 1 month prior to commencing treat-ment with buspirone (DeMartinis et al., 2000). Thus, GAD patients previ-ously treated with benzodiazepines are not necessarily poor candidates for efficacious treatment with buspirone; however, to maximize the effect of buspirone, these patients need to be switched from a benzodiazepine to buspirone very carefully and may need to go through a benzodiazepine-free period. This may not be practical and may be met with resistance. Patients should understand very well the rationale for such a procedure.

Buspirone might be a good choice for nondepressed GAD patients who should not be prescribed benzodiazepines because of dependence or abuse issues. As stated above, buspirone might also be useful for GAD patients who have not been previously exposed to benzodiazepines. Bus-pirone is apparently more efficacious in alleviating cognitive than somatic symptoms of anxiety (Rickels et al., 1982). The treatment usually starts with 5 mg three times a day, and the dose may be increased to 60 mg/day, depending on the patient's response and side effects.

Hydroxyzine

Hydroxyzine is the histamine H_1 receptor antagonist, which can be useful in the short-term treatment of GAD (Lader and Scotto, 1998; Llorca et al., 2002). Its use may be particularly suitable for GAD symptoms such as ten-sion and insomnia. Hydroxyzine appears to exhibit the onset of anxiolytic action fairly quickly (within 1 week), but in a more recent study (Darcis et al., 1995), a significant anxiolytic effect was found only after 4 weeks of treatment. Hydroxyzine can be quite sedating; its optimal dosage for GAD has not been established, as it has been reported to be efficacious in a small dose (50 mg/day) and a fairly high dose (300–400 mg/day).

Other Medications

Beta-adrenergic blockers (propranolol, atenolol) can be used to suppress physical symptoms caused by noradrenergic stimulation—tachycardia, palpitations, and tremor—if these symptoms are particularly prominent or distressing. Beta-adrenergic blockers exhibit a therapeutic effect fairly quickly after their administration, and they can be taken continuously or on an as-needed (prn) basis. However, these medications are not effica-cious for other key features of GAD, such as tension and worrying, and should not be used as the only pharmacotherapy in GAD.

Beta-adrenergic blockers are contraindicated in patients with asthma, bradycardia, heart failure and certain arrhythmias. Caution is required when administering some β-adrenergic blockers (especially propranolol) to patients with a history of depression, as they can precipitate another depressive episode.

Clonidine is another medication that may be used in the treatment of GAD because of its inhibitory effects on the locus coeruleus. It was found to be efficacious in one study (Hoehn-Saric et al., 1981), but its side effects and a tendency for it to lose therapeutic effect over time preclude its frequent use in GAD.

Long-Term Pharmacological Treatment

It is not clear how long pharmacological treatment of GAD should last. In view of the chronic nature of GAD symptoms and possible role of antidepressants in preventing the first episode of depression or recurrence of depression, it is reasonable to administer medications for at least 12–24 months.

Medication used in the treatment of GAD should be discontinued very gradually. As with other anxiety disorders, the cessation of pharmacotherapy is associated with a high risk of relapse of symptoms of GAD. This risk can be decreased somewhat by the use of psychological treatments or some of their techniques (e.g., relaxation).

Treatment-Resistant Generalized Anxiety Disorder

It is not well established what constitutes an adequate medication trial for GAD. However, it is reasonable to assume that approximately 8–10 weeks of treatment with the first-line antidepressant (venlafaxine or an SSRI), given in a maximum tolerable dose, is sufficient to establish whether that medication is efficacious. If there has been some response (Table 3–16), it may be worthwhile to continue treatment with an antidepressant for another 2 or 3 months, as patients may show incremental response over the subsequent several months and achieve remission after 5 or 6 months of treatment. Alternatively, the first-line antidepressant can be augmented with a benzodiazepine, hydroxyzine, a β-blocker, or clonidine.

If there has been no response at all to treatment with a first-line antidepressant (Table 3–16), another first-line antidepressant from a different antidepressant class can be administered. The other possibility is to consider a TCA (alone or with a benzodiazepine) or trazodone. If there is still no response, patients can be switched to buspirone or hydroxyzine.

TABLE 3–16. Pharmacological Options for Treatment-Resistant Generalized Anxiety Disorder

---

A. Partial response to first-line treatment (venlafaxine extended release or an SSRI)

    Continue treatment for 2–3 months

    Augment with a benzodiazepine, hydroxyzine, β-blocker, or clonidine

B. Lack of response to first-line treatment (venlafaxine extended release or an SSRI)

1. Switch to another first-line medication (and augment it, if necessary)

2. Switch to a TCA (and augment it, if necessary) or trazodone

3. Switch to buspirone

4. Switch to hydroxyzine

5. Switch to a benzodiazepine only

SSRI, selective serotonin reuptake inhibitor; TCA, tricyclic antidepressant.

Finally, in some cases, benzodiazepines can be administered for several months or even years as the only pharmacological agents.

PSYCHOLOGICAL TREATMENT

Cognitive, Behavior and Cognitive-Behavioral Therapy

Unlike techniques of cognitive, behavioral, and cognitive-behavioral therapy (CBT) in panic disorder and agoraphobia, which are more firmly linked to corresponding theoretical models and have been used more consistently over more time, cognitive, behavioral, and cognitive-behavioral therapies for GAD are still being developed and their techniques refined. This process is occurring alongside conceptual developments in the areas of pathological worry and GAD. As a result, various "packages" of cognitive, behavioral, and cognitive-behavioral therapies have emerged for GAD. Those that have been most successful or that appear promising are described and reviewed here.

Cognitive Therapy

Cognitive therapy of GAD generally proceeds through the same stages as cognitive therapy of other anxiety disorders: (1) identification of appraisals of threat and beliefs that are associated with worries; (2) challenging of these appraisals and beliefs through evidence seeking and introduction of alternatives; and (3) replacement of dysfunctional appraisals and beliefs with rational approaches (alternatives). In addition, the use of cognitive therapy in GAD is based on various assumptions about how pathological worry is maintained: by avoidance of autonomic arousal and other unpleasant emotions (Borkovec et al., 1991, 1998), by beliefs that worry is beneficial (Rapee, 1991; Freeston et al., 1994), and/or by intolerance of uncertainty (Ladouceuer et al., 1997; Dugas et al., 1998b). Therefore, one of the main tasks of cognitive therapy is to address the factors that maintain pathological worry, with the ultimate goal of alleviating pathological worry.

In the text that follows, several cognitive therapy techniques and procedures specific for use in GAD are briefly described (see also Table 3–17).

Distinguishing between the two types of worries. The first step is to distinguish between the two types of worries: (1) worries that pertain to the "here-and-now" situation and that have some basis in reality (e.g., worry about current marital problems and its consequences), and (2) worries that pertain to a relatively remote future and are of a hypothetical nature (e.g., worry about prolonged suffering from cancer at some point in the future). This distinction is believed to be important (Ladouceur et al., 1993) because of the different treatment strategies used for these two types of worries. Improving "problem orientation" is more helpful for addressing worries about current and relatively realistic issues, whereas "cognitive exposure" is used in the treatment of worries about remote and hypothetical issues.

Improving problem orientation and addressing intolerance of uncertainty. It has been hypothesized that patients with GAD often have poor problem orientation, which is proposed to be different from poor problem-solving (Dugas et al., 1998b; Ladouceur et al., 1998). That is, GAD patients tend to have difficulties in understanding problems (poor problem perception, appraisal or interpretation and attribution) and perceive themselves as

TABLE 3–17. Cognitive Therapy Techniques and Procedures for Treating Generalized Anxiety Disorder

---

- Distinguishing between Type 1 worries (which pertain to the current situation or issues and have some basis in reality) and Type 2 worries (which pertain to a relatively remote future and are of a hypothetical nature)

- Type 1 worries: improving problem orientation (reviewing and correcting steps in the decision-making and problem-solving processes, and helping patients cope with uncertainty)

- Type 2 worries: using cognitive exposure (imagery exposure to the content of worries)

- Identification of specific beliefs about the benefit of worrying, followed by direct and indirect challenging of these beliefs

---

lacking the ability to deal effectively with problems. As a result, they cannot use their problem-solving skills effectively. This is manifested clinically through excessive need for information and reassurance and poor management of time in the problem-solving process, procrastination, indecisiveness, and feeling "paralyzed" by worries. Dugas et al. (1998a; 1998b) believe that poor problem orientation is largely due to intolerance of uncertainty, so that improving patients' "management" of uncertainty would lead to a more effective problem orientation.

Therefore, improving problem orientation involves reviewing and correcting steps in the decision-making and problem-solving processes, and helping patients cope with uncertainty. The latter is facilitated if patients are systematically encouraged to make decisions and deal with problems in the presence of ambiguity and absence of excessive information. Patients may come to terms with uncertainty if it is demonstrated to them that absolute certainty is both unrealistic and unnecessary. Patients are also asked to set limits by prioritizing issues that they take into consideration while making decisions and dealing with problems; furthermore, they need to set deadlines to avert procrastination. Patients will be able to exercise more control over their worries if they can give up the indecisiveness-producing and time-consuming quest for certainty. Worries will also seem less "necessary" if there is less need for certainty.

Cognitive exposure (worry exposure). Cognitive exposure or worry exposure is a good example of blending cognitive and behavioral therapy techniques. It rests on the assumption that worries are maintained by ineffective processing, that is, by avoiding full concentration on worries and experiencing worries as too vague and abstract (cognitive avoidance). Therefore, patients are asked to transform their worries into concrete images and then to process these images without any interruption. In other words, the patients' task is to regularly (on a daily basis for a certain amount of time) visualize in as much detail as possible and under a "worst case scenario" what they worry about (Craske et al., 1992; Brown et al., 1993).

The more accurate characterization of this procedure is imagery exposure to the content of worries, rather than exposure to worries themselves. The rationale for using this technique is twofold. On one hand, it enables the worries to be processed via worry-related images, so that worries can become more concrete; on the other, the rationale is the same as that for using the behavioral technique of exposure to phobic situations and objects—habituation to worry and the underlying anxiety, as represented by the corresponding images.

Challenging beliefs about worry. Challenging the content of worry (i.e., trying to persuade patients that it is unreasonable to worry about matters and issues such as finances or health) may not be helpful, as the content of worry per se is rarely pathological. Therefore, the focus of the challenging effort should be on the reasons for worry and, more specifically, on beliefs about various benefits of worrying. A successful use of this technique first requires identification of specific beliefs about the benefit of worrying. Does the patient believe that worrying prevents the occurrence of the catastrophe that he or she worries about? Or is it that the patient believes that worrying will allow better coping with the problem? It may also be that the patient believes that worrying makes the disappointment less likely.

Whatever the underlying belief is, it should be challenged both directly and indirectly, through behavioral experiments. In the latter case, patients are encouraged to be as "indifferent" as possible about a matter that is otherwise in the focus of their worry. The goal is to demonstrate to patients that a decrease in worry does not make the feared events more likely or the problem-solving process less efficient.

Behavior Therapy

The use of behavior therapy in GAD is based on the hypothesis that pathological anxiety and worry are maintained by symptoms of tension, particularly muscle tension. Therefore, a significant decrease in muscle tension, usually by means of muscle relaxation, leads to a decrease in anxiety in general. Stated otherwise, the goal of behavior therapy in GAD is to achieve good symptom control and, more specifically, control over symptoms of tension.

The rationale for using muscle relaxation is the postulated incompatibility between the state of muscle relaxation on one hand and physiological arousal, tension, and anxiety on the other. Techniques of muscle relaxation have been used in various anxiety disorders, hence, they are not GAD-specific. Relaxation techniques have generally been efficacious in controlling tension and other somatic symptoms of anxiety and may be useful for GAD, especially when combined with cognitive therapy techniques.

The original relaxation technique, called "progressive muscle relaxation," was introduced by Jacobson (1938). It was subsequently modified by Wolpe and Lazarus (1966) and Bernstein and Borkovec (1973), and these modifications have largely been incorporated into the "applied relaxation" (Öst, 1987a) program. Regardless of which version of muscle relaxation technique is used, it rests on alternate tensing and relaxing of each of the 16 muscle groups in a certain order. This procedure helps patients to become better aware of muscle tension as they induce muscle tension and contrast it with muscle relaxation; it also allows patients to exercise control over this tension through relaxation. Furthermore, the effects of muscle relaxation become more obvious if relaxation is preceded by the induced muscle tension. Once patients have learned the basic muscle relaxation technique, it is easier for them to use it quickly, in various situations, and to relax several muscle groups in a well-coordinated fashion.

The use of relaxation can sometimes lead to a paradoxical increase in anxiety because the anxiety-related cognitions have been disinhibited. This should not necessarily be regarded as an adverse effect of relaxation. Indeed, patients should not use relaxation as a way to avoid thinking about the content of their worries. According to cognitive theorists and therapists, this use of relaxation would be just another safety device, designed to shift the attention away from the "dangerous" thoughts and worries, thereby perpetuating the erroneous notion that these thoughts and worries are dangerous.

Muscle relaxation is not the only way of controlling symptoms of anxiety. If GAD patients already have the knowledge of meditation techniques, yoga, or tai chi and practice these with some success, there is no reason to insist that they use muscle relaxation instead of these techniques. It is important, though, that they maximize the benefits derived from their use.

Cognitive-Behavioral Therapy and Treatment Efficacy

In practice, it is usually a combination of psychoeducation, muscle relaxation, and one or more cognitive therapy techniques that is used in the treatment of GAD. Such combinations are now routinely referred to as CBT, which is obviously quite a heterogeneous hybrid in GAD.

Some studies (e.g., Butler et al., 1991; Durham et al., 1994) indicate that CBT of GAD is superior to behavior therapy alone. There have been suggestions (e.g., Barlow et al., 1992; Borkovec and Costello, 1993), however, that there is no advantage of CBT over either behavior therapy or cognitive therapy alone, but that there may be some advantage of CBT over behavior therapy alone 12 months after the end of treatment (Borkovec and Costello, 1993). When CBT with greater emphasis on an earlier version of cognitive therapy was compared with behavior therapy (applied relaxation) alone, they appeared equally efficacious in treating GAD (Öst and Breitholtz, 2000; Arntz, 2003).

Studies of the efficacy of earlier versions of CBT have suggested that a large proportion of GAD patients do not improve with this treatment. For example, at 6-month follow-up after the end of CBT, 58% of patients did not show a clinically significant change in one study (Butler et al., 1991), and 40%–50% were not considered recovered in another study (Fisher and Durham, 1999). The recovery rate at 6-month follow-up after treatment of GAD with an earlier version of cognitive therapy alone and applied relaxation alone was not higher than 55% in a recent study (Arntz, 2003). These findings have all contributed to a search for more efficacious treatments for GAD—treatments that might place greater emphasis on newer concepts about pathological worry and specific inclusion of "worry management" strategies and other, more specific cognitive techniques in the CBT packages for GAD.

A recent study (Ladouceur et al., 2000) has demonstrated efficacy of CBT with a substantial cognitive component that addresses issues of poor problem orientation, intolerance of uncertainty, erroneous beliefs about worry, and cognitive avoidance; moreover, treatment gains in this study were maintained at 12-month follow-up. The same type of CBT, administered in a group format over 14 sessions, has also been efficacious in treating patients with GAD (Dugas et al., 2003). However, it is not yet clear whether this approach to the treatment of GAD might be more beneficial than other treatment modalities within the realm of behavior, cognitive, and cognitive-behavioral therapies.

Supportive Psychotherapy

In supportive psychotherapy, nonspecific psychotherapeutic techniques and procedures are used. Many GAD patients have trouble tolerating stress and report that stressful events often precede exacerbations of GAD. Therefore, it is useful to focus on strategies of coping with stress in the course of supportive psychotherapy, regardless of whether it is administered alone or in conjunction with other forms of treatment. Certainly, some patients need much help and encouragement as they cope with stressful situations and events, especially if they perceive themselves as lacking the confidence and appropriate skills to manage stress.

Psychodynamic Psychotherapy and Psychoanalysis

It is unusual these days to use psychodynamic psychotherapy and psychoanalysis in the treatment of GAD, unless GAD is accompanied by significant character pathology. Because modern psychodynamic thinking tends to emphasize "positive" aspects of anxiety in terms of its facilitating role in accessing intrapsychic conflicts, the goal of psychodynamic psychotherapy in the treatment of GAD is not necessarily a complete disappearance of anxiety; rather the goal is for patients to be able to tolerate anxiety better.

Other specific treatment goals in psychodynamic psychotherapy of GAD depend on the origin of anxiety (Table 3–10). For example, if the fear of punishment (or superego) is the main "driving force" behind the anxiety in GAD, the focus of treatment is on the softening of the rigid, harsh, and punitive superego; that would make it easier for patients to make realistic appraisals of the threats associated with "forbidden" and repressed urges.

A modified, short-term form of psychodynamic psychotherapy, "supportive-expressive psychotherapy," has been specifically developed for GAD and its efficacy was preliminarily tested in one study (Crits-Christoph et al., 1996). This type of treatment is based on psychodynamic assumptions about the role of ambivalent, conflictual attachments and relationships in the development of GAD—not unlike the presumed role of the same factors in the development of panic disorder (see Chapter 2). Within this conceptual framework, an incomplete processing of the trauma(s) is also believed to play an important role in the development of GAD.

COMBINED TREATMENTS

Even more than in other anxiety disorders, there appears to be a discrepancy in GAD between an apparently widespread use of combined (pharmacological and psychological) treatments in clinical practice and very few studies that might support this use. In one study (Power et al., 1990), which compared the efficacy of the combination of CBT and diazepam with the efficacy of CBT alone and diazepam alone in patients with GAD, there were no differences in outcome between patients who received the combined treatment and those who were treated with CBT alone. This finding was interpreted as suggesting both that combining CBT and benzodiazepines is not detrimental and that adding a benzodiazepine to CBT might be superfluous.

As noted in Chapter 2, the issue of combining CBT with pharmacotherapy is highly contentious, with strong views often being expressed about the advantages of CBT alone and the disadvantages of combined treatment. The pragmatic and clinically sound approach is to adapt treatment to the specific characteristics of patients and clinical situations. This may entail initial use of pharmacotherapy followed by CBT, which appears to be the usual sequence of combining these treatments in GAD. In other situations, pharmacotherapy may be instituted to enhance the effects of CBT or following a treatment failure with CBT. It seems that commencing CBT and pharmacotherapy at the same time is the least likely approach, although not one that would be argued against on the basis of the few available data.

4

Social Anxiety Disorder
(Social Phobia)

Social anxiety disorder is conceptualized as an excessive and/or unreasonable fear of situations in which the person's behavior or appearance might be scrutinized and evaluated. This fear is a consequence of the person's expectation to be judged negatively, which would then lead to embarrassment or humiliation. Typical examples of feared and usually avoided social situations are giving a talk in public, performing other tasks in front of others, and interacting with people in general.

Although the existence of social anxiety disorder as a psychopathological entity has been known for at least 100 years, it was only relatively recently, with the publication of DSM-III in 1980, that social anxiety disorder, or social phobia as it was then called, acquired the status of an "official" psychiatric diagnosis. Social anxiety disorder has subsequently attracted much attention from researchers and clinicians, and an impressive body of knowledge about this condition has accumulated. Over the past several years the term *social anxiety disorder* has been increasingly used instead of *social phobia*, because it is felt that use of the former term conveys more strongly the pervasiveness and impairment that are associated with the condition, and it will promote better recognition of this disorder and contribute to better differentiation from specific phobia (Liebowitz et al., 2000).

CLINICAL FEATURES

Features of social anxiety disorder range from very mild, when patients feel apprehensive about one or a few performance-type situations, to quite severe and incapacitating, when patients are socially isolated and impaired in virtually all domains of functioning. In addition to clinical features, social anxiety disorder has subclinical aspects—"stage fright" and shyness—that belong to the realm of normal varieties of behavior (see Stage Fright, Shyness, and Social Anxiety Disorder below).

Two main features characterize social anxiety disorder: excessive and persistent fear of social situations and avoidance of these situations (Fig. 4–1). Social situations are mainly of two kinds. One type is the situations that involve "doing something" (i.e., performing) in the presence of others, and they are referred to as performance-type situations. Examples include speaking in public and eating, drinking, writing, working, and using public toilets in the presence of others (or while others are watching). The other type of situations involves informal and formal interactions with other people, and these are referred to as "interactional situations." Although avoidance of these situations is the most common way of coping with social anxiety, not all patients with social anxiety disorder resort to avoidance. Some may endure social situations with a lot of anxiety or distress.

What Are Patients with Social Anxiety Disorder Afraid of?

Very broadly, patients with social anxiety disorder are afraid of negative evaluation by others; this is usually considered to be the core feature of social anxiety disorder. However, there may be at least two reasons for the

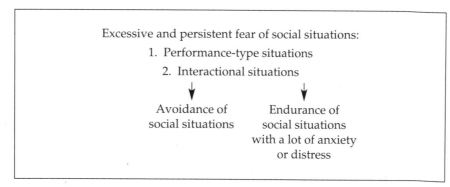

Figure 4–1. Clinical features of social anxiety disorder.

expected negative evaluation, especially in performance-type situations (Starcevic et al., 1994): patients anticipate that they will make a mistake (or generally perform poorly), or they anticipate having visible physical symptoms (such as blushing and trembling) that would reveal their anxiety. Of course, some physical symptoms, such as trembling, may affect performance, so these two reasons for fearing negative evaluation may be interrelated (Fig. 4–2).

A related type of basic fear that can be found in fears of both types of social situations is a fear of being under scrutiny (or sometimes, at the center of attention). Patients then anticipate that they will be judged negatively only because others are looking at them, regardless of what they do and whether they do anything at all. In other words, exposure to the scrutiny of others automatically leads to negative evaluation. The reasons for such fears do vary, but they often have to do with patients' beliefs about being defective or aberrant in some aspects of their personality or behavior. If patients also believe that others are able to "read their mind," a belief that may be quasi-delusional in nature, they end up believing that being under scrutiny reveals these defects or aberrations to others (Fig. 4–3). Such a complex belief system may suggest a more severe underlying psychopathology.

The structure of the fear of interactional situations may be more complex, although the same personality characteristics—feelings of insecurity, low self-esteem, and poor self-confidence—may underlie its various manifestations (Fig. 4–4). Sometimes the fear of interactional situations boils down to a fear of performing poorly in a particular social interaction, and

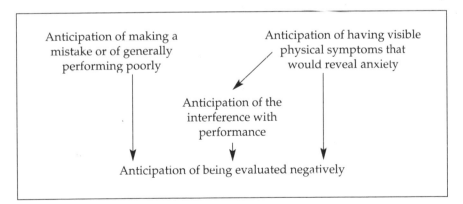

Figure 4–2. Underpinnings of the fear of negative evaluation in performance-type situations.

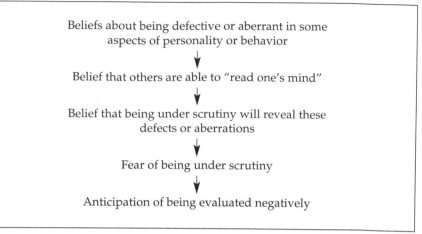

Figure 4–3. Underpinnings of the fear of negative evaluation in relation to the fear of being under scrutiny.

ultimately, to a fear of negative evaluation of such performance by others. For example, patients may feel that they lack the skill of initiating, maintaining, or terminating conversations, that they are "clumsy" when meeting new people, or that they do not know how to talk over the telephone with someone whom they have never met before. In other situations, the underlying fears in interactional situations may have to do more with patients' lack of assertiveness. Examples of such situations include talking to people in positions of authority, expression of disagreement, and returning purchased goods because they are defective.

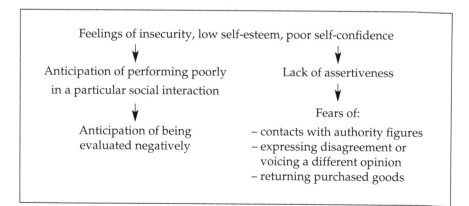

Figure 4–4. Structure of the fear of interactional situations.

Subtypes: Generalized and Nongeneralized Social Anxiety Disorder

Social anxiety disorder encompasses two subtypes—generalized and non-generalized (also referred to as focal, isolated, limited, discrete, circum-scribed, and specific). *Generalized social anxiety disorder* is the term used to characterize fear of numerous social situations, which include both inter-actional and performance-type situations; *nongeneralized social anxiety disorder* pertains to fear of one or just a few such situations, and these are usually (though not invariably) performance-type situations.

The subtypes nongeneralized and generalized social anxiety disorder can be conceptualized on a continuum of severity and features associated with severity (Table 4–1). Stated otherwise, the differences between these subtypes of social anxiety disorder are mainly quantitative in nature (Stein et al., 2000). In view of the relatively few qualitative differences (Table 4–2) and unclear boundaries between the two subtypes in many cases, the ratio-nale for subtyping social anxiety disorder is not unequivocally supported by the existing clinical and research data.

In clinical samples, generalized social anxiety disorder is encountered more frequently than nongeneralized social anxiety disorder, but their prevalence seems to be different in the community, with the ratio of gener-alized to nongeneralized social anxiety disorder being 1:2 (Wittchen et al., 1999; Furmark et al., 2000). The main reason for this difference between clinical and epidemiological samples is the greater severity of the general-ized form of social anxiety disorder; its sufferers are more likely to seek

TABLE 4–1. Dimensional Conceptualization of Subtypes of Social Anxiety Disorder

Characteristics	Nongeneralized Social Anxiety Disorder	Generalized Social Anxiety Disorder
Intensity or severity	Mild	Severe
Co-occurrence with other psychiatric disorders	Less frequent	More frequent
Co-occurrence with personality disorders	Less frequent	More frequent
Complicated by depression and alcohol abuse or /dependence	Less often	More often
Functioning	Less impaired	More impaired
Prognosis	Good	Guarded
Treatment	Relatively simple	More complex

TABLE 4–2. Contrasting Characteristics of Nongeneralized and Generalized Social Anxiety Disorder

Characteristics	Nongeneralized Social Anxiety Disorder	Generalized Social Anxiety Disorder
Age of onset	Variable, not unusual after adolescence	Usually in childhood or adolescence
Mode of onset	Variable, can be abrupt	Gradual
Genetic basis	Weaker	Stronger
Frequency in the community	More frequent	Less frequent
Frequency in clinical setting	Less frequent	More frequent
Gender distribution in clinical setting	Approximately the same in women and men	More frequent among men

professional help. While the prevalence of nongeneralized social anxiety disorder in clinical settings is similar among women and men, there are apparently more men than women with generalized social anxiety disorder in the same setting.

The onset of generalized social anxiety disorder is usually gradual and dates back to patients' adolescence or childhood. Patients typically say that they have always been shy and anxious in social situations. In the nongeneralized subtype of social anxiety disorder, the onset after adolescence is not unusual and it may be relatively abrupt—for example, after an unpleasant or traumatic event, such as suddenly blushing, quivering, losing one's voice, or even having a panic attack while giving a talk.

A genetic link seems to be stronger for generalized social anxiety disorder. Patients with generalized social anxiety disorder were significantly more likely to have a first-degree relative with generalized social anxiety disorder than control group. The frequency of first-degree relatives with social anxiety disorder by contrast, was similar among patients with nongeneralized social anxiety disorder and control group subjects (Mannuzza et al., 1995; Stemberger et al., 1995; Stein et al., 1998a).

Fear of Performance-Type Situations

One of the hallmarks of the fear of performance-type situations is the absence of any problems when patients perform alone or in front of one or only a few persons whom they know well and trust. This suggests that the fear of performance-type situations is generally less about performance itself and more about the performance being watched and judged by others.

Fear of Speaking in Public

Fear of speaking in public is a typical example of the fear of performance-type situations. It is one of the most frequently reported fears in the general population: according to one epidemiological survey in the United States (Kessler et al., 1998), as many as 30.2% of the population reported ever having this fear. Of course, only a small portion of these people—those who avoid public-speaking situations persistently or endure them with inordinate anxiety or distress and are impaired or significantly distressed because of this fear and its consequences—qualify for the diagnosis of social anxiety disorder. The public-speaking fear is the most common type of fear in both subtypes of social anxiety disorder. Because it is so widespread and more often accompanied by high autonomic arousal, the public-speaking phobia has been considered by some (Stein et al., 1994) to represent a distinct and separate type of social anxiety disorder. However, many patients with a fear of public speaking are afraid of other social situations as well.

Patients with fear of public speaking may have various underlying fears: they may be afraid of certain visible symptoms during the talk (e.g., blushing, shortness of breath) or of being under scrutiny by others. These patients are particularly concerned about their performance and often expect to make a mistake, say "stupid" things, or do something embarrassing during the talk. The end result is an expectation that they would be humiliated or ridiculed because of poor performance.

Fear of Taking Tests and Being Examined

A related fear is that of taking tests and examinations, especially when patients are examined orally or while they are performing a certain task as part of their examination. The reactions to tests and examinations may be quite severe, both in the preparation stages and while patients are actually being examined. Just before the exam or in the weeks preceding the exam, patients may have symptoms such as diarrhea, headache, insomnia, and loss of appetite. The symptoms may be so severe that patients decide against taking the exam. During the exam itself, patients may feel that they are about to lose bladder control and have to go to the toilet immediately; sometimes, they become short of breath, experience rapid heart beat, have severe tremor, or develop a full-blown panic attack. Any one of these symptoms may be the reason for them to give up. With such severe physical

symptoms, patients may end up fearing them more than the negative evaluation by their examiners.

Fear of Eating, Drinking, and Writing in the Presence of Others
Patients who are afraid of eating or drinking in the presence of others are
usually concerned that a symptom, such as trembling, would reveal that
they are anxious. The fear of trembling is also prominent among patients
who are afraid of writing in front of others, e.g., when they are signing a
receipt or another document. These fears are usually accompanied by
other social fears. Patients may resort to extensive avoidance of the corresponding situations, which may be quite distressing for them.

Fear of Performing Work Duties under Observation
Some patients are particularly distressed when they have to perform their
job under observation by other people. They are usually concerned that,
under such circumstances, their work-related performance might be inhibited or impaired (e.g., because of poor concentration and/or a greater likelihood of making a mistake). Patients often feel that, in turn, this might
have serious consequences, such as losing a job.

Fear of Using Public Toilets in the Presence of Others
Fear of using public toilets in the presence of others or, more precisely, fear
of not being able to urinate in public toilets or when other people are aware
that the person is urinating is not very common but can be quite disabling.
It is encountered far more often in men and is also referred to as "shy bladder syndrome," or paruresis. The underlying fear of being under scrutiny
by others may lead to an inhibition of urination, even when the urinary
bladder is full. The sufferers usually avoid public toilets and structure their
daily routine around this avoidance. There is a frequent co-occurrence of
paruresis and fears of other performance-type situations, and many sufferers of paruresis are also depressed (Vythilingum et al., 2002).

Fears of Other Performance-Type Situations
Some patients with social anxiety disorder have a particularly strong fear
of entering a room or hall in which people are in a meeting, already seated,
and/or are attending a concert, a lecture, or other public performance.
These patients are particularly concerned that, in this situation, they will
suddenly become the center of attention and be judged with disapproval
or in some other negative way. Patients typically say that the stare of so
many eyes at the same time is deeply disturbing. Although this is not a
prototype of the performance-type situation, sufferers feel that they are

"supposed to act" (i.e., perform) in a certain, prescribed manner. As a consequence of this fear, patients may miss meetings and other important activities, and may ultimately be unable to attend classes regularly or even maintain their jobs.

Fear of Interactional Situations

As already noted, the fear of interactional situations encompasses various fears. In a very broad sense, patients with these fears are concerned about any situation in which they are expected to communicate with others. These situations include simple interactions, such as asking a passerby for directions, as well as more complex interactions, like socializing at a party. The underlying theme in many of these fears is patients' general feeling that they lack basic social skills. The more socially incompetent patients feel, the less important it will be whether they interact in complete anonymity or with someone they know. However, the consequences are likely to be feared more when patients interact with someone known to them; in this situation, patients are particularly concerned about the impression they make and how their current performance will affect their future interactions. They also tend to make negative judgments about their social skills and performance.

Some fears of interactional situations pertain predominantly to certain people and certain situations. This is particularly the case with those situations in which patients are expected to demonstrate some assertiveness. Typical examples include making a complaint about poor service, returning defective items to the store in which they were purchased, or expressing an opinion about an issue that is being discussed, particularly if it is contrary to the prevailing opinion. The corresponding avoidance may be distressing, because it prevents patients from "having things done" or from showing their "true personality." The fear may be in stark contrast to patients' relative calm in "ordinary" social situations in which their insecurity and lack of assertiveness are hidden beneath a well-learned use of social conventions.

Fears of visible and "revealing" physical symptoms that might occur during interpersonal interactions may be so strong that they become the main reason for avoidance of interactional situations or some aspects of these situations. For example, some patients are so terrified about blushing that this particular fear, sometimes referred to as "erythrophobia," drives them to avoid most social contacts. In other cases, patients avoid handshaking because of "showing" that their hands are clammy, or may be afraid of talking because they are concerned that they might start stuttering.

Stage Fright, Shyness, and Social Anxiety Disorder

Social anxiety disorder has an interesting and important relationship with "normal" forms of social anxiety: stage fright and shyness. Stage fright is related to the fear of performance-type situations, whereas shyness is related to generalized social anxiety disorder. Unlike social anxiety disorder, neither stage fright nor shyness are associated with impairment in functioning, and this is the fundamental difference between social anxiety disorder and these two forms of "normal" social anxiety. Assessment of the effects on functioning may be difficult, however, in people who have adjusted their lifestyles to their social anxiety and consequently do not feel that this anxiety interferes significantly with their lives. Moreover, the relationship between shyness and social anxiety disorder is more complex, as discussed below.

The Yerkes-Dodson bell-shaped curve (Yerkes and Dodson, 1908) can help us understand the relationship between the stage fright and phobic fear of performance-type situations. This curve represents a relationship between the degree of anxiety and the quality of performance; whereas mild to moderate anxiety is often stimulating and contributes to better performance, moderate to severe anxiety tends to interfere with performance. Up to a certain point, stage fright may enhance performance, hence the saying that only a bad actor is completely free from stage fright. At the top of the curve (after which the performance declines with increasing anxiety) is a sometimes imperceptible boundary between stage fright and social anxiety disorder.

Unlike stage fright, the phobic fear of performance-type situations is characterized by excessive preoccupation with fear. Although there may be an element of reality in the patients' expectation that their performance will not be good, the performance is not necessarily impaired by the phobia. However, patients avoid "testing" themselves in performance situations, especially if they were disappointed with their performance in the past. Of course, this only perpetuates the phobia, as patients do not have an opportunity to see for themselves what their performance would be like.

Shyness and social anxiety disorder have numerous similarities in terms of their physical, anxiety-related symptoms (e.g., sweating, trembling, tachycardia, blushing), cognitive distortions, and behavioral responses to distressing social situations (Turner et al., 1990). The differences between shyness and generalized social anxiety disorder are believed to pertain mainly to the intensity, frequency, and/or duration of these variables.

Thus, in comparison with shyness, generalized social anxiety disorder can be distinguished in terms of the severity of anxiety. That means that people who are very shy are far more likely to have generalized social anxiety disorder than those who are moderately or minimally shy; this notion is supported by the finding that most shy persons do not have social anxiety disorder (Heiser et al., 2003). However, there does not appear to be a complete overlap between high degrees of shyness and generalized social anxiety disorder, as there are people who are extremely shy but do not qualify for a diagnosis of generalized social anxiety disorder (Chavira et al., 2002). Also, it does not appear that shyness is a necessary factor for the development of generalized social anxiety disorder (Beidel and Turner, 1999). Moreover, there is no strong link between shyness and phobia of performance-type situations, as people with this type of social anxiety disorder are often not shy at all. Recent research (Heiser et al., 2003) suggests that shyness is a very broad construct that is associated not only with social anxiety disorder but also with various anxiety and mood disorders, as well as personality disorders, especially avoidant personality disorder.

Other data also suggest that there are differences between shyness and social anxiety disorder. For example, general population surveys support a very broad conceptualization of shyness, with at least 40% of survey respondents stating that they are shy (e.g., Pilkonis and Zimbardo, 1979). By comparison, lifetime prevalence rates of social anxiety disorder are estimated to be much lower, between 1.6% and 16% (see Epidemiology, below). Further distinctions between shyness and social anxiety disorder are subtler. Thus, shy persons may have a problem at the beginning of social interaction, whereas those with social anxiety disorder experience anxiety throughout the interaction. This may be a consequence of shy persons' higher likelihood of being more attentive to cues from others about their appearance, performance, and behavior, and higher likelihood of responding favorably to positive feedback (Stopa and Clark, 1993).

RELATIONSHIP BETWEEN SOCIAL ANXIETY DISORDER AND OTHER DISORDERS

Social anxiety disorder, particularly its generalized subtype, very often co-occurs with other psychiatric disorders. In the general population, the lifetime rate of the co-occurrence of social anxiety disorder with any psychiatric disorder has been estimated to range between 69% and 81% (Schneier et al., 1992; Magee et al., 1996). Social anxiety disorder often co-occurs with depression, other anxiety disorders, alcohol abuse and dependence, and personality disorders. Clinical implications of the co-occurrence with depression, alcohol-related problems, and personality disorders are summarized in Table 4–3.

TABLE 4–3. Clinical Implications of Relationship Between Social Anxiety Disorder and Depression, Alcohol-Related Problems, and Personality Disturbance

Social Anxiety Disorder and Depression

- Depression frequently co-occurs with social anxiety disorder, particularly in clinical settings.
- Depression usually follows social anxiety disorder and may appear many years after the onset of social anxiety disorder.
- Clinical features are more severe when social anxiety disorder co-occurs with depression and patients are then more likely to seek help.
- Patients are more likely to be suicidal if depression accompanies social anxiety disorder.
- There may be an overlap between social anxiety disorder and atypical depression, which may account for the efficacy of classical, irreversible monoamine oxidase inhibitors in the treatment of social anxiety disorder.
- When patients treated with cognitive-behavioral therapy for social anxiety disorder become depressed, an antidepressant should be added as soon as possible.

Social Anxiety Disorder and Alcohol Abuse and Dependence

- A significant minority of patients with social anxiety disorder abuse alcohol or develop alcohol dependence; excessive use of alcohol usually results from patients' attempts to alleviate social anxiety and improve performance.
- Social anxiety disorder usually precedes alcoholism and generally represents a risk factor for alcoholism. The risk is greater if patients are female, if they have a generalized subtype of social anxiety disorder and/or avoidant personality disorder, and if they had an early onset of social anxiety disorder.
- Some patients are recognized as suffering from primary social anxiety disorder only after they have developed a significant alcohol problem.
- Intensive treatment of alcohol-related problems is a prerequisite for efficacious treatment of social anxiety disorder.
- Benzodiazepines should be avoided in the treatment of social anxiety disorder complicated by excessive use of alcohol.

Social Anxiety Disorder and Personality Disorders

- Personality disorders are far more likely to accompany the generalized type than the nongeneralized type of social anxiety disorder.
- Avoidant, obsessive-compulsive, and dependent personality disorders tend to be most frequently associated with social anxiety disorder.
- There is a significant overlap between generalized social anxiety disorder and avoidant personality disorder, with the latter condition being considered a more severe variant of the same psychopathology.
- The presence of a personality disorder in patients with social anxiety disorder generally implies chronicity and poorer outcome.

Social Anxiety Disorder and Depression

The presence of social anxiety disorder increases the risk of major depression (Nelson et al., 2000; Stein et al., 2001). The frequency of depression among patients with social anxiety disorder tends to be high. In the community, 17%–37% of persons with social anxiety disorder have major depression during their lifetime (Schneier et al., 1992; Magee et al., 1996); in clinical samples, this association is even stronger, with 60%–70% of patients with social anxiety disorder being affected by depression (Stein et al., 1990b; Van Ameringen et al., 1991). Social anxiety disorder seems to be associated not only with major depressive disorder but also with other mood disorders, including dysthymia and bipolar disorder (Kessler et al., 1999b).

Although the sequence may vary, depression usually follows social anxiety disorder and it often occurs many years after the onset of social anxiety disorder. The "demoralization hypothesis" is often used to explain the relationship between social anxiety disorder and depression. That is, because of the chronic and often relentless course of social anxiety disorder, patients feel less and less able to "cope with life," become helpless and hopeless and thus prone to developing depression. But, there may also be a genetic link between social anxiety disorder and depression, with an increased frequency of depression occurring among first-degree relatives of patients with social anxiety disorder.

Generalized social anxiety disorder bears a similarity with the construct of atypical depression, as they both share heightened interpersonal sensitivity and, in particular, hypersensitivity to criticism and rejection. Some support for this association comes from the efficacy of classical, irreversible monoamine oxidase inhibitors in the treatment of both atypical depression (Zisook et al., 1985; Liebowitz et al., 1988; Quitkin et al., 1991) and generalized social anxiety disorder (Gelernter et al., 1991; Liebowitz et al., 1992; Versiani et al., 1992; Heimberg et al., 1998).

Patients with an early onset of social anxiety disorder (before age 15) are more likely to develop depression (Lecrubier and Weiller, 1997). Social anxiety disorder accompanied by depression is associated with greater severity of clinical presentation, and patients are then more likely to be suicidal (Schneier et al., 1992; Davidson et al., 1993a). Major depressive disorder and other mood disorders co-occurring with social anxiety disorder are more severe and have a more chronic course (Kessler et al., 1999b). Patients with social anxiety disorder and depression are more likely to seek help (Lecrubier and Weiller, 1997), and treatment with an antidepressant should commence as soon as possible. This is particularly pertinent to those patients who become depressed while undergoing cognitive-behavioral therapy for social anxiety disorder.

Social Anxiety Disorder and Alcohol Abuse and Dependence

Data from the U.S. National Comorbidity Survey (Magee et al., 1996) suggest that almost 24% of persons with social anxiety disorder develop alcohol dependence in their lifetime, with the corresponding rate for any substance abuse or dependence being almost 40%. Rates of alcohol abuse and dependence in other epidemiological and clinical samples of patients with social anxiety disorder ranged from 15% to 36% (Schneier et al., 1989; Van Ameringen et al., 1991; Davidson et al., 1993a; Weiller et al., 1996). There may also be a significant proportion of patients with alcohol abuse or dependence (16%–25%) who have an underlying and often unrecognized social anxiety disorder (Mullaney and Trippett, 1979; Smail et al., 1984; Thomas et al., 1999). Some patients are identified as suffering from primary social anxiety disorder only after they have developed a significant alcohol problem.

Social anxiety disorder usually precedes alcohol-related problems (Schneier et al., 1992; Lampe et al., 2003), and the presence of social anxiety disorder may generally be regarded as a risk factor for alcoholism (Nelson et al., 2000). Although patients with social anxiety disorder may abuse various substances, alcohol is the preferred substance of abuse, because of its anxiolytic and disinhibiting properties. Indeed, many patients with social anxiety disorder drink alcohol in an attempt to alleviate social anxiety and improve performance in social situations. The use of alcohol is also more likely because of its accessibility and the fact that its moderate use is socially acceptable.

A greater risk of alcoholism in patients with social anxiety disorder has been associated with female gender, early onset, generalized subtype of the condition, and co-occurrence of avoidant personality disorder (Stravynski et al., 1986; Schneier et al., 1989; Morgenstern et al., 1997; Lecrubier, 1998; Regier et al., 1998). The co-occurrence of social anxiety disorder and depression increases the likelihood of alcoholism and suicidality (Nelson et al., 2000).

Patients with social anxiety disorder and alcoholism cannot fully benefit from treatment for social anxiety disorder if they are not treated for their alcohol-related problems first. Only patients who have achieved abstinence from alcohol can be meaningfully engaged in psychological interventions for social anxiety disorder. Benzodiazepines should be avoided in patients who have a history of alcohol or other substance abuse or dependence.

Social Anxiety Disorder and Personality Disorders

Personality disorders are far more likely to accompany the generalized type than the nongeneralized type of social anxiety disorder. Avoidant personality disorder is the most common form of personality disturbance associated with social anxiety disorder, followed by other DSM-IV Cluster C personality disorders—obsessive-compulsive and dependent (e.g., Alnaes and Torgersen, 1988; Turner et al., 1991; Lampe et al., 2003). Less often, patients with social anxiety disorder have other personality disorders; this is understandable, especially for the DSM-IV Cluster B personality disorders (histrionic, borderline, and antisocial types), which seem like an antithesis of social anxiety disorder. Indeed, social anxiety disorder may be conceived of as the direct opposite to histrionic behavioral style: whereas histrionic persons seek attention, patients with social anxiety disorder prefer anonymity and would do anything not to be noticed and not be in the center of attention.

Patients with social anxiety disorder are more likely to exhibit the following personality traits: insecurity, lack of self-confidence, low self-esteem, extreme sensitivity to criticism, feelings of inferiority, unassertiveness, shyness, and tendency toward social withdrawal. Depending on how prominent and pervasive these personality traits are, a diagnosis of avoidant personality disorder may be warranted.

The relationship between avoidant personality disorder and generalized social anxiety disorder has attracted much attention because of their significant phenomenological overlap. The current consensus is that there are few significant differences between avoidant personality disorder and generalized social anxiety disorder, with the former condition being considered more severe (Herbert et al., 1992; Holt et al., 1992; Turner et al., 1992; van Velzen et al., 2000). The rates of avoidant personality disorder among patients with social anxiety disorder vary significantly (from 22% to 89%), which is a consequence of the different diagnostic criteria and different methodology used in various studies.

Patients with social anxiety disorder may exhibit traits of other personality disorders. When their perfectionist tendencies are particularly strong and when they exhibit extremely marked preoccupation with issues of control and rigid attitudes as to what is socially desirable, expected, and allowed, patients may have a co-occurring obsessive-compulsive personality disorder. Others are more passive, as they are extremely afraid of being rejected or abandoned and have an excessive need to please others, are reluctant to express their own opinion or any disagreement, and are unable to make even simple decisions, thus exhibiting features of dependent personality disorder.

Schizoid personality disorder may be encountered in patients with social anxiety disorder who have largely withdrawn from the outside world, possibly because of the disappointing interactions with other people and fear that such interactions might be harmful to them. Patients with paranoid personality disorder and social anxiety disorder are hypervigilant and suspicious about other people's intentions, deeply mistrustful of them, and constantly expecting that others will ridicule them and/or take advantage of them.

The presence of personality disturbance in patients with social anxiety disorder generally implies that the course of social anxiety disorder is likely to be more chronic and its prognosis poorer (e.g., Massion et al., 2002). This has been attributed to avoidant personality disorder, because of its much higher frequency in comparison with the other co-occurring personality disorders. The presence of avoidant personality disorder may not predict the outcome of treatment of patients with the generalized form of social anxiety disorder, however (e.g., Brown et al., 1995).

Social Anxiety Disorder and Other Anxiety Disorders

Social anxiety disorder can co-occur with other anxiety disorders, most commonly with specific phobias, panic disorder with or without agoraphobia, and generalized anxiety disorder. The rates of co-occurrence with these disorders tend to vary significantly, depending on the nature of the sample, diagnostic criteria, instruments used in the study, and the diagnostic thresholds set for these conditions. Approximately one-third of patients with social anxiety disorder have a co-occurring panic disorder with or without agoraphobia, whereas the rates for specific phobias may be higher.

The relationship between generalized anxiety disorder and social anxiety disorder is discussed in Chapter 3. Generalized anxiety disorder may be seen in 33% of patients with the principal diagnosis of social anxiety disorder (Turner et al., 1991). In one study (Mennin et al., 2000), patients with social anxiety disorder and co-occurring generalized anxiety disorder were found to have a more severe illness than patients with social anxiety disorder and no generalized anxiety disorder. Despite this, the response to cognitive-behavioral group therapy for social anxiety disorder was not affected by the presence of generalized anxiety disorder.

Assessment

Diagnostic Issues

The diagnosis of social anxiety disorder can be made on the basis of the same general criteria used to establish a diagnosis of other phobic disorders (Table 4–4). As with other phobic disorders, the most difficult diagnostic criterion pertains to the clinical significance of the disorder. The boundary between "normal" social anxiety and "subclinical" forms of social anxiety disorder on one hand, and social anxiety disorder as a clinical entity on the other, is established by the effects that social anxiety has on functioning. The diagnosis of social anxiety disorder implies that the person is quite distressed about being afraid of certain social situations or that his or her functioning is significantly impaired. Usually, this impairment is generalized and affects relationships, social activities, academic and occupational performance, and functioning within the family. Sometimes the impairment is more evident in certain areas of functioning. For example, students with a paralyzing phobia of examinations may give up their studies, but function fairly well in other social situations.

In DSM-IV-TR, the diagnosis of social anxiety disorder cannot be made if the anxiety in social situations is a consequence of other disorders, such as stuttering and squinting. Likewise, the diagnosis of social anxiety disorder is not to be made if some symptoms usually found in social anxiety disorder—for example, tremor—are a consequence of another condition, such as Parkinson's disease. Some of these distinctions are debatable, as it is not clear, for example, why people who stutter and feel extremely anxious in many social situations should not be considered to suffer from social anxiety disorder in addition to stuttering.

TABLE 4–4. General Characteristics of Phobic Disorders

---

1. There is a fear of *known* objects, situations, activities, or phenomena ("phobic stimuli").

2. Phobic stimuli generally *do not pose a realistic threat*; if they do, the anxiety response is irrational or excessive.

3. There is an *insight* that the fear is irrational or excessive.

4. Exposure to phobic stimuli *elicits an immediate anxiety response*, which may be in the form of a (situationally bound) panic attack.

5. There is *avoidance* of phobic stimuli *or endurance* of phobic stimuli with great distress and/or anxiety.

6. There is *impaired functioning or significant distress* about having the fear.

In ICD-10, attention is drawn to the possibility of misdiagnosing social anxiety disorder in case of an underlying psychotic disorder. Sometimes this is relevant for clinical practice, as some patients who are labeled "socially phobic" feel anxious because of delusions of reference (e.g., they are afraid of a particular group of people because they are convinced that these people talk about them in a derogatory manner and ridicule them). The ICD-10 concept of social anxiety disorder also emphasizes the presence of somatic symptoms that are relatively characteristic of social anxiety disorder (e.g., blushing, tremor, sweating).

The diagnosis of social anxiety disorder is based on information elicited from patients and on psychiatric examination. Patients should be asked questions relevant to all phobic situations, and not just those that they mention spontaneously. When patients with social anxiety disorder are seen for an assessment, they typically lack spontaneity and look inhibited, anxious, and tense. Sometimes they shake or blush, and their hands are often clammy. Being interviewed may seem like a major effort for them. They often avoid eye contact and seem as if the end of an interview cannot come soon enough. However, the appearance and behavior of other patients may be quite different from this stereotype. For example, some patients with social anxiety disorder may be very talkative and difficult to interrupt, usually because they find it difficult to tolerate silence and resort to talking rather than enduring the silence-producing tension. Other patients may seem detached and disconnected, as they attempt to decrease their discomfort in an interpersonal situation. This may be interpreted, however, as lack of interest in other people or even as aloofness.

Although many attempts have recently been made to raise the awareness of social anxiety disorder and improve its detection, it is still often overlooked and neglected (Sheeran and Zimmerman, 2002). This seems to be the case particularly when social anxiety disorder is overshadowed by depression and alcoholism or when patients present with another disorder as their principal psychiatric condition. Also, it appears that many cases of social anxiety disorder are dismissed as "shyness" and are not taken seriously; some clinicians do not believe that the concept of social anxiety disorder is valid and refrain from using it for diagnostic purposes.

Assessment Instruments

The Liebowitz Social Anxiety Scale (Liebowitz, 1987) is a clinician-administered instrument used to measure the severity of social anxiety disorder in terms of both the fear and avoidance of performance-type and interactional situations. Thus it yields separate scores for fear and avoidance of performance and social interactional situations. This instrument is useful for monitoring treatment-related changes in the severity of various aspects of social anxiety disorder.

The Social Phobia and Anxiety Inventory (Turner et al., 1989) is a self-report measure of the severity of psychological and somatic symptoms associated with social situations and avoidance or escape related to social situations. The instrument also yields a total score. The Social Phobia and Anxiety Inventory assesses social anxiety disorder comprehensively, but because of its length and cumbersome scoring, it is not an ideal instrument for routine use, despite its excellent psychometric properties.

Differential Diagnosis

In terms of differential diagnosis, social anxiety disorder should be distinguished from shyness and "normal" social anxiety, other anxiety disorders (especially agoraphobia), body dysmorphic disorder, some types of personality disturbance (e.g., avoidant personality disorder), depression, and psychotic illness (Table 4–5). Distinctions between social anxiety disorder, shyness, and avoidant personality disorder were discussed earlier in Clinical Features and Relationship Between Social Anxiety Disorder and Other Disorders.

Other Anxiety Disorders

The differentiation between social anxiety disorder and some of the other anxiety disorders may sometimes pose problems. For example, patients with agoraphobia may have concerns that are similar to worries of patients with social anxiety disorder: they may be afraid of crowded places not only because of the possibility of having a panic attack and of not being able to escape, but also because of the embarrassment and shame they would experience if a panic attack occurred. Although agoraphobia and social anxiety disorder may co-occur, it is important to ascertain whether features of one disorder are, in fact, a part of the other, as both diagnoses are not warranted in these cases.

TABLE 4–5 Differential Diagnosis of Social Anxiety Disorder

Shyness, "normal" social anxiety

Other anxiety disorders (especially agoraphobia)

Body dysmorphic disorder

Personality disorders (especially avoidant, schizoid, and paranoid personality disorders)

Depression

Psychotic illness (e.g., schizophrenia, delusional disorder)

The structure of fear in agoraphobia is quite different from that in social anxiety disorder (Table 4–6). Patients with agoraphobia are typically concerned about being helpless and alone in case of a panic attack, whereas patients with social anxiety disorder are not at all troubled by being alone, because it is the scrutiny by others that is most troublesome to them. Therefore, situations that provide anonymity and in which there is no expectation to perform, with low likelihood of being under scrutiny (e.g., being in crowded places), do not represent a problem for patients with social anxiety disorder, unlike small groups, where they may be expected to perform and may easily be observed. Also, when in a phobic situation, patients with social anxiety disorder tend to have different physical symptoms from those experienced by patients with agoraphobia (and panic disorder). The former are more likely to blush, sweat, tremble, and have dry mouth and muscle spasms, whereas the latter are more likely to feel dizzy and lightheaded and have palpitations, chest pain or discomfort, and choking feelings (Amies et al., 1983; Reich et al., 1988).

Unlike unexpected panic attacks that occur in panic disorder, panic attacks associated with social anxiety disorder are usually situationally bound or situationally predisposed and have an obvious relationship with the feared social situations. Patients with panic disorder avoid certain social situations, not because they fear that they will be under scrutiny from others but because they feel embarrassed about the possibility of experiencing a panic attack in such situations and then having an urge to escape.

Body Dysmorphic Disorder
Body dysmorphic disorder may sometimes seem like social anxiety disorder, and the two conditions may also co-occur. However, the reason for social discomfort and anxiety in body dysmorphic disorder pertains to the

TABLE 4–6. Distinguishing Between Social Anxiety Disorder and Agoraphobia

Characteristics	Social Anxiety Disorder	Agoraphobia
Main underlying concerns	Scrutiny and harsh judgment by others	Having a panic attack in specific situations
Fear of being alone	Generally rare	Generally frequent
Fear of large crowds	Generally rare	Very common
Anonymity seeking	Present	Usually absent
Type of symptoms in phobic situations	Blushing, sweating trembling, muscle spasms	Dizziness, lightheadedness, choking feelings

imagined bodily defect to which other people are expected to respond negatively, and which the person also finds unacceptable and often repugnant.

Depression
Sometimes it may be difficult to differentiate between social anxiety disorder and depression, as both are characterized by social withdrawal. However, the underlying reason or motive for social withdrawal is what distinguishes these two conditions: in depression, social withdrawal is a consequence of the generalized loss of interest, whereas in social anxiety disorder (not complicated by depression), social withdrawal results from active and specific avoidance of social situations.

Psychosis
Patients with social anxiety disorder may present with a clinical picture that is difficult to distinguish from that of a psychotic illness. In these cases, patients often express fears of other people and attribute to them vicious intentions, sometimes even worrying about their own safety. Patients are typically concerned that others are paying special attention to them, taking every notice of them, talking about them, making derogatory comments, or ridiculing them. Beneath such concerns there may be paranoid delusions, delusions of reference, delusional misinterpretations, and delusions that others are able to read one's mind, suggesting a delusional disorder with a strong paranoid component or schizophrenia (usually paranoid schizophrenia).

EPIDEMIOLOGY

Highlights of the epidemiology of social anxiety disorder are presented in Table 4–7. The National Comorbidity Survey, which was conducted in the United States, using DSM-III-R diagnostic criteria, put the lifetime prevalence of social anxiety disorder at 13.3% (Magee et al., 1996). This finding made social anxiety disorder the third most common psychiatric disorder, after depression and alcohol dependence. One-third of individuals with social anxiety disorder in the community had a phobia of public speaking, another third had a fear of at least one other social situation, and the remaining third had fears of multiple social situations (Magee et al., 1996).

The lifetime prevalence of social anxiety disorder was only 2.7% in the previously conducted U.S. Epidemiologic Catchment Area Study, based on the DSM-III diagnostic criteria (Robins and Regier, 1991). The striking difference in prevalence rates between the National Comorbidity Survey and the Epidemiologic Catchment Area Study reflects different

TABLE 4–7. Epidemiological Data for Social Anxiety Disorder

- Lifetime prevalence rate (U.S.): 2.7% (Epidemiological Catchment Area Study); 13.3% (National Comorbidity Survey)

- Overestimated prevalence rate by the National Comorbidity Survey?

- Prevalence rates quite different in different countries

- More women than man have social anxiety disorder in the community, but the frequency of women and men with social anxiety disorder is approximately the same in clinical samples.

- Persons with social anxiety disorder are more likely to be single, unemployed, and in the lower socioeconomic group, with lower levels of education.

- Age of onset is usually in adolescence (mid-teens to early twenties)

- Mean age of onset: 15–16 years

- Usual period between onset and time of seeking help: more than 10 years

diagnostic criteria and different instruments used to diagnose social anxiety disorder. In an attempt to reconcile these findings and count only those cases deemed clinically significant, Narrow et al. (2002) calculated a 1-year prevalence rate for social anxiety disorder of 3.2%, down from the 7.4% that was reported in the National Comorbidity Survey (corrected lifetime prevalence rate was not reported). Thus, the prevalence of social anxiety disorder might have been overestimated by the National Comorbidity Survey. With a recent estimate of lifetime prevalence of social anxiety disorder of 7.2% in the United States (Stein et al., 2000), social anxiety disorder appears to be one of the most common psychiatric conditions, highlighting its public health significance.

Epidemiological studies in different countries have found strikingly different lifetime prevalence rates of social anxiety disorder, ranging from 0.5% in Korea (Lee et al., 1990a) to 16% in Switzerland (Wacker et al., 1992). These differences can be accounted for by the changing diagnostic criteria over the past 20 years, different diagnostic instruments used in different studies, and cultural differences in the presentation of social anxiety disorder. Not only are there striking differences between Western and Eastern cultures in the concept of social anxiety disorder, but there may also be differences between ethnic groups within Western cultures.

A culturally specific form of social anxiety disorder (taijin-kyofu-shio, or disorder with fear of interpersonal relations) has been described in Japan and Korea. The key feature of this condition is a concern that a person might offend others by blushing, trembling, emitting unpleasant bodily odors, or having other anxiety symptoms, which then leads to avoidance of social situations. This concept of social anxiety is very different from its Western counterpart: the sufferers are not preoccupied with the impact of the anxiety on themselves, but worry about the discomfort that they cause in others by their anxiety.

There are more women than men (the approximate ratio of 1.5:1) with social anxiety disorder in the community (Bourdon et al., 1988; Schneier et al., 1992). In samples of patients with social anxiety disorder, however, the number of women and men tends to be the same, and sometimes there are even more men than women in clinical settings (e.g., Boyd et al., 1990; Degonda and Angst, 1993). This difference may result from several factors. First, women may endure social anxiety disorder without seeking help or may adapt to it more easily, because features of social anxiety disorder are not as incompatible with social roles and expectations for women as they are with the corresponding roles and expectations for men (e.g., a requirement to be assertive). In other words, a failure to fulfill social roles and meet social expectations may be a stronger motivating factor for men with social anxiety disorder to seek professional help than it is for women. Second, the prevalence of social anxiety disorder among men in the community may be underestimated, because social anxiety disorder is often hidden behind its complications, especially alcohol abuse. Finally, men may be more likely to have a more severe form of social anxiety disorder.

Patients with social anxiety disorder tend to be single, marry less often, and have fewer social contacts and fewer friends than comparable groups without social anxiety disorder (Schneier et al., 1992). They are also more likely to remain living with their parents well into their adulthood. As a result of the handicapping effects of social anxiety disorder on their ability to attend school, look for jobs, maintain employment, and advance in their careers, patients with social anxiety disorder are more likely to have lower education, feel frustrated about their professional achievements, be unemployed and financially dependent, rely on social support and welfare agencies, and be in the lower socioeconomic group (Schneier et al., 1992).

It may be difficult to precisely determine the onset of social anxiety disorder, especially in the generalized type. As already noted above in Clinical Features, nongeneralized and generalized forms of social anxiety disorder often differ in terms of the age and mode of onset. The typical onset of social anxiety disorder is in adolescence, with the mean age of onset being between 15 and 16 years (Schneier et al., 1992). Most patients have an onset before the age of 25, and it is unusual for social anxiety disorder to first manifest itself after that age (Schneier et al., 1992; Magee et al., 1996). The early age of onset of social anxiety disorder has important

implications for affecting adversely the development of children and adolescents. Their academic performance may be well below their intellectual
level, they do not develop adequate interpersonal and social skills, and
their interactions with peers are quite limited.

The majority (72%–87%) of persons with social anxiety disorder do
not seek professional help (Magee et al., 1996). When they do seek help, the
time lag between onset of the disorder and onset of treatment is often
longer than 10 years, so that the treatment usually commences when
patients are in their late twenties or thirties. There are many reasons for
this delay: social anxiety disorder sufferers often feel embarrassed about
their fears and are reluctant to disclose them. They may also "adapt" themselves to their fears and accept to a certain extent limitations imposed by
the phobia. Some believe that social anxiety disorder is a part of their personality and that nothing can be done about it.

When social anxiety disorder sufferers seek psychiatric help, more
often than not they do this because of complications of social anxiety disorder (e.g., depression, excessive use of alcohol) or in the context of some
important life change. For example, a new job that demands assertiveness
and effective interpersonal communication makes it very difficult for the
person with a hidden social anxiety disorder to continue avoiding social
activities. Unlike patients with panic disorder and generalized anxiety disorder, those with social anxiety disorder are more likely to initially seek
help from psychotherapists, psychologists, and school counselors than
from primary care physicians (Wittchen et al., 1999).

COURSE AND PROGNOSIS

Most patients with social anxiety disorder have a chronic course, with few,
if any, fluctuations in its intensity. This course creates an impression that
social anxiety disorder is a lifelong condition and is particularly characteristic of the generalized type. The course in nongeneralized social anxiety
disorder may show some variations and be related to the frequency with
which patients have to be in social situations and how skillful they are in
terms of avoiding such situations.

Data on the duration of social anxiety disorder confirm the chronicity
of this condition. In two studies (Heimberg et al., 1990b; Schneier et al.,
1992), 9%–15% of patients had had the illness for most part of their lives;
almost one-third of patients had suffered from social anxiety disorder for
at least 15 years, and the remainder had had social anxiety disorder for at
least 6 years. In another study (DeWit et al., 1999), a median duration of
social anxiety disorder was 25 years.

As already noted, the prognosis of generalized social anxiety disorder is worse than that of nongeneralized social anxiety disorder. This is likely to be a consequence of the difference in severity between these two subtypes. Factors suggesting a poor prognosis of social anxiety disorder (Table 4–8) include an earlier onset (before age 11 [Davidson et al., 1993a] or before age 7 [DeWit et al., 1999]) and longer duration of social anxiety disorder; greater initial severity with greater number of symptoms; presence of other psychiatric disorders, especially depression; various health problems; and lower education (Davidson et al., 1993a; DeWit et al., 1999).

The impairment and disability associated with social anxiety disorder can be quite severe (Schneier et al., 1994; Stein and Kean, 2000; Wittchen et al., 1999, 2000b), as noted above in Epidemiology. In one study (Antony et al., 1998), patients with social anxiety disorder were as impaired as those with chronic, debilitating medical conditions, such as chronic renal failure and multiple sclerosis. Patients' quality of life is severely affected and they often report that they are profoundly dissatisfied with various aspects of their lives (Stein et al., 1999c).

Independent functioning may be very difficult for patients with severe forms of social anxiety disorder, as they tend to perceive every novel social situation as highly distressing and even dangerous. As a result, these patients often have great problems in attending school, in peer and intimate relationships, and in finding and maintaining jobs. Hence, social anxiety disorder is associated with lower academic achievement, increased probability of remaining single or divorcing, and increased likelihood of unemployment (Schneier et al., 1992; Wittchen et al., 1999). Also, patients' work productivity is often reduced and their work performance impaired (Wittchen et al., 2000b). All of these factors have further repercussions in terms of patients' inability to achieve basic goals in life, financial difficulties, and greater social isolation and marginalization. Some patients find the only "refuge" in a quasi-symbiotic clinging to their parents, which can at times appear rather bizarre.

TABLE 4–8. Factors Suggesting a Poor Prognosis of Social Anxiety Disorder

Very early onset (before age 7–11 years)

Greater initial severity, greater number of symptoms

Co-occurring psychiatric disorders

Presence of depression

Presence of health problems

Lower education

Do patients with social anxiety disorder ever recover? It appears that some do, but they are a minority (e.g., Reich et al., 1994; Chartier et al., 1998). Also, recovery may occur after many years of the continuing presence of illness; a study by DeWit et al. (1999) reported that about one-half of patients recovered after as long as 25 years of illness.

ETIOLOGY AND PATHOGENESIS

Many etiological factors contribute to the development of social anxiety disorder. No etiological model can explain by itself all the cases and all the manifestations of social anxiety disorder. It appears that there are several biological and psychological pathways that lead to clinical presentations of social anxiety disorder. The models reviewed below shed some light on these pathways.

BIOLOGICAL MODELS

Genetic Factors

Social anxiety disorder may run in some families. It has been found more often among first-degree relatives of patients with social anxiety disorder than among first-degree relatives of patients with panic disorder and control subjects without mental disorder (Reich and Yates, 1988; Fyer et al., 1993; 1995; Mannuzza et al., 1995; Stein et al., 1998a). The genetic component seems to be stronger in the generalized type of social anxiety disorder (see Clinical Features, above).

Results of twin studies on a genetic component of shyness and social anxiety have been conflicting (Torgersen, 1983; Kendler et al., 1992c; Skre et al., 1993). More recently, one twin study (Kendler et al., 1999) estimated the contribution of genetic factors to the development of social anxiety disorder at 40%–60%, while another twin study (Nelson et al., 2000) among female adolescents estimated the heritability of social anxiety disorder at 28%.

Although family and twin studies do suggest that there is a heritable component in social anxiety disorder, nongenetic patterns of transmission of social fears within certain families (e.g., through modeling) can play a significant role. In addition, a large component of what is inherited in social anxiety disorder may be a nonspecific, general vulnerability to anxiety disorders (Andrews et al., 1990) or depression (Nelson et al., 2000).

Pathophysiological Mechanisms and Neuroanatomy

Little is known about pathophysiological mechanisms in social anxiety disorder, despite a plethora of research over the past 10–15 years. There are three main issues here, and research has yet to find answers to the following questions: (1) Are there any pathophysiological mechanisms specific for social anxiety disorder, that is, mechanisms different from those involved in other anxiety disorders? (2) What is the pathophysiological difference, if any, between the generalized and nongeneralized forms of social anxiety disorder? (3) Which pathophysiological mechanisms play a role in the pathogenesis of social anxiety disorder, and which mechanisms are just correlates of social anxiety disorder?

Neurotransmitter Systems

The serotonin, norepinephrine, gamma-aminobutyric acid (GABA), and dopamine neurotransmitter systems have been implicated in the etiology and pathogenesis of social anxiety disorder. However, data pointing to the abnormalities in these systems have been inconsistent. Also, no transmitter abnormalities have been found to be specific for social anxiety disorder. Hypotheses about the involvement of dopamine and serotonin systems have been partly derived from findings of the efficacy in social anxiety disorder of classical, irreversible monoamine oxidase inhibitors and selective serotonin reuptake inhibitors, respectively.

Patients with prominent performance-type social anxiety may have an underlying norepinephrine dysfunction, so they are either hypersensitive to normal noradrenergic stimulation or they exhibit central and peripheral noradrenergic hyperactivity. This hypothesis is supported by the symptoms (palpitations, tremor, sweating, blushing) that typically occur in performance situations and by the efficacy of β-adrenergic blockers in the treatment of the performance/nongeneralized type of social anxiety disorder.

The dopamine deficiency hypothesis in generalized social anxiety disorder (Liebowitz et al., 1987) is interesting, as the classical, irreversible monoamine oxidase inhibitors are presumed to prevent degradation of dopamine. Also, the convincing efficacy of these medications in generalized social anxiety disorder is rather unique among the anxiety disorders. Furthermore, a substantial number of patients with Parkinson's disease, which is characterized by dopamine deficiency, do have social anxiety disorder prior to the onset of Parkinson's disease (Stein et al., 1990a). Patients with Tourette's disorder, by contrast, were observed to develop social anxiety disorder following treatment with haloperidol, a dopamine antagonist

(Mikkelson et al., 1981). The hypothesis about central dopamine deficiency has recently received further support (e.g., Schneier et al., 2000).

Neuroimaging Studies
A few attempts to tie social anxiety disorder to certain brain structures by means of imaging studies have not produced consistent results. Some studies have reported amygdala abnormalities and/or activation in response to specific, social anxiety–inducing stimuli in the course of imaging (Birbaumer et al., 1998; Schneider et al., 1999), but these findings have yet to be replicated.

Biological "Preparedness" for Social Anxiety (Preparedness Conditioning Theories)

It has been postulated that humans are biologically "prepared" to fear certain stimuli in their environment and that this "preparedness" has a survival value, contributing to the preservation of the species (Seligman, 1971; McNally, 1987). Studies have shown that people are very sensitive to facial expressions of others and are afraid of angry and threatening faces, but only if these facial expressions are directed at them (Öhman, 1986). People respond to such facial expressions in a way that helps them adjust to various interpersonal situations and decrease or avoid danger implied by these expressions. Ultimately, their adequate response helps their own survival and preservation of the species. However, if the person is too sensitive to these facial and other interpersonal and social stimuli so that the fear response appears automatically even when there is no real threat, or if the fear response is excessive, the person may develop social anxiety disorder. This perspective on social anxiety disorder is interesting in view of the poor eye contact exhibited by many patients with social anxiety disorder and their strong fears of being observed.

PSYCHOBIOLOGICAL MODEL—BEHAVIORAL INHIBITION

The behavioral inhibition to the unfamiliar (Kagan et al., 1984, 1987, 1988) was conceptualized as a temporally stable component of inborn temperament that represents a biological basis for shyness. As such, behavioral inhibition has been conceived of as one of the major factors in the pathogenesis of anxiety disorders in general and social anxiety disorder in particular.

Manifestations of behavioral inhibition to the unfamiliar are observable during the first year of life: children of that age have difficulty sleeping in unfamiliar surroundings and often exhibit irritability in novel situations. By 2 years of age, such children tend to avoid contacts with unfamiliar people, places, and objects, and prefer to cling to their mothers. They respond to novel situations with fear, cessation of exploratory and playful activity, and somatic symptoms that are very similar to those seen in anxious adults upon exposure to feared stimuli. This behavioral and physiological pattern at age 2 is predictive of behavioral inhibition at age 7.

In the course of further development, these children often exhibit extreme caution in a range of situations, appear introverted and shy, find themselves at the periphery of social activities, and are likely to become even more isolated. They seem physiologically "overprepared" for danger, as their heart rate is elevated at rest, with further disproportionate increase in heart rate upon exposure to even mild stressors. These children also tend to have elevated blood levels of cortisol and catecholamines.

Behavioral inhibition does not have a unique relationship with social anxiety disorder, but it is most consistently linked with social anxiety disorder (e.g., Mick and Telch, 1998; Cooper and Eke, 1999) and, to a somewhat lesser degree, with panic disorder and agoraphobia (e.g., Rosenbaum et al., 1988). In comparison with uninhibited children, those with behavioral inhibition seem to have a higher risk to develop phobic disorders, including social anxiety disorder (Kagan et al., 1988). When parents of children with and without behavioral inhibition were compared, the former were more likely to have social anxiety disorder or other anxiety disorders, and more often reported anxiety-related problems and anxiety disorders in their own childhood (Rosenbaum et al., 1991). A much higher proportion of children of parents with panic disorder, by contrast, were found to be behaviorally inhibited in comparison with children of normal or depressed parents (Rosenbaum et al., 1988).

Psychological Models

Cognitive and Behavioral Approaches

Aversive Conditioning Model

Traumatic conditioning may play some role in the development of social anxiety disorder, especially the nongeneralized subtype (Stemberger et al., 1995). For example, a sudden blushing or loss of voice during a performance may lead to the perception of a particular social situation as being embarrassing, humiliating, and therefore dangerous. More than one-half of patients may be able to identify an unpleasant or humiliating incident that preceded the onset of social anxiety disorder (e.g., Öst and Hugdahl, 1981). It appears that such a traumatic incident precipitates social anxiety disorder in the context of a specific predisposition, for example, if the person is excessively shy or carries relevant genetic vulnerability. Without a specific predisposition, aversive (traumatic) experiences are rarely sufficient for the development of social anxiety disorder, especially its generalized subtype. According to this model, social anxiety disorder is primarily maintained by the avoidance of relevant social situations, in a fashion similar to the maintenance of other phobias through avoidance.

Cognitive Models
Cognitive models of social anxiety disorder are becoming increasingly important in our efforts to better understand this condition. Patients with social anxiety disorder generally underestimate their social performance, overestimate the probability of poor performance or other adverse social outcome, and overestimate dire consequences of such an outcome (Beck et al., 1985; Lucock and Salkovskis, 1988; Rapee and Lim, 1992). The negative outcome almost invariably has to do with how patients come across to others, and this in turn, is often linked to the occurrence and visibility of the anxiety symptoms: patients overestimate the likelihood of the occurrence of these symptoms, their visibility (McEwan and Devins, 1983), and attention paid to them by others.

Two cognitive models of social anxiety disorder have been formulated (Clark and Wells, 1995; Rapee and Heimberg, 1997). The models have much in common and are based on the idea that the fundamental issue in social anxiety disorder is the fear of negative evaluation by others; according to the cognitive models, social anxiety disorder is a consequence of the expectation that one will be evaluated negatively in social situations. This expectation is regarded as a consequence of certain assumptions and beliefs that patients with social anxiety disorder have about themselves and others (Table 4–9). These assumptions and beliefs lead to an appraisal of social situations as threatening, as a result of which patients experience anxiety. Such appraisals are maintained through avoidance of social situations, use of various safety behaviors, and biases in information processing.

There has been a recent surge in interest in information processing in social anxiety disorder, and studies have found several biases in information processing that appear relatively specific for social anxiety disorder (Table 4–10). A particularly salient aspect of information processing in social anxiety disorder appears to be a combination of decreased attention to external social situations and interpersonal information with increased

TABLE 4–9. Typical Assumptions of Patients with Social Anxiety Disorder

Assumptions About Oneself

1. Negative, social situation–specific beliefs about oneself (e.g., "I am stupid," "I am weak," "I am worthless," "I am boring")

2. Beliefs about social interactions and social evaluation (e.g., "If I have to give a talk and appear anxious, I will humiliate myself," "If I don't do it right, they will laugh at me")

Assumptions About Others

1. Others pay close attention to one's appearance and/or behavior.

2. Others have knowledge of one's thoughts and/or feelings.

3. Others are likely to be harsh and judgmental and quick to reject anyone who makes mistakes or appears inept.

Assumptions About Social Performance

1. Standards of social performance must be strictly adhered to in order to avoid disappointment, humiliation, or rejection.

2. Social performance must be of a high, perfectionist standard to minimize the possibility of making a mistake.

focusing on oneself. Largely as a result of the latter, patients with social anxiety disorder become preoccupied with their physical symptoms and perceive the symptoms as being "responsible" for how they appear to other people. In other words, because they blush or tremble, patients assume that others see them as a failure. This assumption is then difficult to disconfirm, because patients do not generally pay attention to external social information, and they particularly tend to disregard any positive feedback about themselves. Also, the disconfirmation is made difficult by the inherent ambiguity of social interactions so that patients can never be *completely* sure how they are perceived by others. Another potential consequence of preoccupation with oneself may be neglect of the actual social performance, so that the performance itself is compromised (e.g., Woody, 1996). In this case, one's fears about poor performance may to a certain extent be validated.

Another cognitive mechanism in social anxiety disorder involves expectations of anxiety, discomfort, and physical symptoms in social situations. These expectations make it more likely for anxiety, discomfort, and physical symptoms to indeed occur in such situations, thereby strengthening the fear and driving patients to continue avoiding social situations.

TABLE 4–10. Information Processing Bias in Social Anxiety Disorder

Bias	Description
Attention bias	Increased self-focused attention, heightened "public self-consciousness" (Fenigstein et al., 1975; Hope and Heimberg, 1988; Mellings and Alden, 2000)
	Decreased attention to external social situation or information (Chen et al., 2002)
Interpretation bias	Interpretation of physical symptoms as an indication that one appears negatively to others, e.g., as anxious, insecure, and weak (McEwan and Devins, 1983; Amir et al., 1998; Mansell and Clark, 1999; Mulkens et al., 1999; Mellings and Alden, 2000; Roth et al., 2001; Wells and Papageorgiou, 2001)
	Tendency to be more rigid when interpreting one's own anxiety symptoms than when interpretatng the same symptoms in others (Amir et al., 1998; Roth et al., 2001)
	Interpretation of ambiguous, self-relevant social situations and events as negative (Amir et al., 1998; Stopa and Clark, 2000)
	Catastrophic interpretation of mildly negative, but quite innocuous, self-relevant social situations and events (Stopa and Clark, 2000)
Biased self-imagery	Tendency to perceive oneself negatively from an "observer's perspective" rather than watching oneself "with one's own eyes" (Clark and Wells, 1995; Hackmann et al., 1998; Wells and Papageorgiou, 1999)
Memory bias	Defective memory for certain aspects of social situations or interpersonal information or interactions (Kimble and Zehr, 1982; Hope et al., 1990; Mellings and Alden, 2000)
	Memory bias for socially threatening information (Amir et al., 2000)
Biased appraisal of future	Negative expectations from accomplishment and social success (e.g., social success will lead to more social demand and pressure; Wallace and Alden, 1997)

Social Skills Deficits Model

There is an ongoing debate over whether patients with social anxiety disorder lack social skills or whether their anxiety interferes with the use of the otherwise well-developed social skills. Although patients often appear awkward or inept in social situations, that does not necessarily reflect deficiencies in their social skills. Instead, this awkwardness may be more a result of the patients' need to make a certain impression on others, coupled with their insecurity and doubt about being able to do so. This proposition is at the core of the self-presentation theory of social anxiety (Schlenker and Leary, 1982).

A genuine lack of social skills may be observed in patients who report a long-standing lack of knowledge or understanding of some very basic and simple rules of social behavior. These patients usually did not have adequate opportunities to learn social skills or have felt extremely inhibited in their exploratory behavior since early childhood. Hence, their assertion that they do not know how they should behave and what they should do in most social situations does represent a social skills deficiency.

Psychodynamic Approaches

A comprehensive psychoanalytic/psychodynamic account of social anxiety disorder is lacking, mainly because social anxiety disorder tends to be regarded by psychoanalysts as part of a character organization, and not a psychopathological entity per se. Certain psychoanalytic views on social anxiety disorder deserve attention because of their relevance for clinical practice.

Some psychoanalysts relate social anxiety disorder to the feeling of shame and fear of the superego. The feeling of shame and anticipation of humiliation may be a consequence of the projection of harsh, critical, or punitive parental introjects onto others, with the consequent expectation that others treat patients harshly (Gabbard, 1992). The presumed underlying conflict is between a need to compete, achieve, and succeed on one hand, and the fear of success on the other. The success is feared because it is unconsciously equated with "Oedipal victory," whereas punishment is anticipated as the consequence of the latter. In other words, the person is not "allowed" to compete and succeed. Unable to resolve this conflict and striving to avoid the feeling of shame, the person withdraws from social interactions, thereby developing social anxiety disorder.

Another psychodynamic issue in social anxiety disorder pertains to problems in the process of separation–individuation, usually as a result of serious disturbances in the process of attachment and early object relations (Gabbard, 1992; Cloitre and Shear, 1995). In this case, the postulated conflict is between striving toward independence and self-affirmation on one hand, and fear of the loss of love, rejection, and abandonment by primary objects (parents), on the other, as a punishment for such independence. Persons who develop social anxiety disorder give up their pursuit of independence and withdraw from social interactions to appease the primary objects. However, the latter does not eventuate, and they are left with the sense of insecurity and poor self-esteem.

In the psychoanalytic literature, social anxiety disorder has also been linked to exhibitionistic or narcissistic urges to make a "perfect" impression of oneself. A fear of being unable to make such an impression leads the person to anticipate narcissistic injury; to avoid this injury, the person resorts to avoidance of social interactions. This can help explain narcissistic traits in some patients with social anxiety disorder.

Role of Developmental and Childhood Factors

Patients with social anxiety disorder have an increased tendency to perceive their parents as overprotective and rejecting (e.g., Lieb et al., 2000); if the parents' behavior is indeed overprotective and rejecting, that may contribute to the patients' sense of insecurity and inability to rely on themselves and/or trust their own judgment in social interactions. Although such a perception of parents is not specific for social anxiety disorder, it may help account for the development of social anxiety disorder in children who are predisposed to it genetically or through specific temperamental features (behavioral inhibition).

Treatment

The treatment of some forms of nongeneralized, performance-type social anxiety disorder is relatively simple. Treatment of the generalized subtype of social anxiety disorder, by contrast, tends to be challenging. It is in many ways akin to the treatment of personality disturbance, regardless of whether a personality disorder of any kind is formally present or not, because of the negative effects that social anxiety disorder, which usually starts in adolescence, has on virtually all aspects of personality development. The analogy with treatment of personality disorders also means that the treatment is likely to be long, and its outcome in many cases precarious. Furthermore, as with treatment of personality disorders, goals of treatment of generalized social anxiety disorder do not entail a radical change and should more realistically be set to alleviate patients' suffering and their symptoms and improve functioning.

Several efficacious treatment modalities are available for both nongeneralized and generalized social anxiety disorder. They include pharmacotherapy and various forms of cognitive-behavioral therapy. Supportive and psychodynamic psychotherapy can also be helpful to patients with social anxiety disorder, particularly those with the generalized subtype. A combination of pharmacological and psychological treatment may be beneficial to these patients as well.

Pharmacological Treatment

There are several issues in the pharmacological treatment of social anxiety disorder (Table 4–11). First, pharmacological interventions for generalized social anxiety disorder are quite different from those for the nongeneralized subtype. In the latter, pharmacotherapy is distinctly used for fear of performance-type situations, particularly when the feared situations are occasional and for the most part predictable. Second, the choice of a pharmacological agent may largely be determined by the presence of co-occurring conditions, particularly depression and alcohol abuse or dependence. Less often, the co-occurring conditions that influence the choice of medication in social anxiety disorder are personality disorders, generalized anxiety disorder, panic disorder, obsessive-compulsive disorder, and body dysmorphic disorder. Because there is a higher risk of alcohol and other substance abuse in patients with social anxiety disorder than in patients with other anxiety disorders, greater caution should be exercised if benzodiazepines are administered to these patients.

Pharmacotherapy of Nongeneralized Social Anxiety Disorder (Performance Anxiety)

The goal of pharmacological treatment of nongeneralized social anxiety disorder is a substantial decrease in specific physical symptoms that patients find unpleasant or distressing during a particular task or performance. Most commonly, such symptoms are a manifestation of hyperactivity of the sympathic nervous system: tremor, palpitations, tachycardia, and sweating. Hence, the use of β-adrenergic blockers has been very popular for this purpose (Table 4–12), and there is some empirical support for such use (e.g., Brantigan et al., 1982; Neftel et al., 1982; Hartley et al., 1983). It is common for patients to take propranolol (10–40 mg) 30–60

TABLE 4–11. Aspects of Pharmacological Treatment Specific for Social Anxiety Disorder

- The pharmacological approach depends on whether the patient has a nongeneralized or generalized type of social anxiety disorder.
- The choice of medication depends largely on whether there is co-occurring depression or alcohol abuse or dependence.
- Great caution should be exercised if benzodiazepines are administered to patients with social anxiety disorder, as there is a higher risk for alcohol and other substance abuse in these patients than in patients with other anxiety disorders.

TABLE 4–12. Choice of Medication in Treatment of Social Anxiety Disorder

Rank	Medication
Generalized Type	
First-line	SSRIs (especially paroxetine, sertraline, and fluvoxamine)
Second-line	Classical, irreversible MAOIs
Third-line	BDZs (clonazepam)
Fourth–line:	Gabapentin
Nongeneralized Type	
First-line	β-adrenergic blockers (propranolol, atenolol)
Second-line	BDZs

BDZs, benzodiazepines; MAOIs, monoamine oxidase inhibitors; SSRIs, selective serotonin reuptake inhibitors.

minutes prior to a performance situation, such as giving a lecture or performing at a concert. Some patients take atenolol (50–100 mg), a more selective β-blocker. In one survey of musicians, 27% admitted to occasionally using β-blockers before giving a performance, and 96% of them believed that these medications were helpful (Fishbein et al., 1988).

The use of β-adrenergic blockers for fear of performance-type situations is largely based on the assumption that anxiety in some people occurs as a consequence of experiencing (and not misinterpreting) certain physical symptoms. The disappearance of these symptoms (e.g., normalization of the heart rate, removal of tremor and excessive sweating) by means of β-blockers then leads patients to feel that they are not anxious.

The alternative pharmacological treatment of nongeneralized social anxiety disorder, especially if β-adrenergic blockers are contraindicated, is an as-needed (prn) use of benzodiazepines just prior to a performance situation. Usually, a short-acting benzodiazepine (e.g., alprazolam, lorazepam) is taken for that purpose. When benzodiazepines are administered in this context, two issues should be kept in mind. First, benzodiazepines may be sedating and may impair movement coordination, which in turn could interfere with performance; second, benzodiazepines may have an excessively disinhibiting effect on some individuals, which could adversely affect their performance.

Pharmacotherapy of Generalized Social Anxiety Disorder

Goals of Pharmacotherapy and Indications for Use of Medications

Because of the chronic nature of the disorder, relentless anxiety, and frequent presence of issues rooted in personality, pharmacological treatment of generalized social anxiety disorder is much more complex than that of nongeneralized social anxiety disorder. Also, a psychological intervention is usually needed in addition to pharmacotherapy. The pharmacological treatment of generalized social anxiety disorder has immediate to short-term goals of substantially decreasing symptoms and behaviors associated with this disorder. In practical terms, the goals of treatment are to help patients feel less distressed in a range of socially difficult situations, decrease or eliminate symptoms of autonomic hyperarousal upon exposure to these situations, and minimize or eliminate socially driven avoidance. All of these changes lead to an improvement in overall functioning.

On the whole, pharmacological treatment has been moderately successful in achieving these goals; usually a long-term administration of medications is required. Pharmacological treatment does not address the underlying issues of pervasive, negative self-perception and fear of negative evaluation by others. However, medications may indirectly help patients perceive themselves more favorably by improving their performance, strengthening a sense of security in social situations, and boosting their self-confidence. Pharmacotherapy may also be useful in terms of helping patients react with certain indifference to their otherwise distressing concerns about how they appear to others.

In view of these goals of pharmacological treatment, the obvious indication for use of medications in the treatment of generalized social anxiety disorder is a preponderance of distressing somatic symptoms in various social situations. Pharmacotherapy may also be indicated for patients with generalized social anxiety disorder who do not experience prominent physical symptoms but nonetheless are quite disabled by their anxiety. The more severe generalized social anxiety disorder is, the more likely it is that it will be treated with medications, solely or in combination with psychological interventions.

Pharmacological treatment of generalized social anxiety disorder should last for at least 1 year following attainment of a significant response; as with other anxiety disorders, discontinuation of medication is associated with an increased risk of relapse.

Medications for Generalized Social Anxiety Disorder

Three groups of medications have shown efficacy in the treatment of generalized social anxiety disorder: selective serotonin reuptake inhibitors (SSRIs), classical irreversible monoamine oxidase inhibitors (MAOIs), and benzodiazepines. Because of their more favorable side-effect profile, no need for a tyramine-free diet, and fewer interactions with other medications, SSRIs are now considered first-line pharmacological treatment for generalized social anxiety disorder (Table 4–12), whereas classical MAOIs (phenelzine and, to a lesser extent, tranylcypromine) are reserved for treatment-resistant or more severe cases. Benzodiazepines have a limited role in the treatment of generalized social anxiety disorder because of the specific substance abuse vulnerability of patients with this disorder.

Selective serotonin reuptake inhibitors. The use of SSRIs in generalized social anxiety disorder is particularly suitable if there is depression or alcohol-related problems, but also if there is a co-occurring generalized anxiety disorder, obsessive-compulsive disorder, panic disorder, or body dysmorphic disorder. Often significant improvement does not occur after short-term treatment, and there may be further improvement over several months of pharmacotherapy. The latter scenario is similar to the response to SSRIs seen in obsessive-compulsive disorder and suggests that both patients and their physicians should exercise much patience during the course of treatment. Moreover, the longer the patients are treated—for example, for more than 2 years—the greater the likelihood of preventing a relapse.

The initial dosage of an SSRI is the same as in the treatment of depression, unless panic disorder co-occurs with social anxiety disorder. However, higher doses than those used for depression may be required for response (Table 4–13), which tends to occur or start after 8–12 weeks of treatment. Of the SSRIs, evidence of efficacy in generalized social anxiety disorder has been shown for paroxetine (Stein et al., 1998b; Allgulander,

TABLE 4–13. Medication Dosages Efficacious for Generalized Social Anxiety Disorder

Medication	Dose Range
Selective Serotonin Reuptake Inhibitors	
Paroxetine	20–50 mg/day
Sertraline	50–200 mg/day
Fluvoxamine	100–300 mg/day
Classical, Irreversible Monoamine Oxidase Inhibitors	
Phenelzine	45–90 mg/day
Tranylcypromine	40–60 mg/day
Clonazepam	2–6 mg/day
Gabapentin	2900 mg/day

1999; Baldwin et al., 1999), sertraline (Katzelnick et al., 1995; Van Ameringen et al., 2001; Liebowitz et al., 2003), and fluvoxamine (van Vliet et al., 1994; Stein et al., 1999a). The efficacy of sertraline (Walker et al., 2000) and paroxetine (Stein et al., 2002) was maintained over 24-week treatment following a response to acute treatment with these medications, rendering these SSRIs potentially useful in relapse prevention.

Classical irreversible monoamine oxidase inhibitors. The efficacy of phenelzine, a classical, irreversible and nonselective MAOI, in the treatment of social anxiety disorder has been established by several studies (Gelernter et al., 1991; Liebowitz et al., 1992; Versiani et al., 1992; Heimberg et al., 1998). Phenelzine is still regarded by some clinicians as the most powerful pharmacological agent for social anxiety disorder, more efficacious than benzodiazepines (Gelernter et al., 1991) and β-blockers (Liebowitz et al., 1992), and in some aspects even more efficacious than cognitive-behavioral therapy (Gelernter et al., 1991; Heimberg et al., 1998). In one study, as many as 91% of patients with social anxiety disorder were classified as responders to phenelzine (Versiani et al., 1992). A substantial number of patients improve significantly after 8–12 weeks of treatment with phenelzine, and efficacy may be maintained over prolonged periods of time. Tranylcypromine, another classical MAOI, may also be efficacious in treating patients with generalized social anxiety disorder.

The use of classical MAOIs is limited by their unfavorable side-effect profile (hypotension, insomnia, agitation, weight gain, sexual dysfunction), significant interactions with numerous medications (various sympathomimetic amines and dextromethorphan that are contained in many cold and cough over-the-counter medicines, epinephrine, psychostimulants, opioid analgesics, anesthetics, isoproterenol), and the need to avoid all food that contains tyramine (e.g., almost all types of cheese) to prevent an abrupt and large increase in blood pressure. Although the latter restriction represents a significant problem for some patients, others are able to adhere strictly to a tyramine-free diet.

A unique aspect of use of classical MAOIs in generalized social anxiety disorder is a link with atypical depression, for which these medications had demonstrated efficacy (see Relationship Between Social Anxiety Disorder and Other Disorders above). It is not known whether MAOIs are efficacious in treating social anxiety disorder for the same reason or in the same way that they are efficacious in atypical depression, that is, whether they target a feature that the two conditions share—hypersensitivity to interpersonal rejection. This is an interesting possibility and suggests that MAOIs might be a pharmacological treatment of choice when atypical depression co-occurs with generalized social anxiety disorder.

Benzodiazepines. Benzodiazepines can be used in the treatment of patients who have no history of alcohol or other substance abuse and who do not have a co-occurring depression, obsessive-compulsive disorder, or severe personality disturbance. Clonazepam is the only benzodiazepine for which efficacy in social anxiety disorder has been clearly demonstrated (Davidson et al., 1993b). The doses of clonazepam efficacious in the treatment of social anxiety disorder tend to be higher than those used in the treatment of panic disorder (Table 4–13).

Gabapentin. The anticonvulsant gabapentin offers some promise in the treatment of generalized social anxiety disorder (Table 4–12), as its efficacy was demonstrated in one controlled study (Pande et al., 1999). At present, gabapentin should be reserved for pharmacotherapy-resistant patients.

Moclobemide. Moclobemide, a reversible and selective MAO-A inhibitor, initially showed some promise for treatment of generalized social anxiety disorder (e.g., Versiani et al., 1992). Moclobemide is better tolerated than classical MAOIs and its use is not associated with other problems (e.g., a need to have a tyramine-free diet) that make classical MAOIs troublesome in routine clinical practice. However, results of later efficacy studies were not consistent and generally failed to support the initial enthusiasm and expectation that moclobemide might be an adequate substitute for classical MAOIs (Katschnig et al., 1997; Noyes et al., 1997; Schneier et al., 1998).

Pharmacotherapy of Treatment-Resistant Generalized Social Anxiety Disorder

An adequate pharmacological trial in generalized social anxiety disorder consists of 10–12 weeks of treatment with an SSRI, which is given in its maximum tolerated dose.

If the patient responds with some improvement to an adequate trial of an SSRI, further improvement may be observed with continued treatment, as already noted. The other strategy (Table 4–14) is to augment an SSRI with buspirone (e.g., Van Ameringen et al., 1996), clonazepam (e.g., Seedat and Stein, 2004) or gabapentin. At present, there are no guidelines that would assist in making a choice between these options; therefore, a physician has to rely on clinical judgment and consideration of individual patient circumstances.

If there is no response at all to an adequate trial of an SSRI, there are several options for further pharmacotherapy (Table 4–14): first switching treatment to another SSRI, and if the patient still does not respond to treat-

TABLE 4–14. Pharmacological Options for Treatment-Resistant Generalized Social Anxiety Disorder

Partial Response to First-Line Treatment (an SSRI)

Continue treatment with an SSRI

Augment with buspirone, clonazepam, or gabapentin

Lack of Response to First-Line Treatment (an SSRI)

1. Switch to another SSRI (and augment, if necessary)
2. Switch to phenelzine
3. Switch to clonazepam
4. Switch to gabapentin
5. Consider switching to venlafaxine

SSRI, selective serotonin reuptake inhibitor.

ment, considering a switch to phenelzine, clonazepam, or gabapentin. Venlafaxine may also be administered, as one study found that it may be efficacious in treatment of patients who do not respond to SSRIs (Altamura et al., 1999). The choice of medication and the sequence of switching depend on the particular circumstances of each patient. When switching a patient's treatment from an SSRI to a classical MAOI or vice versa, a washout period must be strictly observed (at least 2 weeks for all SSRIs except for fluoxetine, in which case the washout should last 5 weeks). Under no circumstances should an SSRI be combined with a classical MAOI, because of the risk of serotonin syndrome.

PSYCHOLOGICAL TREATMENT

Various techniques of cognitive-behavioral therapy (CBT) have been successfully used in social anxiety disorder. Therefore, they will be presented here in some detail. Psychodynamically oriented psychotherapies also play a role in the treatment of social anxiety disorder, but there is less empirical support for their use.

Cognitive-Behavioral Therapy

Cognitive-behavioral therapy for social anxiety disorder has evolved over the past 20 years and this treatment is now available in three basic forms: exposure-based therapy, social skills training, and cognitive therapy. Research on the efficacy of these treatments has been fruitful in shedding

Table 4–15. Indications for Use and/or Goals of Treatment for Various Techniques of Cognitive-Behavioral Therapy (CBT) in Social Anxiety Disorder

Indications for Use and/or Goals of Treatment	Technique(s)
Technique that should always be used, because of its efficacy, as part of any CBT program	Exposure
Technique that should be used if there is a marked deficit in social skills	Social skills training
Technique that should be used with the goal of directly making relevant cognitive changes	Cognitive therapy
Multiple treatment goals and/or enhancement of treatment effects	Exposure + social skills training Exposure + cognitive therapy Exposure + cognitive therapy + social skills training

more light on how to use them. The recommendations summarized in Table 4–15 are based on research findings and clinical experience. Thus, exposure-based therapy has proved to be very efficacious and should be included in any treatment package for social anxiety disorder. If the patient does have a marked deficit in social skills, it is reasonable to add social skills training, usually before exposure. Finally, cognitive therapy can be added with the goal of directly changing social anxiety–relevant appraisals and beliefs (in addition to favorable cognitive changes produced by exposure or social skills training). All three basic treatment procedures can be combined and administered in an individual or group format.

Exposure-Based Therapy

Exposure to feared social situations in the treatment of social anxiety disorder is based on the same principles as those of exposure-based treatments for other anxiety disorders. Exposure is conducted gradually, in accordance with the hierarchy of phobic situations, so that patients first expose themselves to the least anxiety–provoking situations. They move up the hierarchy of phobic situations as soon as they have habituated themselves to the previously practiced situation and have been able to remain in the situation without feeling anxious. The outcome of exposure-based therapy depends largely on patients' motivation and persistence with the homework, self-directed exposure between sessions with the therapist. There are also some specific aspects of exposure in social anxiety disorder (Table 4–16).

First, in-session exposure should be used as often as possible before in vivo exposure to prepare patients for self-directed exposure in vivo. These

TABLE 4–16. Aspects of Exposure-Based Therapy That Are Relatively Specific for
Social Anxiety Disorder

- In-session (therapist-assisted) exposure should be used before in vivo (self-directed) exposure.
- Role-playing by the therapist is very helpful.
- In vivo (self-directed) exposure should be gradual.
- Exposure should well reflect the reality of social situations, which are often unpredictable; patients have little, if any, control over them.
- More exposure sessions may be needed for successful outcome.

exposure exercises involve role-playing with the therapist, whereby the therapist takes on a role of the person with whom the patient feels anxious and/or has difficulty interacting. The simulation of the real-life social situation allows the therapist to observe patients' behavior first-hand. The therapist can then give appropriate feedback to patients and discuss with them all the relevant aspects of that situation. This is also an opportunity for patients to talk about their feelings and thoughts during the exposure. Some of these thoughts may be challenged by the therapist, who thereby adds a cognitive technique to the basic exposure-based treatment.

Second, conducting exposure-based therapy is more difficult in social anxiety disorder than in agoraphobia or specific phobias, because of the unpredictability of many social situations; neither the therapist nor the patients have much control over them. This unpredictability is particularly anxiety-provoking to patients with social anxiety disorder and calls for a more spontaneous approach when devising specific exposure tasks. For example, patients should plan to attend a meeting as part of their exposure, regardless of whom they might see there, whether they might be called to participate actively in the discussion, how long the meeting would last, and what else might happen. The rationale is that patients should conduct exposure in a way that reflects their encounters with real-life social situations fairly well.

Exposure treatment for social anxiety disorder has been found to be efficacious (Butler et al., 1984), although further treatment gains might be made with the addition of cognitive techniques (see below). Some data (e.g., Scholing and Emmelkamp, 1996) suggest that successful exposure therapy of social anxiety disorder may require more sessions (up to 16). However, the number of sessions needed to bring about a significant improvement does vary from one patient to another.

Social Skills Training

Social skills training is derived from the social skills deficits model of social anxiety disorder and based on the assumption that patients with social anxiety disorder have a basic deficiency in social skills. Although this assumption has never been confirmed, it is often accepted as valid because it has an intuitive appeal and many patients with social anxiety disorder do look socially inept. Also, these patients often report that they "just don't know" what to do or say in social situations and that they have no understanding or knowledge of how some very basic aspects of social communication and interaction are "supposed to proceed" (e.g., not knowing what the sequence of steps is when purchasing or ordering something). Social skills training may be useful for all of these patients, regardless of their level of anxiety (Trower et al., 1978).

Social skills training is used with the purpose of helping patients acquire skills that would be useful in various social situations. There are several components of a typical social skills training program:

1. Providing patients with information on what constitutes successful and effective social behavior
2. Giving instructions to patients on how they should act in a specific situation to learn a particular skill
3. Role-playing and modeling, so that the therapist first shows to patients how to negotiate a specific situation, subsequently asking patients to do the same
4. Giving corrective feedback to patients on how they performed
5. Patients practicing a particular skill in the presence of the therapist (rehearsal)
6. Patients practicing the same skill in real-life situations (homework).

Most social skills, particularly basic and advanced communication skills, can be learned using this sequential approach. If an emphasis is on learning assertive behavior (i.e., how to say "no," how to deal with authority figures, or how to be more effective in a leadership role), the treatment is sometimes referred to as "assertiveness training." It is important that patients adhere to the plan that they have devised together with their therapist. Social skills training can be conducted in both an individual and group format.

While social skills training has been useful in terms of alleviating some symptoms of social anxiety disorder and improving certain aspects of patients' functioning, it has not been as efficacious for other features of social anxiety disorder. It has often been insufficient to significantly decrease avoidance behavior and modify patients' core fears and beliefs (e.g., Marzillier et al., 1976; Trower et al., 1978; Stravynski et al., 1982; Wla-zlo et al., 1990).

Cognitive Therapy

Cognitive therapy is based on the cognitive model of social anxiety disor der, which emphasizes the etiological role of faulty appraisals of oneself (as weak, inadequate, etc.), others (as powerful, negative assessors of the patient), and social interactions and situations (as being inherently dangerous). Therefore, the goal of cognitive therapy is to correct these appraisals and replace them with more accurate alternatives. Cognitive therapy may also aim to change some of the patients' core self-concepts; in this case, treatment is likely to last longer.

As in cognitive therapy for other anxiety disorders, the key components of treatment are identification of automatic thoughts, challenging of their validity, and replacement of these thoughts and the corresponding appraisals with realistic, "normalizing" appraisals.

Identification of automatic thoughts proceeds by asking patients to imagine typical social situations that they are afraid of and then to verbalize or record the thoughts that occur in their mind as they contemplate entering a social situation or as they find themselves in one. More detailed information about automatic thoughts can be obtained through patients' diaries. Eliciting automatic thoughts is also useful for the purpose of understanding what patients with social anxiety disorder are really afraid of. Table 4–17 lists typical automatic thoughts of patients with social anxiety disorder. These automatic thoughts reveal various expectations, pre dictions, and concerns that patients may have about themselves and others, and it is important for the therapist to have as thorough an understanding of them as possible. Patients' grossly unrealistic expectations and anticipation of catastrophic consequences of their performance or behavior in social situations should be the focus of treatment.

The core component of cognitive therapy is challenging the validity of automatic thoughts. This can be done in various ways (Table 4–18): by listing the evidence in support of and against automatic thoughts (and in support of and against everything that such thoughts imply), by identifying cognitive errors that patients are making (e.g., catastrophizing, mind-reading, personalization, "all-or-nothing" thinking [Butler and Wells, 1995]), by conducting behavioral experiments, and, sometimes, by using paradoxical interventions. The goal of the challenging exercises is for patients to understand the basis of their irrational thinking, which would then make it possible for them to change it.

The final component of cognitive therapy is introducing and exploring alternative, more rational ways through which patients might perceive

TABLE 4–17. Typical Automatic Thoughts of Patients with Social Anxiety Disorder

Assumptions of What Patients Might Do or What Might Happen to Them

"I will embarrass myself."

"I won't know what I'm doing."

"I will talk nonsense."

"I will lose control."

"I will start shaking."

"I will blush."

"I will lose my voice."

"I won't be able to say what I wanted."

Assumptions of How Others Will Respond or What Others Might Think

"Everyone will laugh at me."

"They will think I am stupid."

"They will think I am a fool."

"They will see that I am anxious."

"They will think something is seriously wrong with me."

TABLE 4–18. Procedures Used to Challenge Validity of Automatic Thoughts in Social Anxiety Disorder

Procedures	Components or Examples of Procedures
Listing the evidence in support of and against automatic thoughts (and in support of and against everything that such thoughts imply)	Questions that patients need to ask: How do I know that they will laugh at me? Why do I think that I will embarrass myself? What will happen if I do come across as awkward?
Identifying and challenging cognitive errors:	Questions that patients need to ask:
Catastrophizing	What will happen if I make a mistake?
Mind-reading	How do others know how I feel?
Personalization	Why do I think that it all has to do with me?
"All-or-nothing" thinking	What will happen if I don't do it the right way? Will I lose it completely?
Behavioral experiments	Asking for directions and finding out that no one is giving the patient a "strange look"
Paradoxical procedures	Being deliberately clumsy and realizing that nothing catastrophic happens as a result

186

themselves and others and understand social situations more realistically. Alternative interpretations, appraisals, views, and understanding should be subjected to validation in the same way that automatic, dysfunctional thoughts are. Only if the alternatives pass this test and patients are satisfied with their validity will they be fully accepted by patients. An example of this part of cognitive therapy is given in Table 4–19.

Combined Exposure-Based and Cognitive Techniques

Although exposure-based therapy has proved valuable and essential for the treatment of social anxiety disorder, it does not address directly the underlying dysfunctional beliefs and patients' self-perception. Likewise, pure cognitive therapy may be less successful than exposure in reducing avoidance of social situations. Therefore, it appears logical to combine behavioral (exposure-based) and cognitive treatment approaches—a strategy first espoused by Butler et al. (1984) and subsequently supported by reports of the superiority of combined treatment over exposure alone (Mattick and Peters, 1988; Mattick et al., 1989).

Another view, derived mainly from meta-analytic studies, stipulates that adding cognitive therapy techniques to exposure-based therapy in social anxiety disorder does not produce results better than results of exposure-based therapy alone (e.g., Feske and Chambless, 1995; Taylor, 1996). Also, if the cognitive change produced by exposure therapy (Mattick

TABLE 4–19. Example of Replacing Automatic, Dysfunctional Thoughts in Social Anxiety Disorder with Realistic, "Normalizing" Alternatives

Previous Automatic Thought	Alternatives
I will look stupid because I don't know how to ask to buy tickets correctly.	There is no "correct" way of asking for tickets.
	Even if I ask in a way that is unusual, I will still get the tickets.
	If I worry too much about how I look to others, I may not get things done.
	Looking clumsy or inexperienced is not the same as looking stupid.
	I can live with the thought that I may look stupid to some, because I know I am not stupid.
	I will not worry about people who judge others on the basis of their behavior in trivial situations.
	I will not worry too much about how I appear to others.

and Peters, 1988; Newman et al., 1994) is sufficient, the use of cognitive therapy might be superfluous.

Regardless of this controversy, a combined (cognitive-behavioral) approach to the treatment of social anxiety disorder is reasonable, appears complementary, and is widely used in clinical practice. There are encouraging reports (e.g., Turner et al., 1995) that gains with CBT are maintained over prolonged periods of time.

Group Therapy

Cognitive-behavioral therapy for social anxiety disorder may be conducted in group settings, as they offer some distinct advantages over individual treatment. These advantages include simulation of various social situations, greater opportunities for social exposure and different forms of role-play, support from other members of the group, learning through observation of other group members, the giving and receiving of feedback about social performance, and modification of one's own attitudes and views.

Group therapy may also have some disadvantages. For example, many patients with social anxiety disorder initially find groups intimidating. In group therapy, there is also less opportunity for individual members to work through their own, relatively specific problems. Some patients may not be suitable for group therapy programs, because their personality characteristics (e.g., argumentativeness, hostility) might have an adverse effect on group dynamics. A compromise solution for some patients may be to offer them individual therapy first (which might focus on building social skills or on the more personal, specific issues), and then enroll them in a group.

A decision as to whether a patient is to be treated individually or in a group should be based on the specific circumstances of each patient. It has not been demonstrated that group cognitive therapy for social anxiety disorder is more efficacious than the individually based treatment approach (Stangier et al., 2003).

Cognitive-behavioral group therapy for social anxiety disorder, as developed by Heimberg and colleagues, is a highly structured form of treatment, consisting of 12 sessions held once a week and conducted by two therapists in a group of six patients. This form of treatment incorporates most of the ingredients of cognitive therapy and exposure-based treatment discussed above for social anxiety disorder, and has established itself as the standard psychological treatment of social anxiety disorder. It was also found to be efficacious (Heimberg et al., 1990a; 1993). Furthermore, significant clinical improvement was found to persist for 5 years following cessation of cognitive-behavioral group treatment (Heimberg et al., 1993).

Psychodynamic Psychotherapy

The aim of psychodynamic psychotherapy in social anxiety disorder is to uncover and work through the specific, underlying conflicts and issues that underlie this disorder. There is no single type of unconscious conflict that characterizes all patients with social anxiety disorder, as this condition may have different developmental antecedents (see Etiology and Pathogenesis, above). As with psychodynamic psychotherapy in general, the conflicts in social anxiety disorder are uncovered and worked through primarily by means of transference and interpretation.

The relatively specific issues in the course of the psychodynamic psychotherapy of social anxiety disorder include patients' expectations to be judged negatively and harshly by the therapist along with mistrust toward the therapist, patients' feelings of shame for wanting to succeed or win, and various narcissistic issues, such as pursuit of perfection and underlying needs for praise and admiration.

COMBINED TREATMENTS

Combining medications and CBT for social anxiety disorder seems to be common in clinical practice. However, it is unclear how these treatment modalities should be optimally combined—for example, what the sequence of their administration should be. One form of treatment is usually started first (most commonly pharmacotherapy), and then another treatment (usually CBT) is added, particularly if there has been an insufficient response to the initial treatment or if the goal is to enhance the response to the initial treatment by adding another one. General issues that arise in the course of combining pharmacotherapy and CBT are discussed in Chapter 2.

There have been very few studies examining the efficacy of combined treatment in social anxiety disorder. Not unexpectedly, their results are conflicting. In one study (Blomhoff et al., 2001), after 24-week treatment there were no significant differences in efficacy between treatments with sertraline plus exposure, sertraline alone, and exposure alone. However, exposure alone was not more efficacious than placebo, whereas treatments with sertraline plus exposure and sertraline alone were found to be more efficacious than placebo. In an extension of this study (Haug et al., 2003), patients treated for 24 weeks with sertraline alone, exposure alone, and sertraline plus exposure were compared 1 year after the beginning of treatment. Following cessation of treatment, patients treated with exposure alone continued to improve, whereas those treated with sertraline exhibited a tendency toward deterioration. The authors concluded that in the long term, exposure alone was more efficacious than a combination of exposure and sertraline, a finding similar to the long-term effects of combined pharmacotherapy and CBT in panic disorder (see Chapter 2). These discrepant findings clearly call for more research in this area, with the hope that such research would reflect the reality of clinical practice more accurately.

5
Specific Phobias

Specific phobias (also referred to as simple and isolated phobias) represent a heterogeneous group of disorders characterized by excessive and irrational fear of one of relatively few and usually related objects, situations, places, phenomena, or activities (phobic stimuli). These phobic stimuli are either avoided or endured with intense anxiety or discomfort.

CLINICAL FEATURES

As with other phobic disorders (agoraphobia and social anxiety disorder), the main features of specific phobias are excessive, persistent, and irrational fear of certain phobic stimuli and avoidance of these stimuli as much as possible. In contrast to agoraphobia and social anxiety disorder, the nature of phobic stimuli is different; patients with specific phobias are fearful of certain animals, heights, the sight of blood, flying, etc. Also, reasons for the fear of phobic stimuli are usually different from reasons for the phobic fear given by patients with agoraphobia and social anxiety disorder (Table 5–1). One reason has to do with some aspects of the phobic stimulus that may represent a real danger under certain circumstances. For example, people can be bitten by venomous snakes, one can fall from a high-rise

TABLE 5–1. Reasons for Fear and Avoidance in Specific Phobias

- Some aspects of the phobic stimulus represent a real threat under certain circumstances.
- Patients fear certain symptoms and their anticipated consequences (e.g., loss of control), which might occur upon exposure to a phobic stimulus.
- Patients experience a feeling of disgust.

building, and planes do crash occasionally. Patients with phobias of snakes, heights, and flying, however, grossly exaggerate the likelihood of any of this happening to them.

Another reason for fearing certain phobic stimuli in specific phobias is related to the reasons given by patients with agoraphobia and by some with social anxiety disorder (Table 5–1). That is, some patients with a specific phobia may be afraid of certain symptoms that they expect upon exposure to a phobic stimulus. Furthermore, they may be fearful of the anticipated consequences of these symptoms, for example, loss of control or some somatic catastrophe. For example, patients with claustrophobia often say that they are afraid of enclosed places because they will not have enough air and will then suffocate and die. Patients with a phobia of having blood drawn are often afraid that they will faint and "make a scene" in corresponding situations; some feel quite embarrassed about this, in a way that would almost qualify this fear as a form of social anxiety.

Yet another reason underlying some specific phobias is a feeling of disgust (Table 5–1). Some patients may be afraid of snakes not so much because they are potentially dangerous but because they elicit a strong feeling of disgust. Sometimes it is difficult to ascertain whether the primary emotion is fear or disgust, or whether both are present, with avoidance of the phobic stimuli being driven by both feelings.

Of course, two or more reasons for fearing phobic stimuli may be present in patients with a particular specific phobia. For example, patients who are fearful of heights may be afraid of that situation both because they might fall and because they might feel lightheaded and dizzy in high places, and then lose control and fall. Likewise, a patient with a phobia of having blood drawn may anticipate feeling disgusted at the sight of blood, fear the pain involved, and be afraid of fainting. It is important to understand the underlying reasons for any particular phobia, because successful treatment depends in part on this understanding.

Although persistent fear of phobic stimuli is a feature of specific phobias, the intensity of fear varies depending on whether patients are in contact or expect to be in contact with their phobic stimuli. Panic attacks are not rare if the contact with phobic stimuli cannot be prevented and if patients are unable to escape situations in which these contacts do occur. The phobia will not represent a clinical problem as long as its sufferers are able to avoid phobic stimuli without a cost to their functioning. The phobia turns into a psychiatric disorder only when the fear becomes too distressing, avoidance is no longer possible, and/or avoidance starts to interfere significantly with functioning. For example, a person with a long-standing fear of flying and avoidance of air travel who has recently received a job promotion and is now expected to make frequent business trips by plane can no longer resort to avoidance. The person may find it very difficult to cope with the demands of the new situation and seeks professional help for the phobia.

There are several subtypes of specific phobias that were originally proposed on the basis of phenomenology, that is, the nature of phobic stimuli. According to DSM-IV-TR, these subtypes are as follows: phobias of animals, phobias of stimuli (e.g., water, heights) that occur in the natural environment, blood-injection-injury phobia, situational phobias, and other types of phobias (e.g., choking phobia). In addition to phenomenology, these subtypes of specific phobias may also be differentiated on the basis of the usual age of onset, female-to-male ratio, presence of unexpected panic attacks, dominant underlying themes, problems, or issues, degree to which a familial component is present, and other characteristics (Table 5-2).

Phobias of Animals

Although the reason for fearing certain animals lies in their dangerousness (e.g., sharks, lions, crocodiles), many dangerous animals are not objects of an animal phobia, as most people afraid of these animals do not feel impaired by such fear (e.g., they simply avoid places where they might encounter dangerous animals). Indeed, patients with animal phobia are usually afraid of animals such as snakes, dogs, cats, spiders and other insects, rats, and mice. Only a minority of these animals is dangerous, so factors other than danger seem to be more important in determining whether particular animals will be feared and avoided to the extent characteristic of a phobia. The most important of these factors seems to be a feeling of disgust elicited by some animals (e.g., Tolin et al., 1997; Lipsitz et al., 2002). It has been argued (McNally, 2002) that even with animals such as spiders, the main underlying issue is a feeling of profound disgust rather than a perception of danger, considering that only 0.1% of all the varieties of spiders are dangerous to humans.

The universal nature of the feeling of disgust probably accounts for the finding that disgust-relevant animals (e.g., spiders, cockroaches, worms) are feared to the same or very similar extent in different countries

TABLE 5–2. Characteristics of the subtypes of specific phobias

Characteristics	Animal Phobias Subtype	Natural Environment	Blood-Injection-Injury Phobia	Situational Phobias
Onset	Childhood	Variable	Childhood	Adolescence, early 20s
Female-male ratio	Women > men	Women > men	Women = men	Women > men
Presence of unexpected panic attacks	No	No	No	Yes
Dominant theme, problem or issue	Disgust	Exaggerated appraisal of danger	Disgust, concern about fainting	Fear of physical symptoms or panic attack, exaggerated appraisal of danger
Familial component	Less prominent	Less prominent	More prominent	Less prominent
Unique patho-physiology	No	No	Yes	No

(e.g., Davey et al., 1998). Animal phobias typically have an onset in childhood and are more common among women (Table 5–2).

Phobia of Eements in Natural Environment

This is a heterogeneous group of phobias, which includes phobias of heights (acrophobia), water, storms, and thunder and/or lightening. It appears that in many patients with phobias from this group, particularly patients with phobias of heights and water, there is no history of contact or traumatic experience with the phobic stimuli prior to the onset of phobia. This finding may suggest that such phobias have an "innate," survival-relevant character (see Etiology and Pathogenesis, below).

The age of onset of natural environment phobias varies (Table 5–2), but in many cases it tends to be early. The main underlying theme in this subtype of phobia is the danger associated with phobic stimuli (Lipsitz et al., 2002). That is, patients with the phobia of heights are typically afraid of falling off, whereas those with the water phobia are afraid of drowning.

Blood-Injection-Injury Phobia

This is a unique type of specific phobia (Table 5–2). Unlike all other phobias, it is characterized by a pathophysiological reaction to the phobic stimulus which has two phases: after initial and short-lasting tachycardia, there is a parasympathetic activation and vasovagal response, with bradycardia and hypotension, which very often—in more that 75% of cases—leads to fainting (vasovagal syncope). Many patients feel very embarrassed about fainting and sometimes resort to extensive avoidance because they expect to faint when they see blood or when they should have their blood drawn. This avoidance can be so extreme that patients' health is jeopardized because they refuse to undergo the necessary medical procedures.

A feeling of disgust (at the sight of blood or needle injuring a person's physical integrity) has been reported as the main underlying problem (Page, 1994; Tolin et al., 1997; Lipsitz et al., 2002), thus blood-injection-injury phobia can be conceptualized as one of the disgust-driven phobias. Alternatively, the avoidance associated with blood-injection-injury phobia may also be understood as a response to the anticipation of fainting in phobic situations.

It appears that this subtype of phobia has a stronger familial component than other subtypes of specific phobias (e.g., Marks, 1988). Unlike other subtypes of specific phobias, the proportion of women and men with blood-injection-injury phobia is about the same (see Epidemiology, below). Most cases have an onset in childhood.

Situational Phobias

As their name suggests, these phobias denote a fear of certain situations. The most common types of situational phobias are claustrophobia, fear of flying, and phobia of driving. This subtype of specific phobias generally has a later onset than other subtypes (see Epidemiology, below). There is some disagreement as to what the main underlying concern or problem is for patients with situational phobias (Table 5–2); some (Craske and Sipsas, 1992) suggest that it is the fear of physical symptoms and panic-like sensations, while others (Lipsitz et al., 2002) report that the main issue for these patients is an expectation of danger in the specific situations they are afraid of. In any case, unexpected panic attacks seem to occur far more often in patients with situational phobias than in those with other subtypes of specific phobias (Ehlers et al., 1994; Lipsitz et al., 2002), so their preoccupation with or fear of panic and its symptoms is quite understandable.

There is a phenomenological overlap between situational phobias and agoraphobia, and the two may co-occur; other similarities between situational phobias and agoraphobia are reviewed in Relationship Between Specific Phobias and Other Disorders (below).

A typical example of the situational phobia is claustrophobia—fear of small, enclosed places. Being in an elevator is a prototypical claustrophobic situation, but patients with claustrophobia are often afraid of other situations, such as long tunnels, underground passages, subways, cellars, caves, mines, and even airplanes. The essence of claustrophobia is a fear of being confined to a small place from which escape is difficult or impossible. Patients with claustrophobia typically state that they are afraid of being "stuck" or "trapped"; some have frightening images of being "buried alive" in case of an underground accident. They may also voice a concern that there would be no one to help them in a claustrophobic situation. Patients with claustrophobia are often afraid of not having enough air and of choking in a claustrophobic situation. If they have a panic attack in such a situation, their respiratory symptoms (shortness of breath, choking sensations) may be particularly prominent or paid attention to, because of the catastrophic misinterpretations of these symptoms.

Fear of flying is a unique type of situational phobia in that there may be different reasons underlying this fear: (1) confinement, as in claustrophobia; (2) being high above the ground, as in fear of heights; (3) possibility of having a panic attack, as in agoraphobia; and (4) possibility of an accident (plane crash), as in "true" phobia of flying. Sometimes there is more than one reason behind the fear of flying in a particular patient.

Fear of driving or travel is another type of phobia in which it is important to establish the underlying reason for fear. As with patients who fear flying, patients with this type of phobia may be afraid of having a panic attack while being in a car, train, or other vehicle (in which case, this fear may be a part of agoraphobia), or they may be excessively afraid of accidents. Fear of driving or travel sometimes precedes the onset of agoraphobia.

Other Types of Specific Phobias

Phobia of Choking
This type of phobia is less common and is characterized by the fear of swallowing. This fear is usually a result of the belief that swallowing food or even drinking fluids may lead to choking; the fear typically follows accidental choking on food. In the most severe cases, patients may lose much weight or become dehydrated because of their failure to have an adequate intake of food and fluids. In less severe and more typical cases, patients with this phobia may have trouble swallowing medications, are extremely

slow while eating or drinking, and may refuse certain types of food because of the concern that they might choke while trying to swallow it.

Disease Phobia

Disease phobia is characterized by excessive fear of getting a serious, life-threatening disease. It is directly related to the common perception of diseases; the greater the perception of the disease as dangerous and incurable, the higher the likelihood that it will become the focus of a phobia. This helps explain the widespread phobic fear of tuberculosis, syphilis, and other incurable bacterial infections a century ago, and the widespread AIDS phobia and cancer phobia today.

Patients with a disease phobia tend to avoid all situations, people, objects, or other stimuli that remind them of the dreaded disease. This avoidance is rarely incapacitating but may at times be embarrassing or adversely affect treatment-seeking behavior.

Dental Phobia

Dental phobia is a term usually used to denote fear of various dental procedures. However, it is a heterogeneous condition, and upon detailed analysis, it may point to one or more of the following underlying problems: (1) fear of needles, blood, and/or specific dental interventions, which may be indistinguishable from the blood-injection-injury phobia (and include fainting); (2) fear of pain; (3) fear of local anesthesia, which may entail fear of an allergic reaction and/or fear of losing control; (4) fear of becoming infected with a disease, such as HIV/AIDS; (5) fear of being confined to the dentist's chair, which may be a form of situational phobia or a part of agoraphobia (in the latter case, there is a particularly strong fear that a panic attack might occur while the patient is seated in the dentist's chair); and (6) fear of choking during dental intervention.

It is important to understand the nature of the underlying fear and plan treatment accordingly. The avoidance associated with dental phobia may lead to a serious neglect of dental health, thereby making later dental interventions more complicated.

Space Phobia

This is a rare type of specific phobia, characterized by the fear of losing balance and/or falling. Patients with this type of phobia are typically concerned that they might fall if they do not have anything to lean on. Space phobia may have severe consequences in terms of limiting patients' mobility to the extent that they become bed-ridden.

Relationship Between Specific Phobias and Other Disorders

Unlike most other anxiety disorders, specific phobias represent a relatively pure form of psychopathology, which does not occur very often with other psychiatric disorders. Epidemiological findings (Magee et al., 1996) contradict this clinical impression, however, as they suggest that specific phobias do co-occur frequently with other anxiety disorders. When patients with specific phobias suffer from other psychiatric conditions, the co-occurring disorders are usually agoraphobia or social anxiety disorder.

Specific phobias are frequently diagnosed as a co-occurring condition when the principal disorder for which help is being sought is another anxiety disorder (deRuiter et al., 1989; Sanderson et al., 1990; Starcevic et al., 1992b). This suggests that specific phobias may be complicated by other anxiety disorders, especially since in most cases of co-occurrence, specific phobias tend to precede the onset of other anxiety disorders. Alternatively, specific phobias may be overdiagnosed in the context of another anxiety disorder, perhaps because of the lowering of a diagnostic threshold for specific phobias under these circumstances. A diagnosis of a specific phobia co-occurring with another principal anxiety disorder rarely has significant clinical implications.

Specific Phobias and Agoraphobia

There is a significant relationship between a subtype of specific phobia, claustrophobia, and agoraphobia (Table 5–3). The situations feared and avoided by patients with claustrophobia and agoraphobia (e.g., elevators, tunnels, planes, other enclosed places) are often very similar and pertain to confinement. Patients may mention a similar reason for avoidance—fear of certain physical symptoms or panic attack occurring in the phobic situations. Furthermore, both claustrophobia and agoraphobia are more common in women and have an onset at approximately the same age (early twenties).

However, there are also important differences between claustrophobia and agoraphobia (Table 5–3). Patients with agoraphobia typically avoid a wider range of situations (in addition to those typical of claustrophobia), and they are more likely to report symptoms of unsteadiness, dizziness, and fainting feelings upon exposure to phobic stimuli, unlike patients with claustrophobia who are more troubled by breathing problems, "air hunger," and choking-like sensations when they find themselves in claustrophobic situations. Largely as a result of the different symptoms experienced and/or anticipated, patients with claustrophobia and agora-

TABLE 5–3. Similarities and Differences Between Claustrophobia and Agoraphobia

Similarities

Type of situations feared and avoided (confinement-type situations)

Reason for avoidance: fear of certain physical symptoms and/or fear of a panic attack occurring in the phobic situations

More common in women

Onset at approximately the same age (early 20s)

	Differences	
Criteria for Differentiation	*Claustrophobia*	*Agoraphobia*
Range of situations avoided	More constricted	Wider, including non-claustrophobic situations
Symptoms upon exposure to phobic situations	Breathing difficulties, "air hunger," choking-like sensations	Unsteadiness, dizziness, fainting feelings
Catastrophic cognitions	Choking	Fainting, losing consciousness
Intensity of phobic fear over time	More constant	More often tends to fluctuate

phobia have different catastrophic cognitions: claustrophobic patients are more likely to be concerned about suffocation in a phobic situation, whereas those with agoraphobia more often worry about the possibility of fainting and losing consciousness. There are further, more subtle differences between claustrophobia and agoraphobia: for example, the intensity of fear in patients with claustrophobia tends less often to fluctuate in comparison with the intensity of fear in agoraphobia.

Claustrophobia and agoraphobia do not exclude each other as diagnoses and can co-occur in the same person at the same time. However, there is sometimes a tendency to view claustrophobic fears as part of agoraphobia, because the latter is a wider psychopathological entity. Claustrophobia may sometimes precede the onset of agoraphobia.

Other types of situational phobias may also co-occur with agoraphobia, and in these cases it is important to ascertain, on the basis of the reason given for fear and avoidance, whether they should be conceptualized as part of agoraphobia or as disorders in their own right. When patients are afraid of driving, travel, or flying because they are excessively concerned about accidents and the possibility of having panic attacks (and then not being able to escape from a car, bus, train, boat, or plane), they qualify for diagnoses of both specific phobia and agoraphobia. If one of these reasons for fear and avoidance predominates, only one diagnosis should be given.

Still another example of a specific phobia that may co-occur with agoraphobia is the phobia of heights. Patients with this phobia are afraid of heights mainly because they are afraid of falling. The fear of this happening is strengthened by the expectation of having a panic attack in that situation, which is more characteristic of agoraphobia. Again, both diagnoses are warranted if both reasons for fear and avoidance of heights are given, with the diagnosis of agoraphobia being more appropriate if, in addition to heights, patients are afraid of other, more typical agoraphobic situations.

ASSESSMENT

Diagnostic Issues

A diagnosis of specific phobia is made on the basis of the same criteria used for diagnosing phobic disorders in general (see Table 4–4). The most difficult diagnostic criterion is the one pertaining to the impairment in functioning *as a result* of a phobia. This criterion also marks the boundary between normal or diagnostically "subthreshold" fears and a diagnosis of specific phobia. For example, while the fear of flying is very common in the general population and cannot by itself be considered an illness, refusal of an attractive job by a person with a severe fear of flying because that job would involve frequent airplane travel would suggest that this person suffers from a phobic disorder. Because of the relatively circumscribed nature of phobic stimuli and greater ease with which they are avoided, the impairment in a specific phobia is usually not as generalized as it is in agoraphobia and social anxiety disorder; that is, only certain areas of functioning tend to be affected by specific phobias.

If the person is not clearly impaired by the phobia, for a diagnosis to be made, affected persons must be troubled or distressed by their fear and/or avoidance. The wider context of fear and avoidance and the likelihood of exposure to a phobic stimulus also play a role in determining whether any given fear qualifies for a diagnosis of specific phobia—and even when this diagnosis is made, whether it is of clinical importance. For example, a phobia of snakes is not clinically significant if the sufferer is unlikely to come in contact with snakes because of the place where the person resides, his or her lifestyle, and/or type of job.

The diagnostic criteria for specific phobias are essentially the same in DSM-IV-TR and ICD-10. The advantage of DSM-IV-TR is in its subtyping scheme. During the assessment, it is good practice to inquire whether patients have fears other than those that they report spontaneously; many patients tend to have fears of several stimuli within the same subtype of specific phobias. For example, patients with a phobia of elevators often have phobic fears of tunnels, underground passages, subways, cellars, planes, and generally all situations and places from which escape might be difficult. Patients may also have fears from different specific phobia subtypes (e.g., Hofmann et al., 1997; Curtis et al., 1998).

In an interview situation, patients with specific phobias usually do not seem anxious or troubled as long as they do not have to talk about the objects of their phobias and as long as they do not have to face the phobic stimuli. When they do address or face these stimuli, patients have typical physiological and behavioral fear responses, including panic attacks, avoidance, and escape. This contrast in the patients' appearance and behavior, depending on whether they have to face phobic stimuli or talk about them, may be quite striking.

Counterphobic behavior may suggest presence of a phobic disorder, although the phobia has been "disguised." This behavior pertains to excessive confrontation with danger and sources of fear and has the purpose of denying that there is any danger and any fear at all. Such behaviors may be relatively transient or more persistent. The latter is seen in certain professions, for example, among some automobile race drivers.

A diagnosis of specific phobia should not be made if the phobic features can be better accounted for by another, more broadly conceptualized psychiatric condition, such as obsessive-compulsive disorder, agoraphobia, posttraumatic stress disorder, social anxiety disorder, separation anxiety disorder, or even a psychotic disorder.

Assessment Instruments

The assessment instruments for specific phobias are used to ascertain the presence of various types of fears and phobias, assess the severity of fear and/or avoidance, and monitor changes during treatment. The most comprehensive among these instruments is the Fear Survey Schedule (Wolpe and Lang, 1964), but because of its length, it is not particularly suitable for routine use in clinical practice. Several modifications of the Fear Survey Schedule have been developed since its original publication.

Instruments that measure the severity of fear and avoidance in certain types of specific phobia may be more useful for clinical work with patients who suffer from these phobias. An example of such an instrument is the commonly used self-report Fear Questionnaire (Marks and Mathews, 1979), which assesses avoidance associated with agoraphobia, social anxiety disorder, and blood-injury phobia. Another instrument that specifically assesses various aspects of the blood-injection-injury phobia is the Blood-Injection Symptom Scale (Page et al., 1997).

Differential Diagnosis

The most common disorders for consideration in the differential diagnosis of specific phobias include agoraphobia, obsessive-compulsive disorder, and hypochondriasis. The relationship between specific phobias and agoraphobia and criteria for making a diagnostic distinction between the two are presented in Relationship Between Specific Phobias and Other Disorders (above).

Obsessive-compulsive disorder may sometimes resemble a phobic disorder, especially when prominent avoidance is part of its clinical presentation. The differentiation between the two is based mainly on reasons for fear and avoidance. For example, patients who are afraid of heights because they might have an urge to jump off probably suffer from obsessive-compulsive disorder, not a phobia of heights. The same consideration applies to patients who are afraid of driving because they have disturbing images of running off the road, patients who fear needles and all sharp objects (because these could be used to hurt someone), or patients who have distressing thoughts about contamination and infectious diseases and therefore avoid using public toilets and payphones. In these cases, patients are unlikely to have a "simple" driving phobia, blood–injection–injury phobia, or disease/contamination phobia, respectively.

Occasionally, hypochondriasis needs to be differentiated from disease phobia. While patients with hypochondriasis are usually afraid that they already have a serious physical disease, patients with disease phobia fear that they will become a victim of such a disease in the future. In addition, patients with disease phobia are more likely to avoid various disease-related situations, activities, and stimuli (e.g., hospitals, doctors, conversations about health and illness), whereas patients with hypochondriasis make numerous visits to doctors, use health care excessively, and show much interest in all matters related to health and illness.

EPIDEMIOLOGY

The main epidemiological data on specific phobias are presented in Table 5–4. Specific phobias are among the most common psychiatric disorders. The lifetime prevalence of specific phobias in the U.S. National Comorbidity Survey was estimated at 11.3% (Kessler et al., 1994; Magee et al., 1996), whereas their prevalence in the previous Epidemiologic Catchment Area

TABLE 5–4. Epidemiological Data for Specific Phobias

- Lifetime prevalence (U.S.): 11.3%–12.5%
- Prevalence rates are likely to be different in different countries.
- The order of frequency of different subtypes of specific phobias appears to vary, depending on the setting (general vs. clinical population) and cultural and social factors.
- Generally more common among women, with a ratio of 2–2.5:1 (except for blood-injection-injury phobia)
- Usual age of onset depends on the subtype of phobia:

  Animal phobias: (early) childhood

  Blood-injection-injury phobia: (later) childhood

  Situational phobias: adolescence, early 20s

  Natural environment subtype of phobias: variable
- Very few persons with specific phobias (<1%) seek professional help.

study was 12.5% (Regier et al., 1988). It is likely that the prevalence rates of specific phobias in other countries are different, considering the influence of cultural factors on the patterning of phobias (e.g., Raguram and Bhide, 1985; Chambers et al., 1986). The prevalence rate figures may also be affected by the differences in meeting the impairment criterion required for the diagnosis of specific phobias.

In adult clinical populations, the most frequent subtype of specific phobia is situational phobia, followed by the natural environment, blood-injection-injury, and animal subtypes (American Psychiatric Association, 2000). Within these subtypes, claustrophobia, phobia of driving or flying, phobia of heights, and spider phobia are commonly seen in clinical practice. Dental phobia is also not rare in clinical populations. Help-seeking patterns for specific phobias vary from one country to another and are also determined by the degree of dysfunction and impairment caused by the phobias. The order of frequency of the specific phobia subtypes may be different in the general adult population in the United States, as reported by the Epidemiologic Catchment Area study (Eaton et al., 1991): the most common types of phobias in the community are phobias of small animals (e.g., insects) and snakes, followed by phobias of heights, water, storms, closed spaces, and other animals. An earlier epidemiological survey (Agras et al., 1969) found the blood-injection-injury phobia to be the most frequent, followed by the natural environment, and animal and situational subtypes.

All subtypes of specific phobias, except for blood-injection-injury phobia, are more commonly seen among women, with the female-to-male ratio being approximately 2–2.5:1 (Bourdon et al., 1988; Fredrikson et al., 1996; Magee et al., 1996). The prevalence of blood-injection-injury phobia is approximately the same in women and men (Agras et al., 1969; Himle et al., 1989; Fredrikson et al., 1996). Women were also found to be more likely to have several types of specific phobias (Fredrikson et al., 1996). A greater prevalence of phobic fears among women is usually considered a consequence of social and cultural factors; that is, the expression of fear is more socially acceptable in women than it is in men, and there are fewer expectations from women to perform fearlessly.

The age of onset of specific phobias depends on the subtype of phobia. Phobias of animals and blood-injection-injury phobia usually appear in childhood, while the situational phobias occur later, in adolescence or early 20s (Öst, 1987b; Himle et al., 1989; Lipsitz et al., 2002). The mean ages of onset for various types of specific phobias are as follows (Öst, 1987b): for animal phobia, 7 years; for blood-injection-injury phobia, 9 years; for dental phobia, 12 years; and for claustrophobia, 20 years. The onset of phobias encompassed by the natural environment subtype of specific phobias appears to be variable; for example, phobia of heights seems to have a later onset.

The prevalence of specific phobias in clinical populations is lower than that of agoraphobia and social anxiety disorder. It has been estimated that less than 1% of all persons with specific phobias seek treatment (Agras et al., 1969; Regier et al., 1990). This is likely a consequence of less impairment and less distress being associated with specific phobias in comparison with agoraphobia and social anxiety disorder. It is generally easier for the sufferers of specific phobias to avoid their relatively circumscribed phobic stimuli than it is for the sufferers of agoraphobia and social anxiety disorder to avoid their multiple phobic situations.

COURSE AND PROGNOSIS

The course of specific phobias ranges from spontaneous remission to chronicity. Some children with specific phobias seem to grow out of their phobia and experience remission without any treatment. It is not clear whether any particular type of phobia is more likely to disappear, but it has been speculated that this may be the case more with phobias of animals, darkness, thunder, and water. One study (Agras et al., 1972) showed that practically all patients with specific phobias who were younger than 20 reported improvement at follow-up; in contrast, improvement was reported by less than one-half of adults with specific phobias. If a phobia in adults has continuously been present from childhood, its spontaneous disappearance is uncommon and may occur in only 20% of cases.

The course of specific phobias may depend less on the type of phobia than on the mode of its onset and persistence of avoidance. Thus, phobias that appear after traumatic events may be more chronic than phobias that develop as a result of the transmission of information or observational learning (see Etiology and Pathogenesis, below). The most persistent course may be seen in those phobias that were apparently not learned (e.g., some cases of phobia of heights, water, or spiders); the fact that it is difficult for these phobias to be extinguished may suggest that they have survival value. As for the effects of avoidance on the course of specific phobias, the longer patients avoid phobic stimuli, the more likely they are to maintain their phobia for long periods of time. If, however, life circumstances force patients to expose themselves to phobic stimuli, there is greater opportunity for natural habituation of fears to occur and greater likelihood for patients to no longer resort to avoidance behavior.

Disgust driven phobias (e.g., many cases of blood-injection-injury phobia and spider phobia) may be more difficult to extinguish and more likely to have a chronic course.

Psychiatric complications of specific phobias (e.g., depression, alcohol abuse) are rare, and in this respect, specific phobias are different from agoraphobia, social anxiety disorder, and most other anxiety disorders. However, specific phobias may precede other anxiety disorders. Whether the presence of specific phobias should be considered a risk factor for developing other anxiety disorders is not known; even when specific phobias seem to represent this risk factor, it is not clear whether they confer a specific or nonspecific predisposition for developing other anxiety disorders. It appears that some situational phobias (particularly claustrophobia and phobia of driving or traveling) may predispose patients to agoraphobia.

Despite the fact that they often have a chronic course and are unlikely to disappear without treatment, the prognosis of specific phobias is generally good, because they rarely have an incapacitating effect on functioning. In addition, their prognosis tends to be favorable because of fewer psychiatric complications and their fairly encapsulated nature (i.e., lacking the tendency to encompass more and more phobic stimuli over time and to progressively lead to avoidance of an even greater number of phobic stimuli).

ETIOLOGY AND PATHOGENESIS

Specific phobias are a heterogeneous group of disorders unlikely to have common etiology and pathogenesis. Moreover, there are often several etiological and pathogenetic factors operating within the same type of phobia. For example, phobias of certain animals may be innate, have a hereditary component, or appear as a result of traumatic experience, observational learning, and/or transmission of relevant information.

BIOLOGICAL MODELS

Genetic Factors

One family study (Fyer et al., 1990) has found that the first-degree relatives of patients with specific phobia have a three times higher risk for specific phobia than the first-degree relatives of control subjects without any psychiatric disorder. However, this tendency for specific phobias to run in the families may be more a consequence of shared environment (and interactions among various family members) than a consequence of hereditary transmission, as suggested by the results of twin studies (Kendler et al., 1992c; Skre et al., 1993).

There is some indication (e.g., Marks, 1988; Fyer et al., 1990) that blood-injection-injury phobia has a stronger hereditary component than other types of specific phobias.

Neurobiological Factors

Very little is known about the neurobiology of specific phobias, and the few studies that have attempted to elucidate pathophysiological mechanisms and cerebral structures involved in the etiology and pathogenesis of specific phobias have not yielded consistent or significant results.

Nonassociative Theory

Although this theory (Menzies and Clarke, 1995) has emerged from psychological studies of etiological factors in specific phobias, it implicitly suggests some biological mechanism in the causation of certain types of specific phobias. It proposes that these phobias are not learned but are inborn.

The central tenet of the nonassociative theory is that at least some phobias are not acquired through associative learning; that is, for a phobia to occur, it is not necessary that the association be made between the initially neutral stimulus and perception of danger. This link is presumed to be automatic, i.e., innate. What is there to support this theory?

In many instances of phobias, there is no recollection or report of a traumatic or any other contact with the phobic stimulus before the onset of phobia; patients with such phobias or their parents typically state that the phobia has "always" been present or that it has been present from the very first, nontraumatic contact with the stimulus. This pattern was observed in some instances of water phobia, phobia of heights, and spider phobia (Menzies and Clarke, 1993a; 1993b; 1995), but was extended to other types of fear, such as "stranger anxiety" and separation anxiety in infants, and fears of pain, strong noise, and sudden loss of physical balance. The underlying hypothesis invokes the concepts of natural selection, survival, and preservation of the species. In other words, our ancestors developed fears of naturally occurring dangers and these fears were then incorporated into a human genetic code, becoming part of the transgenerationally transmitted genetic material. As a result, the human infant is innately equipped to protect itself from dangers, and therefore avoids potentially dangerous stimuli without previously being in contact with them.

Although humans are "prepared" to fear and avoid stimuli such as water, heights, and the like, most do not develop a phobia because of habituation, i.e., repeated nontraumatic exposure to the potentially phobic stimuli. Those who go on to develop phobias as adults do so because of incomplete habituation, because their fears have been reinforced directly or indirectly by their parents, or as a result of "dishabituation" in the context of stress (Menzies and Clarke, 1995).

PSYCHOLOGICAL MODELS

There are two main psychological models of the origin of specific phobias: the first model encompasses various accounts that have been derived from learning theory, whereas the second is the psychoanalytic account of phobias. The first model has been much more useful for clinical practice. The psychoanalytic model is mentioned for historical reasons and has limited clinical relevance.

Models Derived from Learning Theory

Stated very broadly, all models of specific phobias derived from learning theory postulate that phobic manifestations are a consequence of the learning process. Another characteristic common to these models is a distinction between the factors that give rise to phobias and factors that are responsible for their maintenance. Phobic fears can be acquired through classical (traumatic) conditioning, vicariously (by observing emotional reactions and behavior of others), and by transmission of relevant information

(Rachman, 1991). Phobias are maintained through avoidance by means of operant (instrumental) conditioning.

Classical (Pavlovian, Aversive, Traumatic) Conditioning

This is the oldest learning-theory account of the development of phobias. In essence, it conceptualizes phobia as a conditioned reflex. This was demonstrated through the case of "little Albert" by Watson and Rayner (1920). Albert was an 11-month-old boy who developed a phobia of white rats (initially a neutral, not an anxiety-provoking stimulus) after he had been repeatedly exposed to a white rat together with a loud noise (an aversive, unconditioned stimulus). Because the loud noise elicited an automatic, unconditioned fear response, its pairing with exposure to a white rat made Albert learn to fear white rats through association of the two. This fear then became a conditioned fear response to a newly conditioned stimulus (white rats). Albert not only showed fear every time he saw white rats (without hearing a loud noise at the same time) but also had a fear reaction to other objects that resembled white rats, such as white rabbits and white fur coats. The latter phenomenon came to be known as the *generalization* of the phobic stimuli.

Many people develop phobias after classical conditioning, which often has a form of traumatic experience. A typical example is a phobia of dogs that developed as a result of the specific trauma—an attack by a dog. Likewise, a person who was stuck in an elevator for hours may develop a phobia of elevators, and the person who had a sudden panic attack while driving may develop a phobia of driving. Phobias that occur as a result of traumatic conditioning tend to have an abrupt onset and are usually more severe; unlike phobias that appear through other mechanisms, these phobias occur at any age.

As demonstrated by one study (DiNardo et al., 1988), among people who had had a traumatic experience with dogs, the number of those who did and did not develop a phobia of dogs was approximately the same. This suggests that other factors (e.g., genetic vulnerability, aspects of personality such as neuroticism, negative appraisals of the traumatic situation and/or of one's skills of coping with such a situation) may also contribute to the development of phobias.

Preparedness "Variant" of the Conditioning Theory

Proponents of the classical conditioning model have had difficulty explaining the fact that out of the vast pool of potential phobic stimuli, only relatively few become the focus of phobias. In an attempt to overcome this limitation of the classical conditioning model, Seligman (1971) has suggested that phobic stimuli are not subject to random selection in the process of conditioning: humans are "prepared" to fear certain objects and/or situations because these stimuli indicated physical danger and a threat to survival to our ancestors (even though they do not necessarily represent such a threat today). Because phobias have a survival value, Seligman has also postulated that they are difficult to extinguish. This came to be known as the *preparedness theory* of fear acquisition. Its main tenets have not received sufficient support (e.g., McNally, 1987).

Vicarious (Observational) Learning

Phobias may be acquired through observation of another person's fearful behavior in a particular situation and the corresponding nonverbal cues. This is particularly common with children, who can learn from their parents to be afraid of certain animals or situations. Although parents do not share with their children that they have particular fears, children observe that their parents are afraid and adopt the same fear and fear-related behavior (e.g., avoidance), whether through imitation of or identification with their parents. Phobias that develop through this mechanism are usually less severe and are more easily subject to extinction than phobias acquired through traumatic conditioning.

Learning Through Transmission of Relevant Information

Phobias may also develop through direct transmission of information about the dangerousness of particular objects, situations, or phenomena. For example, many children are not afraid of dogs before their parents specifically tell them that dogs are dangerous. Phobias that develop in this way also tend to be less severe than phobias acquired through traumatic conditioning. They can also be more easily dismissed with the acquisition of new information and maturation.

Operant (Instrumental) Conditioning

As already noted, operant conditioning explains the maintenance of phobias. Mowrer (1960) has formulated a two-factor theory about the formation and maintenance of phobias. According to this theory, fear initially develops as a result of classical conditioning; in the second phase, fear is temporarily reduced or eliminated by avoidance of the feared stimulus, and phobia is thereby maintained (operant conditioning). That is, the fear motivates a person to look for means to reduce fear, and every behavior (e.g., avoidance) that succeeds in reducing fear is reinforced. However, phobic fear can persist even in the absence of avoidance behavior. In these cases, the factors that perpetuate phobic fear include secondary gain, cognitive biases, and specific meaning or significance attached to the phobic stimuli.

Cognitive Factors in the Etiology and Pathogenesis of Specific Phobias
Similar to other anxiety disorders, specific phobias have been found to be
associated with biases in information processing, particularly biases in
attention and judgment. Certain beliefs about phobic stimuli (e.g., beliefs
about their dangerousness as a consequence of the exaggerated perception
of threat) and beliefs that patients have about themselves (e.g., beliefs that
they are not capable of coping with anxiety when facing the objects of their
fears) may play an important role in maintaining phobias (e.g., Thorpe and
Salkovskis, 1995). It is important to identify these beliefs and challenge
them in the course of treatment.

Psychoanalytic Approaches

The main tenet of the psychoanalytic theory of phobias is that there is some
fundamental anxiety behind every fear. Therefore, the therapist's task is to
uncover this fundamental anxiety and the associated intrapsychic conflicts; according to the psychoanalytic theory, without such an uncovering, the understanding of phobias is only superficial. Moreover, if the
conflicts are not resolved, the treatment may lead to a replacement of one
type of phobia with another, a claim that has generally not been supported
by studies and clinical practice.

   Freud (1909/1955a) was the first to illustrate the principles of the psychoanalytic approach to phobias in his case of "little Hans." Freud proposed that Hans, who was frightened of horses, had, in fact, castration
anxiety, and was afraid of his father because of the unconscious sexual
longings for his mother. Thus, the unresolved Oedipal conflict was behind
Hans' phobia of horses. Freud also postulated specific defense mechanisms that are used by people with phobia, with the goal of defending the
ego against the unacceptable sexual urges; these mechanisms are displacement, symbolization, and avoidance. *Displacement* refers to transfer of the
conflictual material to a neutral object, which has no obvious relationship
with the conflict but becomes a focus of the phobia. Through displacement,
the person disguises the true nature of his or her anxiety. The underlying
issues are less concealed by the use of symbolization, whereby some
aspects of the phobic object or situation symbolize the original conflict.

   Post-Freudian psychoanalysis considered some phobias to be related
to conflicts originating from different developmental stages (e.g., pre-
Oedipal) or to reflect superego anxiety. However, the original controversial tenet—that there is something "more fundamental" behind every
phobia—has not changed, despite the general lack of support for it. This
tenet has hindered, rather than fostered, further development of the psychoanalytic theory of phobia, and patients who suffer from specific pho-

bias as their principal or sole psychiatric condition are unlikely to be treated by psychoanalysis or psychodynamically oriented psychotherapy.

TREATMENT

It is practically impossible to treat specific phobias without some form of exposure therapy; if the therapist can succeed in negotiating with patients that they use exposure to the phobic stimuli, then this is likely to be beneficial for them. A combination of exposure-based therapy and medications is used relatively rarely, and only in situations where it is clearly warranted.

The treatment of specific phobias should be strictly individualized and depends on the type of phobia. It relies very much on patients' motivation, as patients may be more tempted than those with other disorders to give up treatment and return to their previous pattern of phobic avoidance and general adaptation of their lifestyle to their phobia. The main goals of treatment of specific phobias are alleviation of fear, disappearance of phobic avoidance, and the consequent improvement in functioning.

BEHAVIORAL TREATMENTS

Several techniques of behavior therapy for use in treating specific phobias have been developed over the last four decades. They include systematic desensitization, other exposure-based treatments (Table 5–5), and modeling. While all of these techniques were found to be efficacious in treating specific phobias, exposure in vivo appears to have advantages over

TABLE 5–5. Characteristics of Systematic Desensitization and Other Exposure-Based Treatments in Specific Phobias

Behavioral Techniques	Nature of Exposure	Rate of Exposure	Use of Relaxation
Systematic desensitization	Imaginal	Gradual	Yes
Standard exposure	In vivo, sometimes combined with imaginal, rarely only imaginal	Gradual	No
Flooding	In vivo	Massive	No
Implosion therapy	Imaginal	Massive	No

imaginal exposure (e.g., Marks et al., 1971; Bourque and Ladouceur, 1980). Also, some behavioral techniques are more suitable for certain types of specific phobias. Cognitive therapy techniques may be added to behavioral treatment; cognitive therapy alone appears to be less efficacious in the treatment of specific phobias, although there are occasional reports of its efficacy in some specific phobias (e.g., De Jongh et al., 1995).

Systematic Desensitization

This technique, introduced by Wolpe (1958), was the first efficacious behavioral technique, but it is rarely used today. It consists of imaginal exposure to the phobic stimulus while the patient is undergoing progressive muscle relaxation. The rationale for the simultaneous combination of this exposure with relaxation lies in the postulated mechanism of reciprocal inhibition. *Reciprocal inhibition* refers to the inhibition of anxiety-associated hyperactivity of the sympathetic nervous system by activation of the parasympathetic nervous system through muscle relaxation. The repeated coupling of imaginal exposure and muscle relaxation leads to counterconditioning, so that the phobic stimulus elicits progressively less fear.

Systematic desensitization uses a hierarchy of phobic stimuli (see Chapter 2, Exposure-Based Therapy for Agoraphobia). The treatment starts with imaginal exposure to the phobic stimulus (or an aspect of the phobic stimulus) that is anticipated to produce the least amount of anxiety, and this exposure continues until the anxiety subsides substantially. The treatment then proceeds with imaginal exposure to the stimuli (or certain aspects of the stimuli) that are anticipated to elicit progressively more anxiety. This gradual approach to exposure, with the prior construction of a phobic hierarchy, has been incorporated into other types of exposure-based treatments.

Exposure-Based Treatments

The type of exposure-based therapy used most commonly in the treatment of specific phobias is gradual exposure in vivo. This exposure is performed in a manner very similar to that used in the treatment of agoraphobia; it is described in more detail in Chapter 2. Progressive muscle relaxation is usually not used in the course of exposure in vivo, unless patients develop severe physical symptoms during exposure (Öst et al., 1982). It is useful to expose patients with specific phobias to various aspects and components of phobic stimuli in the gradual, hierarchy-based sequence. For example, patients with a dog phobia can be exposed to tapes of barking dogs and/or slides and videos in which dogs are presented in situations of increasing degrees of implicit or explicit threat.

Exposure is used because it is essential for the extinction of phobic fear and disappearance of phobic avoidance. Avoidance prevents the person not only from being in contact with the feared stimulus but also from extinguishing the fear by not allowing the person to realize that the stimulus need not be feared because the anticipated, harmful outcomes do not occur (see Chapter 2 for discussion of mechanisms of change in the course of exposure therapy). If the fundamental underlying emotion in a particular phobia is disgust rather than fear, treatment with exposure may not be sufficient or adequate because the feeling of disgust may not effectively habituate during repeated exposure (e.g., Foa and McNally, 1996).

Many variants of exposure-based therapy have been used in the treatment of specific phobias. Recent trends include attempts to shorten the treatment without sacrificing its efficacy. Thus, a single prolonged session (2–3 hours) of therapist-directed exposure, whether conducted individually (Öst, 1989) or in a group setting (Öst, 1996; Öst et al., 1997), was found to be as efficacious as self-exposure conducted over a longer period (Öst et al., 1991b; Hellström and Öst, 1995).

Exposure-based treatment may be modified when used for certain types of specific phobias. This is particularly the case with blood-injection-injury phobia, in which patients fear fainting during exposure as much as they fear the actual phobic stimulus itself. Modifications of the exposure therapy have been developed with the specific aim of minimizing the risk of fainting during exposure. An example of this modification is "applied tension," which requires patients to induce muscle tension during exposure (e.g., Öst and Sterner, 1987; Öst et al., 1991a); fainting is incompatible with the physiological correlates of tension.

Flooding entails a massive in vivo exposure to the phobic stimuli that elicit high levels of anxiety; it is usually conducted in the presence of the therapist. *Implosion therapy* pertains to massive exposure in imagination. Flooding and implosion therapy are rarely used, as they are generally not well tolerated by patients and also appear less efficacious than gradual exposure in vivo.

Finally, a technique of interoceptive exposure (described in Chapter 2) can be used in the treatment of specific phobias if there is a prominent fear of certain anxiety symptoms (e.g., shortness of breath, dizziness, palpitations) occurring in the phobic situation.

Modeling

Modeling (Denney et al., 1977) is used in the treatment of specific phobias usually in combination with exposure-based techniques (e.g., Öst et al., 1997). Modeling consists of the therapist demonstrating to the patient how to approach and contact the phobic stimulus, and then asking the patient to do the same. Modeling also relies on hierarchies of the feared stimuli, and is thus conducted gradually. It is based on the theory of social learning (Bandura, 1977), which emphasizes the role of cognitive factors and observation of fearful behavior in the etiology and pathogenesis of phobias.

Other Forms of Psychological Treatment

Although exposure-based therapies alone or in combination with other behavioral techniques are quite efficacious in the treatment of specific phobias, some patients find this treatment too demanding, are unable to complete the course of therapy, and/or fail to maintain motivation for treatment. It is estimated (e.g., Prochaska, 1991) that as many as 25%–50% of patients drop out of behavioral therapy of specific phobias. For patients who fail behavioral therapy or are not sufficiently motivated for it, it is worthwhile exploring other treatment options.

Hypnotherapy can be attempted, alone or in combination with some behavioral techniques. There are several encouraging reports on the use of hypnotherapy in the treatment of specific phobias, especially dental phobia. However, use of hypnotherapy as the first-line psychotherapeutic modality for specific phobias cannot be recommended at this time.

In addition to its use in posttraumatic stress disorder, eye movement desensitization and reprocessing (EMDR) has been tried in the treatment of specific phobias. However, at least one study (Muris et al., 1997) failed to show its superiority over exposure in vivo. This technique is described in more detail in Chapter 7.

As noted before, psychodynamically oriented psychotherapy and psychoanalysis are now rarely used in the treatment of specific phobias. Not only is there lack of evidence that these types of psychotherapy are efficacious for specific phobias, but they also do not appear to be a rational treatment choice for a relatively circumscribed problem for which brief, well-targeted, and efficacious treatments exist. It should be mentioned in this context that even Freud considered exposure necessary in the psychoanalytic treatment of phobias. The psychoanalytic assumption that phobic fears always have an underlying, "hidden" meaning, different from the one suggested or reported by patients, is on shaky grounds. As a result, insisting that the goal of treatment in specific phobias is to be uncovering of the underlying, unconscious problems and resolution of the corresponding conflicts may not be helpful to many patients, especially if they continue to be fearful and resort to phobic avoidance.

PHARMACOLOGICAL TREATMENT

Pharmacotherapy alone is not the treatment of choice for specific phobias. It may be used if patients cannot tolerate exposure-based treatments or are not interested in other types of psychological therapy. Pharmacotherapy may be useful in the treatment of patients with specific phobias who also have panic attacks, especially unexpected panic attacks. Medications, usually benzodiazepines because of their fast onset of action, may be used on an as-needed basis before exposure to the phobic stimulus. For example, patients with a phobia of flying can take a benzodiazepine before going to the airport. However, when they are used in this fashion, medications are not to be taken frequently, and patients should bear in mind that effects of such pharmacotherapy are only short term.

Even when used in combination with behavioral treatments, medications may not be particularly useful and fail to have long-term effects. The use of benzodiazepines with exposure-based treatments is controversial and many behavior therapists advise against such a combination, for reasons discussed elsewhere in this book (see Chapter 2). However, benzodiazepines may be carefully used during the initial phases of exposure treatment, with the goal of alleviating the overwhelming anxiety and facilitating exposure.

6
Obsessive-Compulsive Disorder

Obsessive-compulsive disorder (OCD) is a unique psychiatric condition in that it is characterized by features—obsessions and compulsions—that are distributed on a continuum from normality to the most severe and incapacitating manifestations. Furthermore, OCD is unique among the anxiety disorders in being related to a large number of psychiatric and neurological conditions with which it may have more in common than with other anxiety disorders. Obsessive-compulsive disorder is often portrayed as an intriguing disorder that tends to represent a treatment challenge.

CLINICAL FEATURES

Typical clinical features of OCD include obsessions and overt (behavioral) compulsions. It was only relatively recently realized that in addition to overt (behavioral) compulsions, patients with OCD may exhibit a range of other behaviors (such as avoidance and reassurance seeking) as well as use covert (mental, cognitive) compulsions (or cognitive rituals) in response to obsessions. All these behaviors and covert compulsions that appear in response to obsessions have been encompassed by the term *neutralization*. The purpose of neutralization is to alleviate anxiety or distress, "undo" obsessions and/or prevent harm associated with obsessions. Thus, it would perhaps be more accurate to rename OCD as "obsessive-neutralizing disorder." The components of OCD are schematically presented in Figure 6–1.

Obsessions

Obsessions are usually defined as recurrent thoughts, impulses, and/or images that are experienced as uncontrollable. Also, they are not just excessive worries about real-life problems, and they cause marked anxiety or distress, so that a person feels compelled to "do something" with them, for example, attempt to ignore, suppress, or neutralize them or resist them in some other way. The other reason for this urge to do something with obsessions is that they are usually, though not invariably, experienced by the person as alien, intrusive, strange, "crazy," senseless, or inappropriate. When obsessions are recognized as such, they are also referred to as "ego-dystonic," and the person experiencing them is thought to have "preserved insight." "Poor insight" is exhibited by individuals who do not experience and recognize obsessions as unacceptable, senseless, or unreasonable ("ego-syntonic" obsessions). In such cases, it is worthwhile exploring whether these phenomena are, in fact, overvalued ideas or even delusions. The characteristics of obsessions are summarized in Table 6–1.

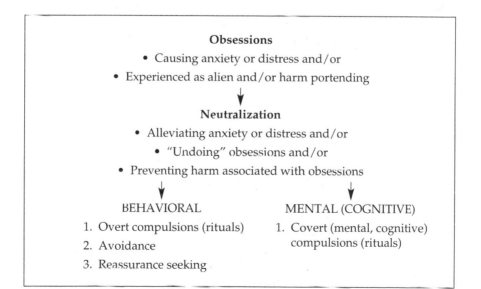

Obsessions
- Causing anxiety or distress and/or
- Experienced as alien and/or harm portending

Neutralization
- Alleviating anxiety or distress and/or
- "Undoing" obsessions and/or
- Preventing harm associated with obsessions

BEHAVIORAL
1. Overt compulsions (rituals)
2. Avoidance
3. Reassurance seeking

MENTAL (COGNITIVE)
1. Covert (mental, cognitive) compulsions (rituals)

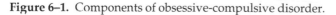

Figure 6–1. Components of obsessive-compulsive disorder.

TABLE 6–1. Characteristics of Obsessions

- Thoughts, impulses, and/or images
- Recurrent and/or repetitive
- Uncontrollable
- Not just excessive worries about real-life problems
- Cause marked anxiety or distress
- Usually (though not invariably) experienced or recognized by the person as alien, intrusive, strange, "crazy," senseless, or inappropriate ("ego-dystonic" or "good-insight" obsessions) and portending harm
- The person feels compelled to "do something" with obsessions—attempt to ignore, suppress, or neutralize them or resist them in some other way—to achieve one or more of the following goals:
  1. Alleviate anxiety or distress
  2. "Undo" obsessions because of their alien or "dangerous" nature
  3. Prevent harm associated with obsessions

It is useful to distinguish between obsessions, normal intrusive thoughts, mental compulsions, worries (such as those found in generalized anxiety disorder), ruminations (e.g., ruminations encountered in depressed persons), other types of intrusive thoughts (such as trauma-related intrusions in posttraumatic stress disorder), overvalued ideas (e.g., those seen in hypochondriasis, body dysmorphic disorder, or anorexia nervosa), and delusions (as part of a psychotic illness). All of these phenomena are often repetitive, some are experienced as intrusive, uncontrollable, and/or distressing, whereas others are associated with an urge to do something in response to their content or as a result of the way in which they are experienced. The features of other phenomena that distinguish them from obsessions are shown in Table 6–2.

Compulsions

Compulsions are defined as repetitive behaviors (overt compulsions) or unobservable mental acts (covert compulsions, mental compulsions, cognitive compulsions) that are performed in response to an obsession and often according to strict rules; the purpose of compulsions is to alleviate anxiety or distress, undo obsessions, and/or prevent harm associated with obsessions. Although compulsions usually produce some relief, they have to be performed over and over again, because this relief does not last very long. Over time, the person may start believing that a dreaded event has not happened because he or she is performing the compulsion. In such cases, the person may ultimately believe that a failure to perform a com-

TABLE 6–2. Distinguishing Between Obsessions and Related Phenomena

Normal Intrusive Thoughts

- Not interpreted as meaning that the person is responsible for having them
- Not experienced so distressingly that the person has to suppress or neutralize them
- More controllable

Mental Compulsions

- Initiated voluntarily and, thus, under the person's control
- Occur in response to obsessions, with the purpose of alleviating anxiety or distress caused by obsessions, "undoing" obsessions, and/or preventing harm

Pathological Worry

- Content pertains to real-life problems, without reference to something abhorrent or shameful and one's personal responsibility for worrying; usually future oriented
- Not experienced as alien, "crazy," or inappropriate

Depressive Ruminations

- Content pertains to themes of loss and personal failure; usually past oriented
- Not experienced as alien, "crazy," senseless, or inappropriate
- No attempt to ignore, suppress, or neutralize them; usually not resisted

Trauma-Related Intrusions (as in posttraumatic stress disorder)

- Monothematic and highly specific: content pertains to a particular traumatic event
- Not experienced as alien, "crazy," senseless, or inappropriate

Overvalued Ideas

- Held with a more firm belief
- Not experienced as alien, "crazy," senseless, or inappropriate
- No attempt to ignore, suppress, or neutralize them; usually not resisted

Delusions

- Fixed, unshakeable beliefs, without the person experiencing uncertainty and doubt about their validity
- Often held on the basis of delusional evidence (explanation for having delusions is not plausible and suggests loss of reality testing)
- Not experienced as alien, "crazy," senseless, or inappropriate
- No attempt to ignore, suppress, or neutralize them; usually not resisted

TABLE 6–3. Characteristics of Compulsions

- Overt behaviors or unobservable mental acts (covert compulsions, mental compulsions, cognitive compulsions) that the person feels driven to perform in response to an obsession and often according to strict rules
- Repetitive
- The purpose of compulsions is one or more of the following:
    1. Alleviation of anxiety or distress caused by obsession (but compulsions are performed excessively and repeatedly, without achieving this goal in the long run)
    2. Undoing of obsession (although compulsions cannot realistically do that)
    3. Prevention of harm associated with the obsession (although compulsions cannot realistically do that)

pulsion would have disastrous consequences, and this belief may then become the main reason for performing the compulsion. Patients with OCD typically report that they feel driven to perform compulsions, but the sense of urge is subjective and patients do not really "have" to perform them. Stated otherwise, unlike obsessions that are intrusive and thus not a product of free will, compulsions are initiated and performed voluntarily and are under patients' control (although on casual inspection it may not seem like that). The term *ritual* is often used interchangeably with *compulsion*, but more precisely, the ritual refers to a stereotyped act (whether overt or covert) that is performed in accordance with strict and rigid rules. Characteristics of compulsions are summarized in Table 6–3.

In recent years, attention has been drawn to the relationship between compulsions, "impulsions" (Shapiro and Shapiro, 1992), and impulsive behavior (Table 6–4).

Mental (covert) compulsions are frequently seen among patients with OCD, but they may be difficult to recognize, because they are unobservable, "invisible" mental acts; hence the term *covert compulsions*. Examples

TABLE 6–4. Distinguishing Between Compulsions, "Impulsions," and Impulsive Acts

"Impulsions"

Occur in response to a sensation or an urge

Performed until the person feels satisfied or "just right"

Performed with the purpose of achieving a sense of completion, relief, or satisfaction

Impulsive Acts

Performed in response to an urge or tension

Performed to provide relief, pleasure, or gratification

include silent counting, performing of various operations with numbers, imagining a particular situation, repeating a thought a certain number of times, recalling the "right" thought, and praying. If patients do not reveal spontaneously that they perform mental compulsions, it is useful to ask how they cope with a particular obsession (which they previously had volunteered to reveal) or what they do to alleviate their distress about having such an obsession. Mental compulsions may be triggered by various types of obsessions and involve very different mental acts, but their common denominator is their purpose to alleviate obsession-induced anxiety or distress, undo obsession, and/or prevent harm by nonbehavioral means.

As is the case with overt compulsions, it is important to understand the purpose of covert compulsions by asking patients why they are performing them. Prevention of harm in the future is a common reason for the use of covert compulsions. For example, a patient with an obsession that her parents would die every time she saw vehicle license plates with digits added up to an even number "had" to look for license plates where the corresponding sum was an odd number. The purpose of this concealed compulsive activity was to prevent her parents' death.

Avoidance

As a way of temporarily alleviating anxiety, avoidance is commonly used for coping with some obsessions, as it is for coping with phobic fears. Unlike compulsions, avoidance cannot undo an obsession and except in relatively few circumstances (e.g., avoidance of driving for fear of having an urge to drive the car off the road), it is not bestowed with the power of preventing some dreadful event in the future. Therefore, avoidance is often used as a first-line response to obsessions that are not experienced as threatening to the extent that further measures need to be taken against them. For example, a regular church-going patient with an obsession involving an image of him shouting blasphemous sentences in church started to avoid church services. When he had to attend a service and could not resort to avoidance, he was compelled to come up with other means of coping with his obsession and developed a covert compulsion.

Reassurance Seeking

Reassurance seeking is also a commonly used measure against obsessions and serves the purpose of alleviating anxiety, albeit temporarily. Like avoidance, it cannot prevent harm, and is often used in a way analogous to that in which avoidance is used. However, obtaining reassurance may undo the reassurance-related obsession, at least temporarily. Another difference is that reassurance seeking depends on someone else—the person willing to provide reassurance—whereas avoidance is independent of others.

Reassurance seeking is often related to checking compulsions and may be resorted to instead of checking or alternatively with checking. Whereas checking can be both past and future oriented and thus used in a variety of situations and serve different purposes (see Pathological Doubt, Checking, and Reassurance seeking, below), reassurance seeking is more restricted in its scope and effects in that it is mainly past oriented (i.e., reassurance is sought about something that has or has not occurred in the past, for example, whether the patient hit a pedestrian while driving or whether he or she was infected with HIV).

Insight

As already noted, a realization by patients with OCD that their obsessions are alien, intrusive, strange, "crazy," senseless, irrational, or inappropriate, is referred to as "insight." Only patients who have good insight will have a need to ignore, suppress, neutralize, or resist their obsessions. Patients who have OCD with obsessional beliefs held with greater conviction, that are not experienced as alien, "crazy," senseless, irrational, or inappropriate and are therefore not resisted may, in fact, have overvalued ideas (see Table 6–2). In DSM-IV-TR, these phenomena are referred to as "poor-insight" obsessions, but that may be a misnomer. For example, a patient who believed that he had to check the locks on the doors and windows three times in one sequence and two times in the opposite sequence to ensure that his home would not be broken into did not resist performing this ritual at all. He could be characterized as having poor insight. He acknowledged, however, that his belief was "unusual," while not finding it unreasonable or senseless, because he thought that his checking compulsion actually prevented burglary of his home. Should this patient be considered to have partial rather than poor insight?

It has been appreciated for some time that the presence of insight in OCD is a matter of degree, with some OCD patients having very good insight on one side of the continuum, and others, at the other extreme, having no insight at all (Insel and Akiskal, 1986; Kozak and Foa, 1994). This distribution of insight in OCD patients has been highlighted by a study (Marazziti et al., 2002) that found excellent insight in 48% of patients, good insight in 21.5%, moderate insight in 15.5%, poor insight in 10%, and no insight in 5%.

While the continuum conceptualization of insight takes into account the multidimensional nature of the very construct of insight, it does not resolve the problem of OCD with poor insight. Do OCD patients with poor insight represent a distinct subgroup of OCD patients who differ from OCD patients with good insight in respects other than insight? Some studies (e.g., Marazziti et al., 2002) have reported that this is not the case, whereas others suggest that OCD with poor insight is more likely to be associated with certain types of obsessions and compulsions, for example, hoarding (Frost et al., 1996). Does OCD with poor insight predict a response to treatment? Again, the answers to this question are equivocal: while hoarding (as a typical representative of poor-insight OCD) suggests a poorer response to treatment (Black et al., 1998; Winsberg et al., 1999), there was no confirmation of the relationship between the degree of insight and treatment outcome in another study (Eisen et al., 2001). Clinical experience does suggest, however, that the treatment of poor-insight patients tends to be more complex, often requiring modifications to the usually administered pharmacotherapy and cognitive-behavioral therapy. Also, OCD with poor insight may imply a less favorable prognosis, perhaps independently from impact of poor insight on treatment. Finally, is OCD with poor insight associated with psychotic illness? While the lack of insight with regard to OCD manifestations is often seen in patients having psychotic illness co-occurring with OCD, OCD patients with poor insight do not necessarily demonstrate an association with psychosis and may have no history of psychotic symptoms at all (e.g., Marazziti et al., 2002). These issues need to be resolved before the status of poor-insight OCD becomes more clear.

Types of Obsessions and Compulsions

The most common types of obsessions and compulsions are listed in Table 6–5. Patients with OCD usually have both obsessions and compulsions, although one or the other phenomenon may predominate at any point in time, giving an impression that a person is experiencing obsessions only or exhibiting only compulsions. In fact, OCD with "pure" obsessions (without compulsions) and OCD with "pure" compulsions (without obsessions) seem to be rare, with the frequency of the former being 8.5% and frequency of the latter being 0.5% in one sample of OCD patients (Foa and Kozak, 1995).

The themes of obsessions and the type of compulsions may vary over time, a pattern reported by 60% of OCD patients in one long-term, follow-up study (Skoog and Skoog, 1999). Sometimes these changing obsessions and compulsions appear to be related; for example, there seemed to be an underlying theme of perfectionism in a patient who presented with paralyzing, doubting obsessions and consequent indecisiveness at one time,

TABLE 6–5. Common Types of Obsessions and Compulsions

Obsessions	Frequency[a] (%)	Compulsions	Frequency[a] (%)
Multiple obsessions	72	Checking	61
Contamination	50	Multiple compulsions	58
Pathological doubt	42	Washing, cleaning	50
Somatic	33	Counting	36
Need for symmetry	32	Need to ask or confess	34
Aggressive	31	Need for symmetry or precision, rearranging objects	28
Sexual	24	Hoarding	18

[a]Frequency data are from Rasmussen and Eisen (1992).

and repetitive rituals of rearranging objects so that they would "look right" at another time.

Multiple obsessions and compulsions are also very common (Table 6–5). Some patients with multiple obsessions and compulsions may seem to have only one type of obsession and/or compulsion because that is the most troubling one to them, they do not mention spontaneously other obsessions or compulsions, and they are not asked about them.

There have been attempts to classify various obsessions and compulsions in several groups on the basis of their theme or content and other characteristics. Some authors have proposed phenomenological subtypes of OCD that also have in common other features and distinct patterns of response to treatment. These attempts at classification have generally been unsuccessful, however, partly because many OCD patients have obsessions and compulsions from various putative subtypes and because the underlying psychopathological mechanisms are the same regardless of the subtype. Still, various types of obsessions and compulsions seem to be associated with certain specific features. The most common obsessions and compulsions are described and their relative specificities reviewed in the text below.

Contamination, Washing, and Cleaning
Contamination obsessions are among the most frequent in patients with OCD. Their main underlying theme is a fear of being contaminated, regardless of whether contamination occurs through germs, dirt, bodily secretions and excretions, or in some other way. Contamination fears may be connected with fears of certain diseases, particularly infectious illnesses, because of the way they spread. These fears may also be related to a strong

feeling of disgust about human secretions and excretions or potentially contaminated objects. Another component of the contamination experience may be a fear of just not feeling clean.

Patients with contamination obsessions are preoccupied with distressing and frightening thoughts or images of being infected or dirty as a result of having been in contact with supposedly contaminated objects or people. As a result of these obsessions, patients become hypervigilant about any possibility of contamination and may first attempt to avoid and prevent every contact with the perceived sources of contamination. Thus, they may try to open the doorknob with gloves on their hands or by using elbows rather than hands; other examples are placing a handkerchief over a payphone while using it or avoiding a handshake. Patients may involve other people in their "preventative measures," for example, by asking them to first wash their hands when they come for a visit or by requesting that their children follow a strict code of hygiene at home.

If patients feel that they have inadvertently been in contact with the contaminated object or person, they will feel even more distress and they usually have an urge to wash or clean to "get rid" of the contaminating material. Thus, washing and cleaning compulsions are usually performed with the purpose of alleviating distress or anxiety caused by the corresponding obsessions. The washing and cleaning compulsions need to be performed for as long as patients feel contaminated or dirty, and this may take a very long time (e.g., several hours). In other cases, episodes of washing are relatively brief, but have to be repeated many times per day.

To ensure getting clean, some patients use strong and obviously inappropriate cleaning devices while washing their hands, such as detergents or bleach; others rub their hands or other body parts so much that they damage the skin, sometimes creating severe lesions and causing dermatitis. In the latter case, it is important to ascertain whether washing compulsions have an additional purpose, for example, self-punishment for imagined or real wrongdoing. Sometimes washing has a symbolic meaning, as an expression of the need to obtain atonement for aggressive, sexually unacceptable, or other inappropriate acts, or to undo such acts, regardless of whether these have been committed in fantasy or reality. Harsh and very concrete washing and cleaning rituals (e.g., cleaning completely, until the skin starts bleeding) often indicate the presence of a significant underlying psychopathology, such as severe personality disturbance or even psychosis.

Although washing and cleaning compulsions are usually related to contamination obsessions, they may subsequently run their own course or be unrelated to such obsessions even from the onset of OCD. Thus, patients may develop a compulsion to wash a certain number of times not necessarily because that would cleanse them from germs, but because that number has a special significance for them and patients fear the consequences of not only washing less but also of washing more. Magical thinking is the basis for such ritualized compulsions, and compulsions then serve the purpose of preventing a dreaded catastrophe.

Pathological Doubt, Checking, and Reassurance Seeking

In very broad terms, obsessional self-doubt pertains to a person's recurrent and tormenting feeling that something about him or her is "not right." This feeling may refer to various aspects of the person's personality, behavior, physical appearance, or health. Self-doubt is often associated with uncertainty as to whether the person has done something or not. This uncertainty and inflated responsibility often lead to checking compulsions, which serve the purpose of alleviating distress or anxiety by "making sure" that there is no reason for further doubting, at least temporarily. More specifically, the underlying purpose of checking compulsions is to abolish uncertainty and reassure oneself that one will not be held responsible if something bad happens. This is particularly evident when checking is future oriented. For example, if a burglary occurs after a person has checked five times that all the doors and windows are locked, the expectation is that the person will be less likely to hold himself or herself responsible; likewise, in case of fire, the person who has made sure that all the electrical and gas appliances have been turned off and unplugged would feel safe in that he or she has not made the fire more likely.

Unless performed ritualistically and driven by magical thinking, future-oriented checking compulsions usually do not serve the purpose of preventing future harm, although on the surface it may seem that this is what they were designed for. Their main purpose is alleviation of anxiety associated with an obsession that one will be held responsible in case of an accident or other mishap.

Other types of checking compulsions that are more past oriented are related to excessive reassurance seeking and serve the purpose of alleviating anxiety and diminishing the burden of responsibility for something that patients suspect they have or have not done. Sometimes, this checking and reassurance have the effect of temporarily undoing the underlying obsession. For example, patients who are uncertain in a quasi-delusional way as to whether they have committed a crime or done something else that is socially unacceptable will constantly check and/or ask for reassurance that they did not do these things. They are relieved when they find out or are told that nothing dreadful happened, and they may also feel that the underlying obsessional doubt is gone, but these effects of checking and reassurance do not last very long. Another example of pathological doubt, intolerance of uncertainty, reassurance seeking, and checking compulsions can be found among some hypochondriacal patients with somatic obsessions, as their doubts and uncertainty pertain to their health.

Like washing and cleaning compulsions, checking compulsions may become increasingly complex over time, so that they must be performed in a certain, strictly specified way and/or a certain number of times. Because of the prominent magical thinking behind such checking, any deviation from the rules of the ritual is believed to be dangerous and to have some dreaded consequence. Again, the patient feels excessively responsible for precise, ritualistic performance of the compulsion, but in these cases, the purpose of the checking rituals is less to alleviate distress or anxiety than to prevent harm or undo the corresponding obsession.

Need for Symmetry, Rearranging Objects, and Perfectionism
The dominant clinical manifestation of some patients with OCD is a preoccupation with rearranging objects so that they follow a certain pattern, usually a symmetrical or balancing one (for example, balancing the shape and color of objects). Thus, the compulsion of rearranging objects occurs in response to an obsession about objects having to be arranged in a certain pattern, order, or sequence. This compulsion is usually preceded by uneasiness and tension about objects not being arranged in the "right" way, and is therefore performed with the purpose of alleviating uneasiness and tension (Rasmussen and Eisen, 1991). Typically, patients say that they have an urge to move objects because the way in which objects are arranged "just doesn't feel right." Likewise, patients continue moving and rearranging objects until they are arranged in a way that "feels right." Therefore, these compulsions often resemble "impulsions" (see Compulsions, above). A related type of compulsion is doing something (typically touching or tapping) or balancing one's movements in a specific pattern or sequence. These obsessions and compulsions are often found in OCD patients who also have tic disorders (Leckman et al., 1994; Miguel et al., 1995).

It is often difficult to understand what constitutes a pattern that is "just right." One possibility is that it reflects a peculiar and highly idiosyncratic tendency toward perfectionism. This is supported by clinical observations that, like perfection, finding the "right" pattern is very hard, with patients spending a lot of time trying to find one with which they would be satisfied. When this type of compulsion is combined with pathological doubting and checking, it may be almost impossible for patients to complete their tasks. Patients may appear extremely slow at whatever they do, a phenomenon referred to as "primary obsessional slowness" (Rachman and Hodgson, 1980). The presence of primary obsessional slowness has been associated with poor response to both pharmacotherapy and behavior therapy.

Less often, when compulsions of rearranging objects are connected through magical thinking with some imagined catastrophic outcome, they are performed with the purpose of preventing harm in the future. This is done in a very ritualized manner and a strictly specified sequence for fear of harmful consequences if the compulsion is not performed correctly. In these situations, patients also have an inflated sense of responsibility for preventing the catastrophe. For example, one patient had an obsession that her parents would die if the plates on the table were not arranged in a symmetrical fashion, with two on each side; therefore, she had to arrange plates accordingly. Over time, this patient became more and more concerned about the manner in which she set the table, as the lack of symmetry was no longer "permitted" at any time during the process of setting the table. Hence, she had to make sure to simultaneously put plates on different sides of the table for symmetry to be maintained at all times.

Sexual, Aggressive, and Religious Obsessions and Compulsions

Sexual and aggressive obsessions are probably the most unpleasant and most frightening of all obsessions. Patients with sexual and aggressive obsessions are usually afraid that they might behave in a sexually inappropriate manner or hurt and even kill their family members, friends, co-workers, or mere bystanders. Patients with sexual obsessions are typically concerned that they might become sexually disinhibited, utter obscenities in public places, behave in a sexually "perverted" manner and have sex with a family member, have sexual contact outside marriage, or have a sexual relationship not consistent with their sexual orientation. The feared aggressive behavior might be only verbal, so that patients are concerned that they might swear at someone or shout. Sometimes, patients are obsessively preoccupied with thoughts or images of harming or killing themselves.

The main theme underlying sexual and aggressive obsessions is a fear of losing control over one's behavior; this possibility of losing control makes sexual and aggressive obsessions so profoundly distressing. Since patients do not trust themselves that they will remain in control, they often take measures to prevent the dreaded sexual or aggressive act. They usually do so by avoiding people with whom they might have a sexual encounter or by removing from their home all objects that could be used as weapons (typically all sharp objects such as knives and scissors).

It is even more troublesome when patients have sexual or aggressive obsessions of a different kind: that they have already committed a crime (e.g., robbed a bank, killed someone, or sexually molested a child), had an extramarital affair, or behaved otherwise in a sexually inappropriate manner. These patients repeatedly ask for reassurance that this did not happen or check whether it did happen. In more severe cases, patients are plagued by guilt and a need to be punished, and may confess their "wrongdoing" to their close friend or turn themselves in to the police, admitting their crime. This type of obsession borders on being delusional, and a possibility of primary psychotic illness should be explored in these cases.

Because of the abhorrent nature of sexual and aggressive obsessions and the fact that themes of most of them are socially unacceptable, patients with these obsessions often feel both responsible and guilty for having them. The guilt often drives patients to come up with compulsions that would effectively undo obsessions: this elimination of obsessions liberates patients from guilt, albeit temporarily. Hence, although some compulsions performed in response to sexual and aggressive obsessions serve the purpose of preventing the harm (loss of control) associated with these obsessions, other compulsions are more radical in that they aim to undo obsessions. For example, a patient who had an obsession that he would resort to exhibitionism developed a mental compulsion that consisted of imagining himself dead; his understanding of this compulsion was as follows: "If I am dead, I can't have these terrible thoughts. Therefore, such thoughts do not exist."

Religious obsessions are related to sexual and aggressive obsessions in that they are usually embarrassing and shameful and embody the notion of the threatened loss of control. Patients with religious obsessions are often concerned that they might utter something blasphemous in public situations and places of worship or during religious ceremonies. The underlying reasons for having these obsessions may or may not pertain to the person's attitudes toward religion and related matters. As is the case with compulsions that arise with sexual and aggressive obsessions, compulsions that appear in response to religious obsessions mainly serve the purpose of undoing these obsessions and thereby preventing harm. Also, such compulsions are not necessarily religious in nature.

Religious compulsions may be difficult to recognize, especially when they resemble sanctioned religious rituals. Although religious compulsions always appear in response to obsessions, these obsessions may not be easily accessible if they pertain to religious matters. Therefore, a clinician has to rely on observation or a description of the religious rituals to ascertain whether they are "normal" or a manifestation of OCD. Religious compulsions are excessive, often far above and beyond everything that institutionalized religions prescribe; also, they tend to be performed in ways that are unusual, even for the most devout worshippers. Religious compulsions are performed for various reasons: their purpose may be to alleviate anxiety, as well as undo the underlying obsession and prevent the imagined harm.

Hoarding

Hoarding is characterized by excessive collection and storage of objects that do not have any market or personal (sentimental or otherwise) value. In addition, persons who hoard are usually unable to discard such objects. As with many other manifestations of OCD, hoarding is encountered on a spectrum from very mild (and not pathological) to very severe and extreme, when the person seems almost totally preoccupied with the hoarding activity. In the most severe cases, the person has no room to store any more objects and hoarding is often accompanied by neglect of cleanliness, with the home of the affected person looking extremely unkempt.

Hoarding is an unusual compulsion in that it is often not preceded by or associated with corresponding obsessions. Also, the act of hoarding does not bring about an obvious relief or decrease in anxiety and discomfort, although attempts to prevent hoarding are usually met with resistance. Unlike some other compulsions, hoarding rarely seems to have a strong symbolic meaning and is not performed with the purpose of averting some catastrophe. The reason for hoarding can sometimes be found in the belief that the collected items will have value in the future or be important in some other way (e.g., in case of shortages). However, many patients who hoard are unable to explain why they do it, other than stating that they "just have to do it." Therefore, hoarding often appears to be an automatic activity.

Hoarding is a less frequent manifestation of OCD. Also, hoarding is not specific for OCD, as it may be seen in persons with obsessive-compulsive personality disorder. It is not always easy to distinguish whether hoarding is a part of the former or the latter condition. In OCD, there are usually other obsessions and/or compulsions and hoarding usually causes impairment, whereas hoarding as part of obsessive-compulsive personality disorder does not tend to contribute significantly to the overall impairment associated with that condition. Hoarding is usually accompanied by relatively poor insight and, therefore, patients do not tend to resist it.

Hoarding appears to have unfavorable treatment implications, as it is unlikely to respond to treatment with selective serotonin reuptake inhibitors or clomipramine (Black et al., 1998; Mataix-Cols et al., 1999). Augmentation of a selective serotonin reuptake inhibitor or clomipramine with first-generation antipsychotic medication may be useful in the treatment of hoarding. A possible involvement of dopamine system abnormalities in the pathophysiology of hoarding is also suggested by the finding that hoarding may be related to Tourette's disorder.

RELATIONSHIP BETWEEN OBSESSIVE-COMPULSIVE DISORDER AND OTHER DISORDERS

Obsessive-compulsive disorder tends to co-occur or be associated with several other disorders. The relationship with depression and psychotic illness is particularly important, because of the implications for routine clinical practice. In addition, OCD may co-occur with tic disorders, personality disturbance, and several other anxiety disorders. The concept of obsessive-compulsive spectrum disorders was proposed to emphasize the similarities and interrelatedness between OCD and a number of quite different disorders. Clinical implications of the relationship between OCD and other disorders are summarized in Table 6–6.

Obsessive-Compulsive Disorder and Depression

Obsessive-compulsive disorder and depression commonly occur together and depression is often seen many years after the onset of OCD. One study (Rasmussen and Eisen, 1988) showed that 67% of patients with OCD had a lifetime diagnosis of major depression, whereas 31% were currently depressed. In most patients, depression seems to follow OCD, perhaps as a result of the debilitating effects of long-lasting OCD and the accompanying demoralization, with feelings of hopelessness and helplessness. Consequently, patients with an early onset and chronic course of OCD may be more likely to develop depression.

The relationship between OCD and depression may be more complex. Some patients develop symptoms of OCD only after they have had recurrent major depressive disorder for some time. Also, obsessions and compulsions may become more prominent or appear less intense during a major depressive episode. Depressive ruminations may sometimes resemble obsessions, and it is important to distinguish between the two (Table 6–2). When OCD patients become clinically depressed, the treatment of their depression is often not efficacious if OCD is not treated at the same time (Fineberg, 1999), and with the same antidepressant used in the treatment of OCD (see also Pharmacological Treatment, below). Patients with co-occurring depression may respond less well to combined pharmacotherapy and behavior therapy than those without depression (Overbeek et al., 2002).

TABLE 6–6. Clinical Implications of the Relationship Between Obsessive-Compulsive Disorder and Other Disorders

Obsessive-Compulsive Disorder and Depression

- Depression is likely to co-occur with OCD at some stage in the course of OCD.

- Depressive ruminations sometimes need to be distinguished from obsessions.

- When OCD patients become clinically depressed, treatment of their depression is more likely to be efficacious if OCD is treated at the same time and if the same antidepressant used in the treatment of OCD is also used for treatment of depression.

- When OCD patients treated only by behavior therapy or cognitive-behavioral therapy become depressed, an antidepressant should be added.

- Co-occurring depression may have a negative effect on the outcome of treatment of OCD.

Obsessive-Compulsive Disorder and Psychotic Illness

- Some patients with OCD eventually develop psychosis or already have an underlying psychotic illness.

- It is important to predict which OCD patients are more prone to develop a psychotic illness or already harbor one (patients with poor insight and complex or bizarre obsessions and/or compulsions?).

- Obsessions, overvalued ideas and delusions need to be distinguished.

- For diagnostic and treatment purposes, it is important to distinguish between "delusional OCD" or "obsessive-compulsive psychosis" on one hand, and OCD that co-occurs with or is part of schizophrenia and schizotypal personality disorder on the other; the former appears to have better prognosis than the latter.

Obsessive-Compulsive Disorder and Tic Disorders

- Some patients with OCD have a tic disorder and a sizeable proportion of patients with tic disorders also have OCD or obsessions and compulsions.

- OCD patients with symmetry obsessions and compulsions involving ordering, rearranging objects, and hoarding are more likely to have tic disorders.

- Patients with OCD and Tourette's disorder have more family members with both OCD and Tourette's disorder, and an earlier onset of OCD.

- OCD patients with a co-occurring tic disorder are more likely to respond to a combination of a selective serotonin reuptake inhibitor or clomipramine and antipsychotic medication.

Obsessive-Compulsive Disorder and Personality Disturbance

- Although there is some overlap between OCD and obsessive-compulsive personality disorder, the relationship between them is not unique.

- Presence of severe personality disturbance, especially schizotypal personality disorder, suggests poorer prognosis and poorer response to treatment.

Obsessive-Compulsive Disorder and Psychotic Illness

Obsessive-compulsive disorder is unique among the anxiety disorders in that in a significant minority of patients there is an overlap between OCD and psychotic illness. This relationship appears particularly strong in some adolescent patients who initially present with OCD or OCD-like picture, but then go on to develop a psychosis. It comes as no surprise, then, that it was believed that OCD might be a prodrome of schizophrenia; however, comparisons with the general population and longitudinal studies have shown that OCD patients do not have a higher risk of developing schizophrenia (Goodwin et al., 1969; Black, 1974).

Most commonly, patients with psychosis-related OCD ("delusional OCD" or "obsessive-compulsive psychosis") have OCD with poor insight (they do not believe that their obsessions and/or compulsions are irrational, although they may be distressed by them) and tend to exhibit complex or bizarre obsessions and/or compulsions. Some types of obsessions and compulsions have a strong "flavor" of psychosis, with the underlying delusional strength and quality of obsessional beliefs. For example, a patient had a delusional obsession that he had committed a criminal act for which he repeatedly requested to be punished.

In one study (Eisen and Rasmussen, 1993), psychotic symptoms were found in 14% of OCD patients; almost one-half of these patients had delusional OCD as the only psychotic manifestation, whereas the remainder received diagnoses of schizophrenia, schizotypal personality disorder, and delusional disorder. It appears important to make a distinction between delusional OCD on one hand and OCD that co-occurs with psychotic disorders and schizotypal personality disorder on the other, because the former may have a better prognosis than the latter. Indeed, delusional OCD was found to be related to "classical" (nondelusional) OCD in terms of epidemiological and clinical features (Eisen and Rasmussen, 1993), and OCD patients with poor insight (conceptually related to delusional OCD) were just as likely to respond to a selective serotonin reuptake inhibitor, as were OCD patients with good insight (Eisen et al., 2001). Co-occurring schizotypal personality disorder (which is believed to be related to schizophrenia), by contrast, was clearly identified as indicating poor prognosis in OCD (Jenike et al., 1986; Baer et al., 1992; Moritz et al., 2004). Also, schizophrenia co-occurring with OCD appears to be associated with a generally poorer response to treatment of OCD.

Obsessions and compulsions may be seen among patients with a primary diagnosis of schizophrenia. The proportion of these patients varies from one study to another, with 8%–41% of schizophrenic patients having symptoms of OCD or meeting the diagnostic criteria for OCD (Fenton and

McGlashan, 1986; Berman et al, 1995; Eisen et al., 1997). When these patients were compared with schizophrenic patients who had no obsessions and compulsions, they were more likely to have a more chronic course and greater impairment (Fenton and McGlashan, 1986).

Obsessive-Compulsive Disorder and Tic Disorders

Tic disorders and OCD have an interesting relationship. Clinical and research interest has been focused mainly on Tourette's disorder, a condition with prominent motor and vocal tics. There is a similarity between OCD and Tourette's disorder in that both are characterized by repetitive behavior; tics in Tourette's disorder are involuntary only to a certain degree, and are often performed to provide relief and until patients "feel right" (Leckman et al., 1994). There are several other important aspects of the relationship between OCD and Tourette's disorder.

First, OCD is encountered in a significant proportion of patients with Tourette's disorder; symptoms of OCD and/or a full-blown OCD have been reported in 30%–40% of patients with Tourette's disorder (Leckman et al., 1993). Conversely, 20% of OCD patients had a lifetime history of multiple tics, and 5%–10% of OCD patients had a lifetime history of Tourette's disorder (Leckman et al., 1994). Second, patients with OCD co-occurring with Tourette's disorder have more family members with both OCD and Tourette's disorder and an earlier onset of OCD (Pauls et al., 1995). Third, OCD patients with symmetry obsessions and compulsions involving ordering, rearranging objects, and hoarding, who may in fact exhibit "impulsions" (Table 6–4), are more likely to have Tourette's disorder (Leckman et al., 1994; Miguel et al., 1995). Finally, OCD patients with co-occurring Tourette's disorder are more likely to respond to a combination of a selective serotonin reuptake inhibitor or clomipramine and antipsychotic medication.

Obsessive-Compulsive Disorder and Personality Disturbance

For quite a long time it was believed that OCD and obsessive-compulsive personality disorder have a unique relationship. It was postulated that obsessive-compulsive personality disorder predisposes to OCD, that personality attributes associated with OCD are invariably those of obsessive-compulsive personality disorder, and/or that in comparison with obsessive-compulsive personality disorder, OCD is just a more severe variant of the same underlying psychopathology. These beliefs about the relationship between OCD and obsessive-compulsive personality disorder have not been confirmed. In fact, one study (Baer et al., 1990) found obsessive-compulsive personality disorder in a minority (6%) of OCD patients, whereas other personality disorders were more common (dependent and histrionic) than obsessive-compulsive personality disorder or almost as common (avoidant, schizotypal, and paranoid) as obsessive-compulsive personality disorder.

Nevertheless, the relationship between OCD and obsessive-compulsive personality disorder remains intriguing, particularly from a developmental point of view. To a certain extent, developmental pathways to OCD and obsessive-compulsive personality disorder may be common to both, but then they diverge (see Etiology and Pathogenesis, below).

The presence of severe personality disturbance (particularly schizotypal, paranoid, and borderline personality disorders) is associated with poorer prognosis of OCD and a less favorable outcome of treatment (Jenike et al., 1986; Baer et al., 1992; Moritz et al., 2004).

Obsessive-Compulsive Disorder and Anxiety Disorders

Obsessive-compulsive disorder co-occurs less frequently with anxiety disorders than with depression. Among patients with the principal diagnosis of OCD, the lifetime rates of specific phobia, social anxiety disorder, and panic disorder have been reported to be 22%, 18%, and 12%, respectively (Rasmussen and Eisen, 1988). The current rate of OCD in patients with panic disorder was 17% (Breier et al., 1986). This co-occurrence of OCD with several other anxiety disorders suggests that there may be a common diathesis among some individuals to develop OCD and/or another anxiety disorder; whether they develop one or more of these conditions simultaneously or over time may be a matter of varying genetic and developmental influences. The implications of this co-occurrence are not clear at this time, but they seem to carry less significance for clinical practice than implications of the relationship with depression.

Obsessive-Compulsive Spectrum Disorders

The concept of "obsessive-compulsive spectrum disorders" (Hollander, 1993; Hollander and Wong, 1995) arose from observations of certain similarities between OCD and a number of quite diverse conditions (Table 6–7). These similarities pertain to repetitive behaviors, hardly resistible or irresistible urges to perform certain acts, and/or intrusive thoughts as a prominent component of clinical presentation. The concept of the spectrum has received a lot of attention over the past decade. In addition, the concept was boosted by findings that some of the spectrum disorders respond favorably to selective serotonin reuptake inhibitors, as in OCD.

TABLE 6–7. Disorders Included in Obsessive-Compulsive Spectrum Disorders

Impulse-Control Disorders

Trichotillomania

Onychophagia (nail-biting)

Pathological gambling

Kleptomania

Compulsive buying

Sexual Disorders

Sexual addiction

Paraphilias

Eating Disorders

Anorexia nervosa

Bulimia nervosa

Binge-eating disorder

Somatoform Disorders

Hypochondriasis

Body dysmorphic disorder

Somatization disorder

Personality Disorders

Borderline personality disorder

Obsessive-compulsive personality disorder

Neuropsychiatric Disorders: Tic Disorders and Other Movement Disorders

Tourette's disorder

Sydenham's chorea

Pervasive Developmental Disorders

Autistic disorder

Asperger's disorder

Repetitive Self-Mutilation

Dermatological Conditions

Dermatitis artefacta

Psychogenic excoriation (compulsive skin-picking)

Several dimensions of psychopathology have been proposed within the spectrum: a compulsive–impulsive continuum or overestimation of harm–underestimation of harm continuum, compulsion–impulsion–tic continuum, and approach–avoidance continuum.

The concept of obsessive-compulsive spectrum disorders is too broad and has been criticized (e.g., Rasmussen, 1994; Crino, 1999) on grounds that there are important differences between the conditions included in the spectrum and between OCD and some of these conditions, that OCD itself is quite a heterogeneous condition, and that many of the spectrum disorders have a broader relationship with anxiety and depressive disorders in general, rather than with OCD in particular. It is also possible (Jaisoorya et al., 2003) that some of the disorders within the putative spectrum (e.g., tic disorders, hypochondriasis, body dysmorphic disorder, trichotillomania) are more closely related to OCD than others (e.g., eating disorders, pathological gambling, depersonalization disorder, sexual compulsions).

Assessment

Diagnostic Issues

Unlike some of the other anxiety disorders (e.g., generalized anxiety disorder, social anxiety disorder, posttraumatic stress disorder), OCD has not been a controversial diagnostic category. That is, the existence of OCD and the validity of the diagnosis of OCD are hardly doubted or disputed in the professional community. Obsessive-compulsive disorder is also perceived as real by the lay public. There are several reasons for this status. First, it is a condition with long tradition, having been described and recognized as an illness a long time ago. As such, there is no risk of OCD being regarded as an artificial product of diagnostic and classification schemes or as some sort of voguish diagnosis. Second, unlike many psychiatric disorders, OCD possesses a degree of longitudinal stability (e.g., Mataix-Cols et al., 2002) that reinforces its perception as real. That is, OCD tends to persist for many years despite seemingly efficacious treatment, and also tends to be present in various subthreshold, subdiagnostic, and subclinical forms in persons who appear recovered and with little or no OCD-associated impairment (see Course and Prognosis, below). Third, the finding of a low placebo response rate in OCD, compared to that of other psychiatric disorders, also strengthens the perception of OCD as being real.

Thus, controversies regarding OCD are not about its validity as a psychopathological and diagnostic entity. Questions remain about the heterogeneity of OCD and about how this condition, and its potential sub-types, should be classified. The current classification of OCD among the anxiety disorders in the DSM system is not satisfactory; it may be adequate only for some types of OCD, perhaps those that are characterized by over-whelming anxiety and that resemble anxiety disorders, such as phobias and generalized anxiety disorder. Patients with other types of OCD appear to have more in common with sufferers of schizophrenia and other psy-chotic disorders, while some OCD patients seem to have a neurological rather than a psychiatric condition. The introduction of the concept of obsessive-compulsive spectrum disorders has not resolved these issues (see Relationship Between Obsessive-Compulsive Disorder and Other Dis-orders, above), but it has highlighted multiple links between OCD and a variety of other conditions.

At this stage, it seems reasonable to leave the issue of classification of OCD open. That is, the current placement of the heterogeneous syndrome of OCD among the anxiety disorders should not preclude us from under-standing and treating individual cases of OCD as if OCD were classified elsewhere—for example, among the mood or psychotic disorders.

The key component in the diagnosis of OCD is the presence of obses-sions and compulsions. The DSM-IV-TR and ICD-10 diagnostic criteria for OCD emphasize the definitions of obsessions and compulsions that are pre-sented with some modification in Clinical Features (above; see Tables 6–1 and 6–3). The current diagnostic manual definitions of obsessions and com-pulsions could be expanded in a manner that would further clarify these concepts and highlight the links between obsessions and all behaviors that appear in response to obsessions, not just compulsions (see Fig. 6–1).

The main uncertainty in the area of OCD diagnosis (according to DSM-IV-TR) is about the distinction between OCD with poor insight and "classical" (good insight) OCD. Indeed, this is a crucial issue, which is likely to play an important role in future conceptualizations of OCD and some of the OCD-related disorders. For example, there is a need to clarify whether OCD with poor insight might be better conceptualized as a con-dition that is essentially different from classical OCD. If so, it might be use-ful to establish a separate group of OCD conditions with varying degrees of insight on the dimension of certainty or conviction; such a group might include OCD with overvalued ideas and delusional OCD, making the rela-tionship with obsessive-compulsive spectrum disorders more meaningful. The issue of insight in OCD and the status of OCD with poor insight are further discussed in Clinical Features (above).

The ICD-10 diagnostic criteria for OCD are quite similar to those in the DSM system. However, the proposed subtypes of OCD in ICD-10 include "predominantly obsessional thoughts and ruminations" and "predominantly compulsive acts (obsessional rituals)." In view of findings that most patients with OCD present with both obsessions and compulsions, such subtyping seems superfluous.

Assessment Instruments

The Yale-Brown Obsessive Compulsive Scale (YBOCS; Goodman et al., 1989a) has been the most widely used instrument for measuring the severity of obsessions and compulsions in OCD already diagnosed by other means. It is administered by clinicians as a semistructured interview, and is quite comprehensive because it assesses obsessions and compulsions in terms of time spent on them, their interference with functioning, distress caused by obsessions and compulsions, resistance to them and ability to control these features of OCD. The YBOCS has been used to monitor changes during the treatment of OCD and has therefore been invaluable in treatment outcome studies, acquiring the status of a gold standard measure. It can also be used as a screening instrument, although its administration for this purpose is rather cumbersome.

The Padua Inventory (Sanavio, 1988) is a comprehensive, 60-item, self-report instrument for measuring the severity of OCD and for monitoring changes during the treatment of OCD. Versions with 39 and 41 items have also been developed, but because of its length, this instrument is generally not suitable for screening purposes.

The Maudsley Obsessional-Compulsive Inventory (Hodgson and Rachman, 1977) is another self-report instrument, containing 30 true–false items. While this instrument is not suitable for measuring the severity of OCD, it may be useful as a screening tool and for the purpose of assessing the most salient features of OCD (e.g., washing and checking compulsions).

Differential Diagnosis

In the differential diagnosis of OCD, the most important step is to make a distinction between obsessions and compulsions on one hand, and phenomena and behaviors that may resemble obsessions and compulsions on the other (see Tables 6-2 and 6-4). Once obsessions are distinguished from depressive ruminations, overvalued ideas, delusions, and pathological worry (Table 6-2), the distinction between OCD and depression, hypochondriasis or body dysmorphic disorder, psychotic illness, and generalized anxiety disorder, respectively, will generally not represent a problem. Likewise, if compulsions are correctly distinguished from impulsive acts (Table 6-4), the distinction between OCD and various impulse control disorders will not be difficult.

The questions that need to be asked in the differential diagnosis of OCD are as follows:

• What is the content of the psychopathological (obsession-like) phenomenon?
• Is the psychopathological (obsession-like) pheno nenon experienced as ego-dystonic?
• What is the degree of certainty and conviction with which the psychopathological (obsession-like) phenomenon is experienced?
• What is the behavioral response to the psychopathological (obsession-like) phenomenon, if any?
• How can the compulsion-like activity be described?
• Does the compulsion-like activity appear in response to a psychopathological (obsession-like) phenomenon or in response to a particular feeling or urge?
• What is the goal or purpose of the compulsion-like activity?

Another important consideration in the differential diagnosis of OCD is the fact that many disorders that resemble OCD and may be mistaken for it often coexist with OCD (see Relationship Between Obsessive-Compulsive Disorder and Other Disorders, above). Therefore, the main question in the differential diagnosis of OCD is not necessarily "Is it OCD *or* something else?", but "Is it OCD *and* something else?"

Keeping in mind that OCD is related to several other disorders, and that it bears similarities with them and often co-occurs with these conditions, Table 6–8 presents the most important criteria for distinguishing between OCD and these disorders.

It should be specifically emphasized that OCD and obsessive-compulsive personality disorder differ crucially in that there are no obsessions and compulsions in the latter condition. Some characteristics of obsessive-compulsive personality disorder may represent features of OCD, for example, tendencies toward perfectionism and pathological indecisiveness. Other areas of overlap between OCD and obsessive-compulsive personality disorder include preoccupation with control, a tendency to hoard, and spending a lot of time rearranging objects in certain order and "getting things right"; these are often not experienced as ego-dystonic and can be a part of either condition. In such cases, a definite differentiation should be made on the basis of other features in the patients' clinical presentation.

Finally, OCD should be differentiated from "normal" obsession-like phenomena and compulsion-like activities. Examples of the latter include certain superstitious beliefs, checking behaviors, and religious rituals. Although the demarcation line between OCD and "normality" sometimes

TABLE 6–8. Criteria for Distinguishing Between Obsessive-Compulsive Disorder and Other Disorders

Disorders	Criteria for Distinguishing
Psychosis (e.g., schizophrenia, delusional disorder)	Loss of reality testing Presence of delusions (any obsession-like phenomenon is espoused with firm conviction and is not experienced as ego-dystonic)
Depression	Obsession-like phenomena (depressive ruminations) are congruent with depressed mood and are not experienced as ego-dystonic
Hypochondriasis, body dysmorphic disorder, anorexia nervosa	Obsession-like phenomena (overvalued ideas) are held with a more firm belief, they are monothematic (preoccupation with health and disease, body image, weight and intake of food) and not experienced as ego-dystonic
Generalized anxiety disorder	Obsession-like phenomenon (pathological worry) pertains to real-life problems and is not experienced as ego-dystonic
Specific phobia	Obsession-like phenomenon (preoccupation with specific fears) is not experienced as ego-dystonic and is responded to by avoidance, not compulsions
Impulse control disorders (e.g., trichotillomania, impulsive buying, impulsive sexual activity)	Compulsion-like activity (impulsive acts) is performed in response to an urge or tension (not in response to obsession), with the goal of obtaining relief, pleasure, or gratification (not with the goal of decreasing anxiety or preventing harm)
Tic disorders	Compulsion-like activity (tics) consists of relatively simple motor movements or vocalizations, which are not performed with the goal of decreasing anxiety or preventing harm
Stereotypic movement disorder	Compulsion-like activity (stereotyped movements) consists of a seemingly driven, purposeful motor behavior, which may be performed with the goal of obtaining self-stimulation (not with the goal of decreasing anxiety or preventing harm)
Obsessive-compulsive personality disorder	Absence of obsessions and compulsions Excessive devotion to work, frugality, stubbornness, rigidity, excessive need to control interpersonal situations, lack of warmth

seems to be very thin, there are fairly clear criteria for making this distinction. As long as the obsession-like phenomena are not taken too seriously by the person and do not cause distress, as long as the compulsion-like activities are not too time consuming, and as long as both the obsession-like phenomena and compulsion-like activities do not interfere with functioning and the person is not concerned about them, they remain within the realm of normality.

EPIDEMIOLOGY

The highlights of the epidemiology of OCD are presented in Table 6–9.

Until the 1980s, OCD was thought to be a rare condition. With the introduction of more precise diagnostic criteria and more sensitive assessment instruments, which made it less likely for cases of OCD to be missed, OCD emerged as one of the most common psychiatric disorders. Therefore, it is not that OCD has become more prevalent over the past several decades; it is only our ability to detect it that has improved.

In the U.S. Epidemiological Catchment Area (ECA) Study, OCD was found to be the fourth most common mental disorder, with a lifetime prevalence rate of 2.5% (Robins et al., 1984). The same methodology used in the ECA study was applied to an epidemiological survey conducted in several countries (Weissman et al., 1994), and lifetime prevalence rates were remarkably similar in different socioeconomic settings: 1.9%–2.5%. The only exception was Taiwan, where the prevalence rate of OCD was much lower, but so were the rates for other psychiatric disorders. The finding of this survey suggests that the prevalence of OCD is largely independent from the social, cultural, and economic context.

The prevalence rates based on the ECA study have been called into question, mainly because the study relied on a diagnostic instrument that was used by lay interviewers. Thus, the prevalence of OCD might have been overestimated and cases without clinically significant manifestations might have ended up being counted (Nelson and Rice, 1997; Stein et al., 1997a). Although there is no full agreement on what the corrected preva-

TABLE 6–9. Epidemiological Data for Obsessive-Compulsive Disorder

- Lifetime prevalence in the U.S. ECA study: 2.5%
- Similar prevalence rates in different countries
- The corrected prevalence rates may be lower (e.g., lifetime prevalence rate between 1.5% and 2%)
- Practically no difference in prevalence between women and men
- Age of onset is earlier in males
- OCD in children and adolescents is more common among males than females
- Mean age of onset: 21–22 years (range: 18–24 years), with a substantial proportion having onset in childhood
- Onset is usually insidious, with few, if any stressful or other events preceding it
- Average period between onset and time of seeking help: 7.5 years

ECA, Epidemiological Catchment Area.

lence rates of OCD might be, it is estimated that the lifetime prevalence rate is between 1.5% and 2%.

There appears to be a continuum of severity between *subthreshold* OCD (with relatively minor obsessions and/or compulsions) and *fully diagnosable* OCD (with clinically significant obsessions and/or compulsions, which are associated with distress or impairment). The frequency of individuals (adolescents) in the community with the subthreshold form of OCD was estimated at 8% (Apter et al., 1996). It is not clear what proportion of individuals with subthreshold OCD go on to develop a full-blown OCD.

Obsessive-compulsive disorder is insignificantly more frequent among women than among men (Black, 1974; Noshirvani et al., 1991; Rasmussen and Eisen, 1992; Foa and Kozak, 1995), but there are several differences between women and men with OCD. First, OCD in children and adolescents is more often encountered among males than among females (Hollingsworth et al., 1980; Leonard et al., 1989), and it starts earlier in boys than in girls (Swedo et al., 1989a). Second, the onset of the adult form of OCD is also earlier in men than in women (Rasmussen and Eisen, 1990). Third, men may be more likely to have a co-occurring psychotic disorder or schizotypal personality disorder (Eisen and Rasmussen, 1993). Finally, the prognosis of OCD may be generally worse in men, possibly because an earlier onset of OCD and co-occurrence of psychotic disorders and schizotypal personality disorder are associated with poor prognosis.

As for demographic factors other than gender, none have been consistently associated with OCD. Patients with OCD may be less likely to marry (Rasmussen and Eisen, 1991). They also tend to be impaired in various domains of functioning (social, occupational, academic), and direct and indirect cost of OCD to the society is estimated to be very high (Hollander et al., 1996).

Obsessive-compulsive disorder often begins in childhood and adolescence, with more than 20% of patients reporting onset before age 14 (Rasmussen and Eisen, 1990). Many children exhibit superstitious behavior or have obsessions and compulsions, but subsequently grow out of them. Only a minority of children with obsessions and compulsions actually develop OCD (Riddle et al., 1990). The prevalence of OCD among adolescents appears to be as high as it is among adults (Flament et al., 1988). The disorder may continue into adulthood in a substantial number of children with OCD, but the childhood and adult forms of OCD differ in several important aspects. The usual mean age of onset of the adult form of OCD is around 21–22 years, and ranges between ages 18 and 24 (Bland et al., 1988a; Karno et al., 1988; Rasmussen and Eisen, 1992; Degonda et al., 1993;

Lensi et al., 1996). In the minority of OCD sufferers, less than 15%, the illness first manifests itself after age 35 (Rasmussen and Eisen, 1992).

The onset of OCD is usually insidious, with few, if any stressful or other events preceding it. Sometimes, the onset of OCD is sudden. For example, OCD may first appear during pregnancy (Neziroglu et al., 1992), in men following childbirth (Abramowitz et al., 2001), or after a streptococcal infection (Leonard and Swedo, 2001).

Patients with OCD often have the illness for a long time, an average of 7.5 years (Rasmussen and Tsuang, 1986), before seeking help. An important reason for waiting so long before seeking help and treatment seems to be the shame and secrecy surrounding OCD. Many patients are puzzled by their obsessions and compulsions, often feel that they are "crazy," and go to great lengths to hide their symptoms. There are also problems with recognizing OCD (e.g., Fireman et al., 2001), which contributes to the time lag between the onset of OCD and its correct diagnosis.

The diagnosis of OCD is still missed, particularly when patients present to nonpsychiatric physicians for problems that are apparently unrelated to OCD. For example, patients who wash compulsively may develop dermatitis or even eczema and seek help from primary care physicians or dermatologists. In fact, a recent study (Fineberg et al., 2003) showed that almost 20% of patients in a dermatology outpatient clinic suffered from a clinically significant OCD, and almost all of these patients had not been previously recognized as having OCD. It is important to continue raising the awareness of OCD, to promote its early detection and accurate diagnosis. Another initiative is to educate mental health professionals and primary care providers about efficacious treatments for OCD, because the data suggest that even patients who are correctly diagnosed do not receive adequate treatment for 6–7 years (Hollander and Wong, 1998).

COURSE AND PROGNOSIS

It has been clearly established by numerous studies (Ingram, 1961; Kringlen, 1965; Black, 1974; Rasmussen and Tsuang, 1986; Rasmussen and Eisen, 1992; Demal et al., 1993; Skoog and Skoog, 1999; Steketee et al., 1999) that OCD tends to be a chronic condition in most patients. However, the length of follow-up periods, description of chronicity, and related terminology have varied from one study to another, contributing to some confusion about the course of OCD. Also, some of these studies were conducted when few efficacious treatments for OCD were available, which was likely to affect the course of illness. It appears that three general types of chronicity have been noted in OCD:

- A fluctuating chronic course, in which there are exacerbations and periods of complete or partial remission, observed in 2% (Rasmussen and Tsuang, 1986; Rasmussen and Eisen, 1992), 25% (Kringlen, 1965), 37% (Demal et al., 1993), 46% (Ingram, 1961), and 35%–47% (Black, 1974) of patients
- A steady (constant, continuing) chronic course, without significant fluctuations, observed in 15% (Ingram, 1961), 28% (Demal et al., 1993), 30% (Kringlen, 1965), 54%–61% (Black, 1974), 84% (Rasmussen and Tsuang, 1986), and 85% (Rasmussen and Eisen, 1992) of patients. The last two figures (84% and 85%) include patients who apparently also had some fluctuations.
- Progressive, deteriorating course, observed in 5% (Kringlen, 1965), 10% (Rasmussen and Eisen, 1992; Demal et al., 1993; Skoog and Skoog, 1999) and 14% (Rasmussen and Tsuang, 1986) of patients.

Spontaneous and enduring remissions of OCD occur rarely. The proportion of OCD patients who achieve a lasting remission or recovery (complete absence of symptoms) has been consistently small across studies, reaching 20% at the most (Skoog and Skoog, 1999; Steketee et al., 1999).

Data on the course of OCD are summarized in Table 6–10.

The longest (40 to 50 year) prospective follow-up study of patients with OCD (Skoog and Skoog, 1999) reported several interesting findings. First, patients relapsed after being symptom-free for 10 or even 20 years, which suggests that OCD may be dormant for long periods of time and patients may never lose a propensity to relapse. If the relapse of illness does occur even after 20 years of remission, the characterization of the course cannot be reliable and patients can never be considered fully recovered or cured. Second, the findings of this study belong to the categories of both "good news" and "bad news" with regards to outcome.

TABLE 6–10. Course of Obsessive-Compulsive Disorder

Course	Percentage of patients
Lasting remission or recovery	Maximum 20%
Fluctuating chronic course, with exacerbations and periods of complete or partial remission	2%–47%
Steady (constant, continuing) chronic course, without significant fluctuations (no clear-cut exacerbations and remissions)	15%–61%
Progressive, deteriorating course	5%–14%

After a 40 to 50 year follow-up, 83% of patients showed general improvement and 48% were clinically recovered. However, 60%–67% of patients continued to experience symptoms of varying severity and 37% had diagnosable OCD.

Exacerbations in the course of OCD often occur at times of stress, but cannot be reliably predicted by stressful events. Some exacerbations are relatively mild, below the diagnostic threshold for OCD, and are not registered as true relapses of the original illness.

Predictors of poor prognosis of OCD have been identified by several studies (Table 6–11). These include early age at onset, not being married, greater initial severity of illness, longer duration of illness and chronicity, presence of both obsessions and compulsions, prominent magical thinking, presence of delusions, presence of severe personality disturbance (particularly schizotypal, paranoid, and borderline personality disorders), co-occurrence of bipolar disorder and eating disorder, and poor social adjustment and inadequate social skills.

ETIOLOGY AND PATHOGENESIS

Obsessive-compulsive disorder has attracted the attention of researchers and clinicians of various backgrounds and theoretical orientations and persuasions. Although we still do not have a comprehensive account of the causes and origins of OCD, it is useful to look at the contributions of major schools of thought to our current understanding of this illness.

TABLE 6–11. Predictors of Poor Prognosis of Obsessive-Compulsive Disorder

- Early age at onset (Skoog and Skoog, 1999)
- Not being married (Steketee et al., 1999)
- Greater initial severity of illness (Steketee et al., 1999)
- Longer duration of illness and chronicity (Skoog and Skoog, 1999; Hollander et al., 2002)
- Presence of both obsessions and compulsions (Skoog and Skoog, 1999)
- Prominent magical thinking (Skoog and Skoog, 1999)
- Presence of delusions (Hollander et al., 2002)
- Presence of severe personality disturbance, particularly schizotypal, paranoid, and borderline personality disorders (e.g., Jenike et al., 1986; Baer et al., 1992; Moritz et al., 2004)
- Co-occurrence of bipolar disorder and eating disorder (Hollander et al., 2002)
- Poor social adjustment and inadequate social skills (Skoog and Skoog, 1999)

BIOLOGICAL MODELS

The last two decades have witnessed an explosion of research into biological origins of OCD. The results of this research activity do not point to any pathophysiological mechanism as being unique to OCD, suggesting that OCD is a heterogeneous condition with different etiological and pathogenetic factors involved. Although the full picture is still missing, at this stage we do have a better understanding of some of the pathophysiological processes implicated in the etiology and pathogenesis of OCD, and we know more about brain structures in which these processes take place. Table 6–12 presents findings of biological and neuroimaging studies that are relatively specific for OCD. The findings of genetic, pathophysiological, pharmacological, brain imaging, and neuropsychological studies in OCD are summarized in the text below.

Genetic Factors

Family studies of OCD have consistently demonstrated that there are more first-degree relatives with OCD among children with OCD and adult patients who had an early onset of OCD than among patients with a later onset of OCD (Lenane et al., 1990; Riddle et al., 1990; Bellodi et al., 1992; Pauls et al., 1995; Nestadt et al., 2000). Patients with late-onset OCD may not differ from persons without OCD in terms of the proportion of first-degree relatives who have OCD. Therefore, it appears that childhood OCD and early-onset adult OCD have a stronger genetic component than late-onset OCD. Consequently, in those cases where the risk of developing

TABLE 6–12. Findings of Biological and Neuroimaging Studies That Are Relatively Specific for Obsessive-Compulsive Disorder

- Dysfunction of the serotonin neurotransmitter system (hypersensitivity of postsynaptic serotonin receptors?)
- Increased dopaminergic function in some OCD patients, particularly those with co-occurring tic disorders
- Brain structures implicated in the etiology and pathogenesis of OCD:
  Limbic system: orbitofrontal cortex, cingulate, amygdala, thalamus
  Basal ganglia: striatum (caudate nuclei)
- Dysfunction in the orbitofrontal (limbic)-basal ganglia circuits
- Dysfunction in the cortico-striato-thalamo-cortical circuits
- Certain forms of OCD in childhood: autoimmune processes following an infection with group A β-hemolytic streptococci, with OCD occurring in conjunction with choreiform movements (Sydenham's chorea) or tics

OCD is inherited, OCD tends to start in childhood or adolescence. At this stage, however, it is unclear what is inherited in OCD.

Results of twin studies of OCD have not been consistent and unequivocal in terms of pointing to a significantly higher concordance rate of OCD symptoms among monozygotic than among dizygotic twin pairs.

Although the relationship between genetic factors in OCD and Tourette's disorder is not clear, it appears that a sizeable number of patients with OCD and Tourette's disorder have more family members with both OCD and Tourette's disorder; these patients also tend to have an earlier onset of OCD (Pauls et al., 1995). One study (Bienvenu et al., 2000) found a higher frequency of certain obsessive-compulsive spectrum disorders (hypochondriasis, body dysmorphic disorder, and eating disorders) among the relatives of patients with OCD.

Pathophysiological Mechanisms and Neuroanatomy

Neurotransmitter Systems

The serotonin hypothesis of OCD has been most influential, mainly because of the efficacy of serotonergic antidepressants in the treatment of OCD (and the striking lack of efficacy of noradrenergic antidepressants). Numerous studies with agents that either block or stimulate serotonin receptors have confirmed the role of the serotonin neurotransmitter system abnormalities in the etiology and pathogenesis of OCD. The hypersensitivity of postsynaptic serotonin receptors has been hypothesized as an underlying abnormality in most cases of OCD (Hollander et al., 1988; Zohar et al., 1988), but the precise nature of serotonin involvement in the pathogenesis of OCD is not clear. It appears that several pathophysiological mechanisms involving various serotonin receptors in various areas of the brain may lead to OCD.

In addition to dysfunction of the serotonin system, various other neurotransmitters have occasionally been implicated in the pathogenesis of OCD. Of clinical relevance is increased dopaminergic function in some OCD patients (Goodman et al., 1990a), particularly those with co-occurring tic disorders (e.g., Tourette's disorder). Because first-generation antipsychotics block dopamine receptors, dopaminergic hyperactivity may account for the efficacy of these medications in OCD, when they are used in combination with serotonergic antidepressants.

Brain Structures Involved in Obsessive-Compulsive Disorder

Results of brain imaging and neuropsychological studies as well as experience with neurosurgical procedures have all suggested that certain brain structures are involved in OCD. These structures include the limbic system (orbitofrontal cortex, cingulate, amygdala, thalamus) and parts of the basal ganglia (striatum, and more specifically caudate nuclei) (Baxter et al., 1987; Swedo et al., 1989b; Rauch et al., 1994; Breiter et al., 1996; Rosenberg et al., 1997; Szeszko et al., 1999; Adler et al., 2000; Gilbert et al., 2000). It has been speculated that OCD symptoms are a consequence of functional alterations and possibly hyperactivity of the orbitofrontal (limbic)-basal ganglia circuits.

The corticostriatal hypothesis of OCD postulates very broadly that there is a dysfunction in the cortico-striato-thalamo-cortical circuits. According to this model, disturbances in the pathways between the cortex and the thalamus may be implicated in the pathogenesis of obsessions and obsession like phenomena, whereas abnormalities in the striatum are involved in the pathogenesis of compulsions and repetitive motor acts (Insel, 1992; Rauch and Jenike, 1993).

Neuroimaging studies have also demonstrated functional and structural changes in the orbitofrontal cortex, cingulate, and caudate nuclei in patients who responded to clomipramine, selective serotonin reuptake inhibitors, or behavior therapy (Benkelfat et al., 1990; Baxter et al., 1992; Swedo et al., 1992; Perani et al., 1995; Schwartz et al., 1996; Rosenberg et al., 2000).

Other Neurobiological Aspects

Some types of OCD, particularly those that appear in childhood, may be caused by immunological mechanisms. For example, children with Sydenham's chorea (a disorder of the basal ganglia like Tourette's disorder) very often have symptoms of OCD, and some children with OCD exhibit choreiform movements (Swedo, 1994; Swedo et al., 1994). Because Sydenham's chorea is believed to be a consequence of autoimmune disturbances following an infection with group A β-hemolytic streptococci, it was speculated that at least some forms of OCD in childhood (particularly those with an abrupt onset) might also be a manifestation of bacteria-induced autoimmune processes (Allen et al., 1995; Murphy et al., 1997). This condition, characterized by OCD and/or neurological abnormalities in childhood, has been referred to as **P**ediatric **A**utoimmune **N**europsychiatric **D**isorder **A**ssociated with **S**treptococcal infection or PANDAS (Swedo et al., 1998). A hypothesis about autoimmune etiology was supported by a magnetic resonance imaging (MRI) finding of enlarged basal ganglia in children with OCD or tics who also had a streptococcal infection (Giedd et al., 2000).

PSYCHOLOGICAL MODELS

In view of the centrality of cognitions (obsessions and obsessional thinking) in the clinical picture of OCD, psychological models of OCD attempt
primarily to give an account of why and how OCD patients find themselves so engaged in the specific, anxiety-laden pattern of "thinking about
thinking." Hence, the cognitive account of OCD has now become the dominant psychological explanatory model of OCD.

Cognitive Model

The cognitive model of OCD (McFall and Wollersheim, 1979; Salkovskis,
1985, 1989, 1999; Freeston et al., 1996; Obsessive Compulsive Cognitions
Working Group, 1997; Rachman, 1997, 1998) broadly postulates that OCD
occurs as a result of activation of certain dysfunctional beliefs and schemas
about one's own style of thinking and coping with such thinking. These are
postulated to include beliefs that certain thoughts are dangerous because
they suggest catastrophic scenarios; that these catastrophes might be prevented by the person who is experiencing such thoughts; that prevention
of catastrophes involves further cognitive activity, i.e., both more thinking
and "correct" thinking; that because of insufficient efficacy, such cognitive
activity has to be augmented by certain harm-preventing behaviors (compulsions). Within this general cognitive framework of OCD, specific explanations of some of its components have emerged. They fall into two
general categories: (1) dysfunctional appraisals of intrusions and (2) erroneous or maladaptive beliefs about thoughts and thinking processes, with
prominence of certain cognitive patterns.

An example of the first category of cognitive accounts of OCD is the
model put forward by Salkovskis (1985, 1989, 1999). He has proposed that
intrusive thoughts about unacceptable, disturbing, or repugnant events
are not by themselves pathological, and lead to obsessions only if they are
appraised in a specific way. For OCD to develop, this appraisal involves
the person's exaggerated sense of responsibility for having intrusive
thoughts, for harm that is associated with these thoughts, and/or for preventing harm to oneself or others. Salkovskis et al. (1999) have suggested
that the origin of such responsibility appraisals can be found in strict
upbringing and rigid codes of conduct required by schools or certain religious institutions.

A dysfunctional appraisal of intrusive thoughts may also occur as a
result of attention disturbances in OCD; that is, OCD patients may be
unable to ignore intrusive thoughts, paying inordinate, selective attention
to them (Clayton et al., 1999).

In the second category of cognitive accounts of OCD are those that emphasize erroneous or maladaptive beliefs about thoughts and thinking processes, as well as certain cognitive patterns. These were identified in OCD by Purdon and Clark (1994), Freeston et al. (1996), Shafran et al. (1996), the Obsessive Compulsive Cognitions Working Group (1997), and Rachman (1997; 1998). Some of these patterns appear to be moderately to highly specific for OCD (exaggerated importance of thoughts, concern about control over one's thoughts), others are relatively specific for OCD, as they are also seen in other anxiety disorders (thought-action fusion, intolerance of uncertainty, perfectionist tendencies), and some are common to all anxiety disorders (exaggerated perception of threat, overestimation of danger). The beliefs and cognitive patterns that are relatively specific for OCD, along with corresponding examples, are shown in Table 6–13.

TABLE 6–13. Beliefs About Thoughts and Thinking Processes and Cognitive Patterns That Are Relatively Specific for Obsessive-Compulsive Disorder

Beliefs and Cognitive Patterns	*Examples of Beliefs or Thoughts*
Exaggerated importance of thoughts (Freeston et al., 1996; OCCWG, 1997; Rachman, 1997; 1998)	"If I think about something, it has to be important."
Concern about inability to control one's own thoughts and the anticipated consequences of failed control, whereby such control is considered very important (Purdon and Clark, 1994; Freeston et al., 1996; OCCWG, 1997)	"I should always be in control over what goes through my mind. That I continue to have these crazy thoughts despite my efforts to get rid of them, will have some dire consequences."
Thought-action fusion (TAF) (Shafran et al., 1996)	"Having thoughts about doing something is the same as doing it."
Likelihood TAF (thinking about a disturbing event makes it more probable for the event to occur)	"It will happen just because I think about it."
Moral TAF (having a thought about something unacceptable or disturbing is the same as carrying out that unacceptable or disturbing act)	"Thinking about something so awful means that I am a bad person."
Overvaluing the need for certainty, intolerance of uncertainty (Freeston et al., 1996; OCCWG, 1997)	"I can't stand any ambiguity about the situation. Uncertainty is dangerous."
Excessive need for perfectionism, tendencies towards perfectionism (Freeston et al., 1996; OCCWG, 1997)	"It has to be 100% good, otherwise there is no value in it."

OCCWG, Obsessive Compulsive Cognitions Working Group.

The cognitive model also postulates that OCD is maintained by various neutralizing activities: compulsions, avoidance, and reassurance seeking. Within the model proposed by Salkovskis (1996), neutralizing activities occur because of the patients' need to prevent harm or liberate themselves from the tormenting responsibility for preventing harm. The effect of the neutralizing activities is temporary, however, and patients repeatedly resort to these activities attempting to attain the sense of safety, while paradoxically increasing the perception of threat and preoccupation with danger.

Although often considered separately, the postulated memory disturbances in OCD are, in fact, a part of the cognitive model of OCD. One such disturbance is the possible memory biases toward specific themes and issues that are distressing to OCD patients (Radomsky and Rachman, 1999; Radomsky et al., 2001); for example OCD patients with contamination obsessions and washing and cleaning compulsions may have better memory for contaminated objects and situations. Another interesting hypothesis involving memory postulates that OCD patients with checking compulsions feel insecure about their own memory (Macdonald et al., 1997), which may be the main reason for their repetitive checking rituals. This hypothesis has recently been elaborated (van den Hout and Kindt, 2003) with the proposition that OCD patients with checking compulsions have two primary problems. The first is their excessive need for certainty (as confirmed independently in a study by Tolin et al., 2003), and the second is a critical attitude toward their own memory performance; both of these lead these patients to distrust their memory, so that they resort to checking. However, instead of decreasing memory distrust, repeated checking only increases it, thus creating a vicious circle.

The cognitive model of OCD has given novel, interesting, and convincing insights into the most salient features of OCD and various types of obsessions and compulsions. However, the cognitive model illuminates the psychopathology of OCD better than it does the etiology and pathogenesis of OCD. Various components and aspects of the model have received considerable empirical support. A more broad cognitive account of OCD seems better suited to improve our understanding of OCD than the one that overemphasizes the importance of the concept of inflated responsibility.

Behavioral Model

The behavioral model of OCD is somewhat simplistic, but it is a foundation on which an efficacious treatment, exposure with response prevention, has been developed. The model is based on Mowrer's (1960) two-factor theory of fear acquisition and maintenance. According to this theory, obsessions are seen as unconditioned, fear-inducing stimuli, which are maintained by operant conditioning: by temporarily alleviating fear produced by obsessions, compulsions prevent habituation to the obsession-related feared stimuli and thereby maintain obsessions, while at the same time reinforcing themselves as means of reducing fear. In other words, compulsions are conceptualized as a maladaptive response to obsessions. This response may be useful in the short term, because it alleviates anxiety, but in the long term, its anxiety-alleviating function maintains both the obsessions and the compulsions.

Psychoanalytic Contributions

The psychoanalytic account of OCD is schematically presented in Figure 6–2. The central tenet of the psychoanalytic theory (Fig. 6–2) is that OCD results from regression to the anal-sadistic stage of development (Freud, 1909/1955b; 1913/1958; Nemiah, 1988), as all the other features of OCD are a consequence of this regression.

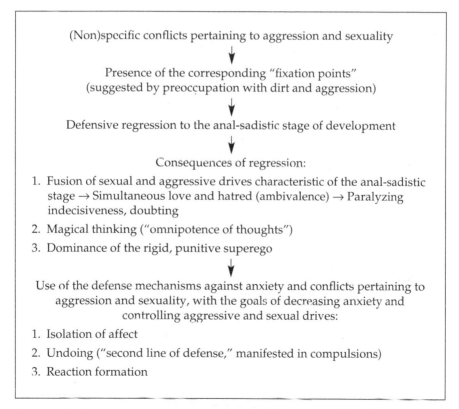

Figure 6–2. Psychoanalytic account of obsessive-compulsive disorder.

The psychoanalytic theory of OCD represents a coherent explanatory model, that offers understanding of OCD on the basis of key psychoanalytic concepts. Although the concepts of conflicts, fixation points, and regression are currently not as widely accepted, the lasting achievement of the psychoanalytic model is its provision of valuable insights into the psychopathology of OCD, particularly the role of underlying aggressive themes, ambivalence, and magical thinking. There may be no agreement among clinicians as to why so many OCD patients seem troubled by aggressive urges, doubting, and indecisiveness, but there is no question that these features are recognized by most as being important in OCD. Moreover, the postulation that magical thinking plays an important role in the psychopathology and pathogenesis of OCD has been very influential, with its implicit suggestion that OCD may be primarily a disorder of the thinking processes. Although the cognitive model of OCD is derived from a different theoretical framework, it is largely an outgrowth and further elaboration of the concept of magical thinking.

The psychoanalytic theory is also helpful in illuminating the similarities and differences between OCD and obsessive-compulsive personality disorder. As a comparison, the psychoanalytic account (Freud, 1908/1959; Abraham, 1921/1942; Shapiro, 1965; Salzman, 1968) of obsessive-compulsive personality disorder is schematically presented in Figure 6–3.

(Non)specific disturbances in relations with primary objects
(e.g., "cold parents")

↓

Low self-esteem + conflicts pertaining to aggression:

↓

A. Consequences of low self-esteem:

1. Need to "conquer" superego → Tendencies toward perfectionism → Fear of making a mistake → Rigid and dogmatic cognitive style
2. Tendency to control others to prevent their loss
3. Difficulty with (fear of) interpersonal intimacy

B. Consequences of conflicts pertaining to aggression:

1. Fear of losing control
2. Ambivalence and indecisiveness
3. Use of the defense mechanisms (reaction formation, isolation of affect)

Figure 6–3. Psychoanalytic account of obsessive-compulsive personality disorder.

TREATMENT

It is a truism that treatment of OCD is often difficult and challenging, putting to test therapeutic skills, patience, and perseverance of many therapists. There is no place for therapeutic nihilism, because efficacious treatments for OCD do exist. Too much optimism is not justified either, however, because current treatments for OCD rarely bring about a complete disappearance of symptoms, and a substantial proportion of patients respond poorly or only partially to almost all treatment modalities. Still, with the more realistic goals of treatment of OCD—e.g., alleviation of symptoms and improvement in functioning—current treatments hold promise for many patients.

Pharmacological treatment and cognitive-behavioral therapy in OCD will be presented separately, followed by a brief discussion of combined treatments, mainly pharmacotherapy in conjunction with cognitive-behavioral therapy. The use of electroconvulsive therapy and neurosurgery in treatment-resistant OCD will also be discussed.

PHARMACOLOGICAL TREATMENT

There are several aspects of pharmacological treatment of OCD that are specific for this condition. These are listed in Table 6–14. During the past

TABLE 6–14. Aspects of the Pharmacological Treatment Specific for Obsessive-Compulsive Disorder

---

- Only medications with specific serotonergic effects (clomipramine, SSRIs) have been efficacious in OCD.

- Criteria for response to medications are less strict for OCD than for other anxiety disorders (e.g., 25%–35% decrease in the score on a rating scale); as a result, many responders to pharmacotherapy are still quite symptomatic.

- Even with the less stringent criteria for response, only 40%–60% of patients with OCD respond to clomipramine or SSRIs.

- Longer duration of treatment (at least 12 weeks) and higher doses of medications (usually higher than doses used in the treatment of depression) are needed for response to occur.

- Slow and gradual response to pharmacotherapy over weeks and months is often observed.

- When compared to other psychiatric disorders, the placebo response rate in OCD is lower.

SSRIs, selective serotonin reuptake inhibitors.

10–15 years, there have been significant advances in the pharmacological treatment of OCD. Patients with OCD are no longer treated nonspecifically with benzodiazepines or other medications. Obsessive-compulsive disorder was the first among the anxiety disorders for which it was demonstrated that selective serotonin reuptake inhibitors (SSRIs) are efficacious. Prior to that, clomipramine, a tricyclic antidepressant with predominant serotonergic activity (inhibition of serotonin reuptake), had established itself as a pharmacological gold standard for treatment of OCD. Despite this progress, there are still many patients with OCD who represent a therapeutic challenge, with about one-half being resistant to any pharmacological treatment.

Medications are used in OCD with the goals of alleviating obsessions and compulsions, decreasing impairment, and improving functioning. A complete and permanent disappearance of obsessions and compulsions occurs rarely and is not a realistic goal of pharmacological treatment. Pharmacotherapy is indicated in almost all cases of OCD, regardless of its severity. While mild to moderate OCD is usually treated with pharmacotherapy, cognitive-behavioral therapy, or a combination of the two, moderate to severe OCD is almost always treated with pharmacotherapy.

At present, there are no clear predictors of good response of OCD to pharmacotherapy—apart from general predictors of good response to any treatment of OCD (e.g., a less pronounced severity of OCD, later onset and shorter duration of illness, episodic course of OCD symptoms, and absence of severe personality disturbance). Obsessive-compulsive disorder with more prominent and disabling obsessions may be more likely to respond to pharmacotherapy or pharmacotherapy combined with cognitive-behavioral therapy, whereas OCD with relatively simple compulsions (particularly washing and cleaning and checking compulsions) may be more amenable to behavior therapy (exposure and response prevention). Certainly, a history of good response of OCD to a particular medication in the past suggests that another trial with the same medication is warranted.

First-Line Pharmacotherapy for Obsessive-Compulsive Disorder: Clomipramine and Selective Serotonin Reuptake Inhibitors

The first-line medications for OCD are clomipramine and SSRIs. The efficacy in OCD has been demonstrated for clomipramine (Thoren et al., 1980; Ananth et al., 1981; Insel et al., 1983; Clomipramine Collaborative Study Group, 1991), fluoxetine (Montgomery et al., 1993; Tollefson et al., 1994), fluvoxamine (Perse et al., 1987; Goodman et al., 1989b), sertraline (Greist et al., 1995a; Kronig et al., 1999), and paroxetine (Hollander et al., 2003). For all practical purposes, there is no difference between them in terms of efficacy, although some reports (e.g., Stein et al., 1995) suggest that clomipramine may be slightly more efficacious. Studies (e.g., Pigott et al., 1990; Freeman et al., 1994; Koran et al., 1996; Bisserbe et al., 1997; Mundo et al., 2000) in which the efficacy of clomipramine was directly compared to that of the SSRIs showed no significant difference. Therefore, the choice between clomipramine and SSRIs is based on the expected side-effect profiles and presence of any contraindications.

Since SSRIs are usually better tolerated than clomipramine, using one of the SSRIs as initial treatment is a reasonable choice (Table 6–15). No medication among the SSRIs has emerged as more efficacious for OCD (except for citalopram, which has not been well studied in OCD). However, certain SSRIs may be used more often for OCD in some settings or may be perceived by some clinicians as being more useful for OCD. Apart from clinician preference and experience, the selection of an SSRI depends on factors such as half-life of the medication and the corresponding ease of ceasing and switching it. Side effects of SSRIs and other issues that emerge in the course of the pharmacotherapy with SSRIs are discussed in Chapter 2.

TABLE 6–15. Choice of Medication in Treatment of Obsessive-Compulsive Disorder

---

First-Line

SSRIs (especially fluoxetine, fluvoxamine, sertraline, and paroxetine)

Second-Line

Another SSRI (if no response at all to the first SSRI)

Third-Line

Clomipramine (if no response at all to the two SSRIs)

Partial Response to First-, Second-, or Third-Line Pharmacotherapy

Augmentations and combinations

1. SSRI or clomipramine + antipsychotic
2. SSRI + clomipramine
3. SSRI or clomipramine + clonazepam
4. SSRI or clomipramine + pindolol

Special Monotherapy Considerations

1. Intravenous clomipramine (if no response or partial response to oral clomipramine)
2. Phenelzine (if no response to all psychopharmacological strategies)

SSRIs, selective serotonin reuptake inhibitors.

In addition to the anticholinergic side effects produced by all tricyclic antidepressants, clomipramine is associated with an increased likelihood of sexual dysfunction. Seizures are more common with clomipramine in higher doses, which are often needed for OCD. The cardiotoxicity and death from overdose represent an additional risk with clomipramine. For these reasons, the maximum dose of clomipramine is set at 250 mg/day, but many patients are unable to tolerate doses higher than 150 mg/day. The initial dose of clomipramine is 25 mg at bedtime; this dose can subsequently be increased by 25–50 mg every 4–7 days, as tolerated. The contraindications for the use of clomipramine include prostatic hypertrophy, closed-angle glaucoma, and cardiac arrhythmias. The presence of other heart problems and a history of seizure disorder dictate that clomipramine be avoided or perhaps used only with utmost caution.

Two practical considerations are important in the treatment of OCD with SSRIs. First, the dosage of an SSRI needed to produce a response is often higher than the dosage used in depression, although some patients may respond to the usual antidepressant dosages of SSRIs. This was clearly demonstrated for paroxetine and fluoxetine. In one study (Hollander et al., 2003), the usual antidepressant dose of paroxetine (20 mg/day) was not better than placebo, whereas OCD patients who were administered 40 or 60 mg/day responded significantly better than those who were on a placebo. Another study (Tollefson et al., 1994) almost found a dose–response relationship for fluoxetine: a better response was reported in OCD patients taking 60 mg/day than in those taking 40 mg/day, whereas those taking 40 mg/day still did better than patients taking 20 mg/day. Therefore, after initiating treatment at standard antidepressant doses (e.g., 20 mg/day of fluoxetine), the doses should be increased as quickly as it is possible. The highest recommended doses of SSRIs and clomipramine in OCD are shown in Table 6–16.

The second practical consideration pertains to the pattern of response of OCD to pharmacological treatment. Although OCD patients may respond to pharmacotherapy early in the course of treatment, it is more usual to observe a slow and gradual response over weeks and months (e.g., de Haan et al., 1997). For this reason, much patience may need to be exercised when patients embark on pharmacotherapy. For example, if the symptoms of OCD have been only slightly alleviated after 3 months of treatment at the highest dose of medication, it is possible that there will be further improvement over the subsequent 3 months. Depending on the circumstances of particular patients, they may then be encouraged to continue taking the medication rather than advised to switch to another one. This makes it difficult to establish more precisely the end point of a phar-

TABLE 6–16. The Highest Recommended Doses of Clomipramine and Selective Serotonin Reuptake Inhibitors in Obsessive-Compulsive Disorder

Medication	Doses
Clomipramine	250 mg/day
SSRIs	
Fluoxetine	80 mg/day
Fluvoxamine	300 mg/day
Paroxetine	60 mg/day
Sertraline	200 mg/day
(Citalopram	60 mg/day)

SSRIs, selective serotonin reuptake inhibitors.

macological trial in OCD: it is uncertain whether there will be further treatment gains after 3, 4, or even 6 months of treatment.

Mechanism of Action of Pharmacological Agents in Obsessive-Compulsive Disorder

How do the efficacious pharmacological agents work in OCD? In an attempt to answer that question, one has to remember that only clomipramine, a serotonergic tricyclic antidepressant, and SSRIs have demonstrated efficacy in OCD. In fact, comparisons between medications with serotonin reuptake blocking properties and antidepressants that lack serotonin reuptake blocking properties, such as amitriptyline (Ananth et al., 1981), clorgyline (Insel et al., 1983), and desipramine (Leonard et al., 1989; Goodman et al., 1990b), showed that the former were superior in the treatment of OCD. These findings suggest that inhibition of serotonin reuptake is a necessary precondition for antiobsessional effects. If so, OCD may be a unique condition in that in most other mental disorders (e.g., panic disorder, generalized anxiety disorder, depression, bipolar disorder), different classes of medications, which have different mechanisms of action, show efficacy. It was originally hypothesized on the basis of the response of OCD to agents that block serotonin reuptake that OCD is specifically related to serotonin dysfunction (see Etiology and Pathogenesis, above).

However, 40%–60% of all OCD patients do not respond to SSRIs or clomipramine. Is there a different pathophysiological mechanism involved in these patients? As already noted (see Obsessive-Compulsive Disorder and Tic Disorders, and Etiology and Pathogenesis, above), OCD patients with co-occurring Tourette's disorder are more likely to respond to a combination of an SSRI or clomipramine and a first-generation antipsychotic, which blocks dopamine receptors. Thus, there may be an increased dopaminergic activity in these OCD patients, in addition to serotonin dysfunction. Interestingly, no success has been reported when using antipsychotics alone in the treatment of OCD.

It was initially believed by some (e.g., Marks et al., 1980) that clomipramine owes the efficacy in OCD to its antidepressant properties, but it was later demonstrated that clomipramine is efficacious in OCD regardless of the presence of depression (Thoren et al., 1980; Ananth et al., 1981; Insel et al., 1983; Flament et al., 1985; Clomipramine Collaborative Study Group, 1991). When OCD patients exhibit clinically significant depression, the latter is likely to respond to the same antidepressant that is efficacious in the treatment of OCD—an SSRI or clomipramine. Antidepressants with a different mechanism of action, such as desipramine, seem to be ineffective in the treatment of both OCD and depression co-occurring with OCD (Goodman et al., 1990b). This suggests that depression co-occurring with OCD may also be characterized by serotonin dysfunction and raises a possibility that depression in OCD can be better conceptualized as part of OCD rather than an independently co-occurring condition.

Long-Term Pharmacological Treatment of Obsessive-Compulsive Disorder

Medications efficacious in the short-term treatment of OCD maintain efficacy over prolonged periods of time (Greist et al., 1995b; Rasmussen et al., 1997). It is now recommended that maintenance pharmacotherapy of OCD be continued for at least 1–2 years after achieving response. The maintenance dosage of an SSRI or clomipramine should be the same as the one with which response was attained during acute treatment.

As with other anxiety disorders, there is a substantial risk of relapse—up to 90% (Pato et al., 1988; Leonard et al., 1991)—if the medication is discontinued. This means that especially for severe and disabling OCD that responded to pharmacotherapy, medication(s) should be used for a very long time, perhaps even indefinitely. If cessation of pharmacotherapy is contemplated at all, it should be done very carefully and gradually. The risk of relapse may be decreased by the use of psychological treatment, especially cognitive-behavioral techniques. In case of relapse, the medication to which the patient responded previously should be administered, but it is uncertain whether the patient will respond to it again.

Pharmacotherapy of Treatment-Resistant Obsessive-Compulsive Disorder

As already noted, the proportion of OCD patients who do not respond to the pharmacological agent of choice, an SSRI, or who respond only partially tends to be high. Therefore, further treatment of these patients is a frequent issue in clinical practice (Table 6–17).

TABLE 6–17. Pharmacotherapy Options for Patients Who Do Not Respond to an Adequate Trial of an SSRI and/or Who Respond Only Partially

Pharmacotherapy options	Reason(s) for considering the treatment option	Likelihood of success
Switching to another SSRI	No response to first SSRI	++/+++
Switching to clomipramine	No response to two SSRIs	++/+++
Intravenous clomipramine	No response (or partial response?) to oral clomipramine	+/++
SSRI or clomipramine plus second-generation antipsychotic	1. Partial response to either an SSRI or clomipramine	++/+++
	2. Complex and/or poor-insight cases of OCD	+/++
SSRI or clomipramine plus first-generation antipsychotic	1. Presence of tic disorders	++/+++
	2. Presence of severe (schizotypal) personality disorder	+/++
	3. Complex and/or poor-insight cases of OCD	+/++
SSRI plus clomipramine	Partial response to either an SSRI or clomipramine	++
Augmenting an SSRI or clomipramine with	Partial response to either an SSRI or clomipramine	
Clonazepam		+/++
Pindolol		+/++
Buspirone		+
Fenfluramine		+
Tryptophan		+
Lithium		+
Trazodone		+
Desipramine		+
Inositol		+
Clonidine		+
Switching to phenelzine	Failure of all previously used psychopharmacological strategies	+

SSRI, selective serotonin reuptake inhibitor. Likelihood of success: +++, fairly high; ++, intermediate; +, fairly low.

An adequate trial of pharmacotherapy for OCD consists of at least 12 weeks of treatment with an SSRI at a maximum dose. As noted before, the duration of pharmacological trial in OCD should be flexible, because of the tendency of some patients to show further treatment gains beyond the initial 12 weeks of treatment. Therefore, some clinicians continue to administer medication for another 12 weeks before deciding that a patient has had an adequate trial.

If there has been no response at all to an adequate trial of one SSRI, the patient's therapy should be switched to another SSRI (Tables 6–15 and 6–17). The failure of one SSRI in OCD may be followed by a dramatic response to another SSRI, a situation quite different from that in most other anxiety disorders. If there is no response to the second SSRI, the patient's medication should be switched to clomipramine (Tables 6–15 and 6–17), unless there are contraindications for its use. If tolerability of these medications is not an issue, only after the patient has completely failed to respond to two different SSRIs plus clomipramine can he or she be declared treatment-resistant.

It is difficult to precisely characterize partial response to pharmacotherapy, because response in pharmacological studies of OCD is defined as a relatively small decrease (25%–35%) in the score on the relevant rating scale, such as the Yale-Brown Obsessive-Compulsive Scale (Y-BOCS). If the clinician were to adhere to these standards, then a partial response would mean that there has been only 10%–20% improvement in symptoms. Most physicians do not have time to administer lengthy instruments such as the Y-BOCS, and their conclusions as to whether the patient has shown partial response are likely to be based on global impression. Hence, it is conceivable that the symptomatic status of OCD patients who are deemed partial responders varies from one clinical setting to another.

Various augmentation strategies have been proposed for OCD patients who respond partially to an SSRI (or clomipramine). Thus, clonazepam, buspirone, pindolol, fenfluramine, tryptophan, lithium, trazodone, desipramine, inositol, and clonidine have all been added to an SSRI or clomipramine (Table 6–17); some of these medications were also used as monotherapy for OCD. Unfortunately, these strategies generally failed to produce encouraging results, except to a certain extent, for augmentation with clonazepam (Hewlett et al., 1992) and pindolol (Dannon et al., 2000).

An SSRI can be combined with clomipramine in treatment-resistant OCD (Table 6–17). This combination requires caution, however, because plasma levels of clomipramine can be raised to the toxic range, with an increased possibility of seizures and cardiac problems. If this combination is used, the patient's ECG and plasma levels of clomipramine and its metabolite should be monitored carefully, and the lowest possible dose of clomipramine administered, usually not more than 100 mg/day (Szegedi et al., 1996).

Another option is to administer clomipramine intravenously to treatment-refractory patients with OCD. A significant proportion of patients who do not respond to oral clomipramine may respond to the same medication when given intravenously (Fallon et al., 1998). This treatment is administered through daily infusions for a period of about 2 weeks, with the doses of clomipramine reaching and even exceeding 300 mg/day (Koran et al., 1997).

A common augmentation strategy (Table 6–17) is to add to an SSRI a small dose of a first-generation antipsychotic (usually haloperidol, up to 5 mg/day); this may be particularly useful for patients with co-occurring tic disorder (McDougle et al., 1994). The SSRI–haloperidol combination may also be helpful in the treatment of OCD patients who have severe personality disturbance from the "odd," DSM Cluster A personality disorders (particularly schizoid or schizotypal personality disorder). Some clinicians endorse the practice of combining an SSRI with a small dose of a first-generation antipsychotic in all complex and poor-insight cases of OCD, regardless of the presence of tics, severe personality disturbance, or quasipsychotic symptoms.

More recently, second-generation antipsychotics have been used in combination with an SSRI or clomipramine (Table 6–17). This combination is also of theoretical interest, because several second-generation antipsychotics act as serotonin–dopamine antagonists. There have been several reports and one controlled trial (McDougle et al., 2000) of risperidone augmentation of SSRIs and clomipramine in treatment-refractory OCD. The results were generally encouraging, as previously refractory patients tended to respond to this combination, regardless of whether they had a co-occurring tic disorder. Interestingly, the dose of risperidone was lower (0.25–3 mg/day) than the dose usually used in the treatment of psychotic disorders. The augmentation with olanzapine and quetiapine is less well studied, with one recent study (Shapira et al., 2004) failing to show advantage of olanzapine augmentation of fluoxetine. It is unknown whether OCD patients might respond to a combination of an SSRI and clozapine, but treatment with clozapine alone does not appear to be efficacious (McDougle et al., 1995).

Yet another possibility for treatment-refractory OCD patients is to try phenelzine, a classical, irreversible monoamine oxidase inhibitor. This strategy does not appear to be very promising, despite a few encouraging reports of efficacy of phenelzine in the treatment of OCD (Vallejo et al., 1992; Jenike et al., 1997).

The treatment-refractory OCD patient who has also failed to respond to augmentation and combination strategies, as well as to alternative pharmacotherapy strategies and psychological interventions, should be referred to a highly specialized center for diagnostic reevaluation and consideration of further treatment options. In terms of biological treatment, these options include electroconvulsive therapy and neurosurgery.

ELECTROCONVULSIVE THERAPY AND NEUROSURGERY

It does not appear that, in the absence of severe depression, electroconvulsive therapy is efficacious for treatment-resistant OCD. If electroconvulsive therapy shows efficacy, it is usually for depressive symptoms, whereas symptoms of OCD respond insofar as they are related to depression.

Neurosurgery has shown some success in treatment of the most difficult and treatment-resistant patients with OCD. Between 25% and 40% of patients have been reported as improved up to 10 years after neurosurgery (Jenike et al., 1991; Hay et al., 1993; Baer et al., 1995; Dougherty et al., 2002). However, many patients who have undergone surgical intervention do not necessarily get better as a result of neurosurgery and still need ongoing treatment with SSRIs, clomipramine, and/or behavior therapy, but they may respond to it more readily.

Most surgical procedures disrupt connections between the basal ganglia and frontal cortex. Although the techniques have been improved considerably over the past two decades, neurosurgery for OCD is still performed in few centers around the world. Also, the most suitable surgical technique remains unknown. Anterior cingulotomy has apparently been the preferred procedure, followed by various capsulotomy techniques, subcaudate tractotomy, limbic leucotomy, and, most recently, gamma knife surgery.

Possible long-term effects and consequences of neurosurgery for OCD have not been studied sufficiently and remain largely unknown. Some of these include weight gain, various cognitive problems, lack of initiative, disinhibition, impulsive and aggressive behavior, and suicide (Jenike et al., 1991; Hay et al., 1993; Sachdev and Hay, 1995; Irle et al., 1998; Dougherty et al., 2002). A recent editorial (Bejerot, 2003) has drawn attention to the many potential adverse effects of neurosurgery in treating OCD, concluding that it should only be performed in highly specialized research settings where its clinical benefits might be weighed extremely carefully against the adverse effects.

In view of the controversial status of neurosurgery in the treatment of OCD and its use as the last resort, indications for it should be strict and clear. At present, a minimum of 5 years of treatment with little or no response is necessary for consideration of neurosurgery. This treatment has to include documented trials of *all* SSRIs and clomipramine, augmentation with antipsychotics and other agents, and behavior therapy (Jenike, 1998).

PSYCHOLOGICAL TREATMENTS

Various psychotherapeutic approaches have been used in OCD, including psychoanalysis, psychodynamic psychotherapy, supportive psychotherapy, and cognitive-behavioral therapy (CBT). Of these, evidence of efficacy exists only for CBT. That does not mean that other types of psychotherapy have absolutely no role to play in the treatment of OCD, as they can be useful for some patients and in certain clinical settings. However, their role is usually limited to that of an adjunct to CBT. Therefore, psychotherapeutic approaches other than CBT cannot be recommended as the standard or sole treatment for OCD.

Cognitive-Behavioral Therapy

Cognitive-behavioral therapy encompasses various combinations and proportions of the techniques of behavior and cognitive therapy. At present, the best evidence of efficacy in OCD exists for the behavioral technique of exposure and response prevention. More recently, the use of cognitive approaches has been on the rise.

Behavior Therapy—Exposure and Response Prevention

Exposure and response prevention (Table 6–18) is based on the behavioral model of OCD and general principles of behavior therapy. It was introduced in the 1960s and over the subsequent two decades became the most widely used behavioral technique for OCD, especially OCD characterized by washing and cleaning and checking compulsions. It appears to be less useful in treatment of OCD with predominant obsessions and few compulsions.

The technique has two components: (1) exposure (used more to alleviate obsessions) and (2) response prevention (used more with the goal of removing compulsions). Patients expose themselves to the feared, obsession-related situations that provoke or intensify anxiety or discomfort, and then refrain from performing a compulsion that they would have otherwise performed to decrease anxiety or discomfort. For example, patients with contamination obsessions and washing compulsions are instructed to

TABLE 6–18. Aspects of Behavior Therapy That Are Relatively Specific for Obsesive-Compulsive Disorder

Exposure

- Use of both in vivo exposure and imaginal exposure is preferable.

- Gradual exposure is better tolerated than flooding.

- There is a greater degree of therapist participation, with use of modeling during therapist-assisted exposure sessions.

- Therapist-assisted exposure sessions should be prolonged (1–2 hours per session) and frequent (preferably conducted more than once a week).

- Intensive (at least 1 hour per day) and frequent (daily) self-exposure plays a crucial role.

- Assistance from family members, partners, or friends in conducting exposure is very important.

Response Prevention

- Response prevention is not time limited and continues as long as possible after the end of an exposure session.

- Complete response prevention (including prevention of mental compulsions) may not be realistic initially.

- Partial response prevention (with precise limit-setting) should be negotiated with the patient.

- The therapist must carefully monitor whether the patient is using any other type of concealed neutralizing activity (e.g., mental compulsions) to decrease anxiety or distress.

- It should never be carried out through coercion or physical prevention of a compulsion by the therapist or someone else.

- Assistance from family members, partners, or friends in conducting response prevention is very important.

touch objects that they consider "dirty" or contaminated (e.g., pieces of clothes and personal belongings that were in contact with the seat on the train), and then they are asked to refrain from washing their hands. With repeated exposure, the obsession elicits less and less anxiety as a result of habituation; such a decrease in anxiety level also leads to a decrease in the patients' need to perform compulsions. Response prevention serves the purpose of demonstrating to patients that an urge to perform a compulsion can be successfully resisted, which boosts the sense of self-efficacy.

There are different ways in which exposure and response prevention can be used, and over the years the technique has undergone various modifications.

Psychoeducation. The use of exposure and response prevention depends crucially on educating patients about OCD and on explaining to them why exposure and response prevention is used and how it should be used. Before any exposure and response prevention commences, it is useful to explain to patients what constitutes normative behavior and standards in those realms affected by patients' obsessions and compulsions (e.g., it is sufficient to take a shower once or twice a day, unless it is a very hot day, and the person perspires a lot). The patients' strict standards of cleanliness or safety or their rigid moral attitudes often obfuscate their understanding of what is normal, sufficient, and appropriate.

Exposure. The exposure component is usually performed by in vivo exposure to fearful stimuli whenever possible. In vivo exposure may be combined with imaginal exposure, depending on the specific nature of obsessions. Imaginal exposure is usually used for obsessions with aggressive and sexual themes and involves activation (that is, visualization) of the corresponding imagery, often with therapist-assisted manipulation of the feared outcomes. Gradual exposure seems to be better tolerated than flooding and thereby strengthens patients' motivation for treatment. Gradual exposure in OCD can be conducted in a way similar to that used in the treatment of agoraphobia and other phobias (see Chapters 2 and 5), with the construction of hierarchies of situations and stimuli to which patients are then gradually, but progressively exposed (starting from the situations that elicit the least amount of anxiety).

In comparison with exposure-based treatment for other anxiety disorders, there is usually a greater degree of therapist participation in the course of exposure for OCD. Thus, in-session, therapist-assisted exposure, which relies on modeling, is often used. Taking as an example contamination obsessions and washing compulsions, modeling is provided by the therapist who touches his or her shoes without washing the hands afterwards, and then asks the patient to do the same in the presence of the therapist.

The duration of therapist-assisted exposure sessions depends on the time that patients need to habituate to the feared situation and thus experience a substantial decrease in anxiety or distress. These exposure sessions usually last 1–2 hours; the frequency of more than once a week apparently produces better results. Thus, for therapist-assisted exposure to be efficacious in the treatment of OCD, it should be intensive—prolonged, repeated, and frequent.

Patients should engage in self-exposure and response prevention exercises between therapist-assisted sessions; these homework exercises should be conducted daily and should last at least 1 hour per day. They should be carefully recorded in terms of the level of anxiety and distress experienced and the feelings and thoughts that appeared in the course of these exercises. Partners and family members can play a vital role in this portion of treatment, and their cooperation and support should be sought whenever possible.

Response prevention. Often the response prevention component is not precisely described and not well understood by patients. Even more than exposure, it relies heavily on patients' motivation and self-discipline—in this case, to refrain from performing a compulsion when they feel the greatest urge to do so. In addition, response prevention is not time limited, but continues as long as possible after the end of exposure. This means that patients are expected to refrain from performing the compulsion not only during and immediately after the exposure but also for as long as possible after the exposure. The therapist has two main tasks. The first is to encourage and support patients as they make an effort not to succumb to an urge to perform compulsion. Second, the therapist must carefully monitor patients to check whether they are using any other type of the concealed neutralizing activity (e.g., mental compulsions) to decrease anxiety or distress. Using such neutralizations might defeat the purpose of response prevention, as one type of neutralizing activity would be substituted for another.

Ideally, patients should aim for complete response prevention from the very beginning of treatment. In reality, a step-by-step approach may need to be taken. For example, limits may be set on compulsions, so that patients initially spend a certain maximum amount of time performing compulsions (e.g., no more than 2 hours/day) or they agree to a maximum number of compulsions allowed (e.g., not washing more than two times per episode or not washing more than 20 times a day). These limits are used to facilitate response prevention, they should always be negotiated with patients (whereby patients' partners or family members can also be involved), and they become increasingly stricter in the course of treatment.

It should be emphasized that response prevention will not be efficacious if it is attempted through coercion or physical prevention of a compulsion by the therapist or someone else—for example, if a family member locks the bathroom and thereby attempts to prevent excessive washing. This is only likely to create or increase patients' resistance. Family members, partners, or friends are often key players in conducting response prevention. Their cooperation with the therapist may be crucial for the outcome of treatment, in terms of their consistent refusal to participate in patients' compulsions, refusal to provide unnecessary, repetitious reassurance, or refusal to continue to be involved in patients' rituals in any other way.

Problems encountered during treatment. Difficulties in the course of exposure and response prevention usually arise from this technique's provocation of anxiety and distress and prevention of immediate relief that would have been obtained from a compulsion or other neutralizing activities. A failure to perform compulsion is particularly frightening to patients who strongly believe that it will lead to something dreadful. Therefore, patients can fully engage in exposure and response prevention only if they have basic trust in their therapist and if the therapist has succeeded in enlisting patients' active collaboration.

It is self-evident that patients need to be highly motivated to succeed in the program of exposure and response prevention. Not surprisingly, a substantial proportion of OCD patients refuse treatment with exposure and response prevention, and approximately 25% fail to adhere to it (Foa et al., 1985). Of those who comply with the treatment requirements, a certain proportion does not improve. Throughout the treatment, patients need to be continuously supported by the therapist and all others who are involved in treatment, particularly partners and family members. Interestingly, it may take longer for exposure and response prevention to show its effects (de Haan et al., 1997), just as it usually takes longer for pharmacotherapy to work in OCD.

Efficacy. Keeping in mind that complete and permanent recovery from OCD is rare, exposure and response prevention has proved to be efficacious for this condition. This was documented in numerous controlled studies (e.g., Marks et al., 1975, 1988; Boersma et al., 1976; Foa and Goldstein, 1978; Foa et al., 1984; Emmelkamp et al., 1989). One early review (Foa et al., 1985) reported that 90% of patients responded to exposure and response prevention, with response being defined as more than 30% reduction in symptoms. A decade later (Foa and Kozak, 1996), 83% of patients across a number of studies were found to be responders to behavior therapy immediately after completion of treatment.

A significant advantage of behavior therapy appears to be the maintenance of treatment gains over long periods of time: in long-term outcome studies, 76% of patients remained treatment responders over a mean period of almost $2\frac{1}{2}$ years (Foa and Kozak, 1996). Despite this, OCD patients have a tendency to relapse, and booster sessions of behavior therapy and maintenance, relapse-prevention programs based on exposure and response prevention (e.g., McKay, 1997) may be very helpful.

Predictors of outcome. The predictors of outcome of exposure and response prevention, regardless of whether exposure and response prevention was administered alone or in conjunction with medications, have been identified by numerous studies. The results of these studies were often conflicting (Table 6–19), but a few factors have been more consistently or more strongly associated with poor outcome: greater severity of initial OCD symptoms, presence of *severe* depression, prominent avoidance of the feared stimuli, unemployment, living alone, lack of compliance with treatment during the first week of therapy, and presence of severe personality disturbance, especially schizotypal personality disorder (Foa et al., 1981, 1983; Minichiello et al., 1987; Cottraux et al., 1993; Castle et al., 1994; Keijsers et al., 1994; Buchanan et al., 1996; de Araujo et al., 1996; de Haan et al., 1997; Moritz et al., 2004). Less consistently or less strongly, poor outcome of exposure and response prevention has been predicted by longer duration of OCD symptoms, absence of overt compulsions, excessive arousal in the presence of the feared stimuli, and previous (unsuccessful) attempts to treat OCD (Foa et al., 1983; Keijsers et al., 1994; Buchanan et al., 1996).

Issues regarding the prediction of outcome of exposure and response prevention pertain to the effects of co-occurring depression, personality

TABLE 6–19. Predictors of Outcome of Behavior Therapy of Obsessive-Compulsive Disorder

More Consistently or More Strongly Shown To Be Predictors of Poor Outcome

- Greater severity of initial OCD symptoms (Keijsers et al., 1994; de Haan et al., 1997)
- Presence of *severe* depression (Foa et al., 1981; 1983; Keijsers et al., 1994)
- Prominent avoidance of feared stimuli (Foa et al., 1983; Cottraux et al., 1993)
- Unemployment (Castle et al., 1994; Buchanan et al., 1996)
- Living alone (Castle et al., 1994; Buchanan et al., 1996)
- Lack of compliance with exposure homework during the first week of therapy (de Araujo et al., 1996)
- Presence of severe personality disturbance, e.g., schizotypal, schizoid, and paranoid personality disorders (Minichiello et al., 1987; de Haan et al., 1997; Moritz et al., 2004)

Less Consistently or Less Strongly Shown To Be Predictors of Poor Outcome

- Longer duration of symptoms (Keijsers et al., 1994)
- Absence of overt compulsions (Buchanan et al., 1996)
- Excessive arousal in the presence of feared stimuli (Foa et al., 1983)
- Previous (unsuccessful) attempts to treat OCD (Buchanan et al., 1996)

disturbance, and poor insight. These issues are important, as they may influence a decision to use exposure and response prevention.

It appears that the presence of mild to moderate depression does not affect the outcome of exposure and response prevention (Foa et al., 1984; Basoglu et al., 1988; Hoogduin and Duivenvoorden, 1988; O'Sullivan et al., 1991). However, there are also reports (e.g., Cottraux et al., 1993) that depression may predict failure of exposure and response prevention, and the negative impact of depression seems to be related to its severity (Foa et al., 1981, 1983; Keijsers et al., 1994). The clinical implication of these findings is that exposure and response prevention may still be used if depression co-occurs with OCD, unless the patient is severely depressed.

The power of personality disorders in predicting the outcome of treatment of OCD with exposure and response prevention is not clear, as the presence of personality disorders has been associated with both poorer response to such treatment (Minichiello et al., 1987; de Haan et al., 1997; Moritz et al., 2004) and lack of effect on treatment outcome (Dreessen et al., 1997). Moreover, some studies have shown beneficial effects of OCD treatment on the co-occurring personality disturbance, regardless of whether behavior therapy (McKay et al., 1996) or pharmacotherapy (Baer et al., 1992) was used. Still, a prudent clinical approach is to use exposure and response prevention with great caution in OCD patients with *severe* personality disturbance, particularly those with schizotypal personality disorder and personality traits.

The issue of the use of exposure and response prevention in OCD patients with poor insight remains unresolved. Although OCD with poor insight, overvalued ideas, and fixed obsessional beliefs is often considered to imply a poor outcome of exposure and response prevention (e.g., Foa, 1979; Kozak and Foa, 1994), one study found that OCD patients with fixed and bizarre beliefs responded well to behavior therapy (Lelliott et al., 1988). On balance, it seems that exposure and response prevention needs to be modified for use in OCD patients with poor insight, so that the underlying beliefs and prominent magical thinking, if present, are addressed. Otherwise, poor-insight patients are likely to have difficulties, especially with response prevention.

Another clinically relevant predictor of the outcome of behavior therapy may be the type of obsessions and compulsions. Certain obsessions or compulsions, for example, those derived from fears of contamination, may be more suitable for treatment with exposure and response prevention (Buchanan et al., 1996). Compulsions such as hoarding, and rearranging objects, however, do not seem to respond well to exposure and response prevention, but they may be inherently more treatment-resistant, regardless of the type of treatment used. The suitability of exposure and response prevention may be determined more by the purpose of compulsions than by the type of obsessions and compulsions. Thus, it appears that exposure and response prevention works better for cases of OCD in which compulsions mainly serve the purpose of alleviating the anxiety produced by obsessions. In contrast, this technique appears to be far less efficacious in OCD patients who are driven to perform compulsions more automatically or as a result of vague discomfort, and who perform compulsions to undo obsessions or prevent future catastrophe.

Cognitive Therapy and Integrated Cognitive-Behavioral Approaches

Ultimately, for psychological treatment to be efficacious in OCD, the belief system that underlies many obsessions and compulsions may need to be modified (although this is not accepted by all the therapists in the field). In other words, removal of obsessions and compulsions may not be possible without addressing, challenging, and modifying the specific beliefs that give meaning and purpose to obsessions and compulsions. This task is within the realm of cognitive therapy.

Cognitive therapy is based on the cognitive model of OCD. It may be particularly suitable for the treatment of obsessions. In clinical practice, cognitive therapy techniques are usually combined with behavioral approaches that may be more efficacious for compulsions; this represents a truly integrated "brand" of CBT.

The specific goals of cognitive therapy in OCD are as follows: (1) elimination of misinterpretations and other dysfunctional appraisals of intrusive thoughts; (2) liberation from excessive responsibility for obsessions and for the harm associated with these obsessions; and (3) elimination of neutralizing activities that arise in response to the inflated sense of responsibility and other negative or catastrophic appraisals. These goals cannot be achieved without also decreasing the importance that patients attach to their obsessions and thoughts in general. Once patients no longer feel obliged to take their thoughts too seriously, their sense of responsibility for having such thoughts is likely to diminish. In turn, the patients' need to perform compulsions or engage in other neutralizing activities is also likely to decrease.

In the course of cognitive therapy, other beliefs and thinking patterns that are relatively specific for OCD are also addressed: beliefs that lack of control over one's thoughts is dangerous and that having a thought about doing something is the same as doing it (thought–action fusion), intolerance of ambiguity, newness and uncertainty, and rigid, perfectionist tendencies.

Cognitive therapy of OCD consists of several procedures: identification of misinterpretations, faulty appraisals, and abnormal thinking patterns and belief systems; their questioning and challenging; behavioral experiments; and provision of alternative, more adaptive, and more realistic appraisals.

In order to identify erroneous appraisals and abnormal thinking patterns, patients need to record every thought, interpretation, and belief that they may have in connection with their obsessions. These thoughts, interpretations, and beliefs are subsequently challenged by asking patients to give evidence "for and against." Behavioral experiments are set up with the goal of testing the validity of patients' beliefs; for example, a belief that their "aggressive" thoughts can kill are challenged by asking patients to check whether deliberately having such a thought does indeed lead to a death of a family member or a neighbor. Demonstrating to patients that their predictions are based on magical thinking—and not on logical and rational reasoning—makes it possible for the therapist to introduce alternatives. For example, an alternative appraisal of aggressive thoughts might be that they are dangerous only insofar as patients allow them to be dangerous by automatically linking them in a magical or superstitious way with the highly unlikely, frightening outcomes.

Another component of cognitive therapy is addressing various "safety behaviors," i.e., neutralizing activities. It is particularly important for patients to understand how a range of behaviors and mental activities adopted in response to obsessions has the ultimate effect of maintaining these obsessions and feeding the anxiety created by the obsessions. This understanding of the neutralizing activities also makes it easier for patients to engage in response prevention.

Cognitive therapy for OCD has been developed relatively recently, and exposure and response prevention remains the psychological treatment of choice for OCD. There is some uncertainty about the value and efficacy of cognitive therapy when compared with that of exposure and response prevention (e.g., James and Blackburn, 1995). Cognitive therapy of OCD needs to undergo further testing lest it become irrelevant for clinical practice despite being based on what seems to be sound theory. Evidence of the efficacy of cognitive therapy in OCD—equal to that of exposure and response prevention—has only started to accumulate (e.g., van Oppen et al., 1995).

Supportive Psychotherapy

There is little that may be specific for supportive psychotherapy of OCD. General supportive measures used in the treatment of other anxiety disorders and, for that matter, other psychiatric disorders may be applied to the treatment of OCD, regardless of whether the primary treatment modality is pharmacotherapy or CBT. Examples of these supportive measures are psychoeducation, help in coping with stressors that may exacerbate clinical features of OCD, and attention to OCD-related family dynamics.

Psychoanalysis and Psychodynamic Psychotherapy

Psychoanalysis and psychodynamic psychotherapy are currently hardly used for the treatment of OCD, because they have generally been unable to alleviate obsessions and eliminate compulsions. Some of the insights of the psychoanalytic theory of OCD now seem more applicable to the treatment of obsessive-compulsive personality disorder, insofar as there are shared features between obsessive-compulsive personality disorder and OCD and despite significant differences between these two conditions (see Figs. 6–2 and 6–3).

COMBINED TREATMENTS

Combining CBT and pharmacotherapy for OCD is apparently very common. It is also logical to combine them, considering that OCD may be difficult to treat with either modality alone and treatments with exposure and response prevention, clomipramine, and SSRIs show approximately equal efficacy (e.g., Kobak et al., 1998). Also, effects of CBT and pharmacotherapy may enhance each other. Medications may make it easier for patients to accept some of the discomforts associated with CBT, and CBT may have longer-lasting effects than those of pharmacotherapy upon cessation of treatment. There is no established sequence of combining the two treatments. Some clinicians prefer to commence pharmacotherapy, adding CBT later (and this may be the more common sequence), whereas others are more inclined to use CBT first and then add a medication in case of an insufficient response to CBT. The general issues arising from the combination of CBT and pharmacotherapy are presented in Chapter 2. Combining these treatment modalities for OCD appears less controversial than for panic disorder.

There have been few studies examining the efficacy of combined treatments in OCD, especially in comparison with CBT alone and pharmacotherapy alone. Two studies showed that adding exposure and response prevention (Simpson et al., 1999) or exposure and response prevention plus cognitive therapy (Kampman et al., 2002) to patients who only had a partial response to pharmacotherapy produced further treatment gains, suggesting that combination treatment might be superior to pharmacotherapy alone. Another study (van Balkom et al., 1998) compared CBT alone to the initial treatment with medications that was followed by CBT, and found no differences between the two approaches, a finding interpreted to suggest that CBT alone might be sufficient. In contrast, two studies (Cottraux et al., 1990; Hohagen et al., 1998) found some advantage for combined treatment (CBT plus fluvoxamine) over CBT alone, but in one of these studies (Cottraux et al., 1990), the advantage was lost at follow-up.

Although more research is clearly needed, preliminary data suggest that combining medications with CBT may be warranted in some clinical situations. Just what the combined approach adds to either treatment alone and when the combined treatment should be used remains to be established by large, carefully designed studies.

7
Posttraumatic Stress Disorder

Posttraumatic stress disorder (PTSD) is characterized by a number of more or less specific symptoms that appear some time after the person has been exposed to a trauma. It represents a complex response to trauma in which anxiety plays only a limited role. Various manifestations of PTSD have led to its also being considered primarily a disorder of memory, a dissociative disorder, one of the "trauma spectrum" disorders, or a condition more closely related to depression. Given its clear etiological link with a traumatic event, PTSD presents a rare opportunity among psychiatric disorders for implementation of programs that might be efficacious in preventing the development of PTSD.

CLINICAL FEATURES

Posttraumatic stress disorder is a very heterogeneous condition, and its clinical features may vary dramatically from one patient to another. The most common manifestations of PTSD are various ways through which the trauma is being reexperienced (symptoms probably most characteristic of PTSD), avoidance of certain situations, places, people, and/or conversations that remind patients of the trauma, decreased emotional reactivity, difficulties in remembering all the details and aspects of the trauma, irritability, tension and almost constant hypervigilance, and negative expectations. Some of these features may appear relatively quickly after the traumatic event, whereas others develop later. A full clinical picture of PTSD is usually present several weeks or months after the trauma. With the more chronic course of PTSD, clinical presentation tends to be more complex, and PTSD is often complicated by depression, substance abuse, and/or personality changes, which lead to further impairment in various areas of functioning.

There are three main groups of symptoms and clinical manifestations of PTSD, as described in DSM-IV-TR. These are symptoms of reexperiencing of the trauma, avoidance and numbing of general responsiveness, and increased arousal. The understanding of clinical features of PTSD first entails conceptualization of what constitutes a traumatic event.

Traumatic Event

In DSM-IV-TR, a *trauma* that may lead to PTSD has been defined as experiencing, witnessing, or being confronted with an event that involves actual or threatened death or serious injury to oneself or others, with the person responding with intense fear, helplessness, or horror. In other words, the life of the patient is directly jeopardized by the traumatic event or the patient has actually witnessed someone's suffering or death. This conceptualization of the traumatic event is still very broad and encompasses very different situations and experiences; it also means that traumatic events that precede PTSD do not include stressful events that are not (directly) life threatening, such as loss of job or divorce. Although this distinction is relatively sharp, there are still events that might be difficult to classify as traumatic, and not just stressful, which are nevertheless considered traumatic by DSM-IV-TR. These include finding out that someone close to the person has died suddenly, has had a serious injury, or has become ill with a life-threatening disease. This tendency to widen the concept of trauma may be related to a growing use of PTSD in litigation processes.

Different traumatic events have different impacts not only because of the very nature of these events, but also because of the specific reactions of persons exposed to them and specific meanings attached to these events by different people (Fig. 7–1). For example, traumatic events in which the life of a person was directly threatened are likely to be experienced differently from the person's witnessing of someone's torture or violent death. A sexual assault may be experienced as more traumatic than an armed robbery. A traumatic situation from which escape was possible or in which the person was able to fight for his or her life is likely to be experienced less

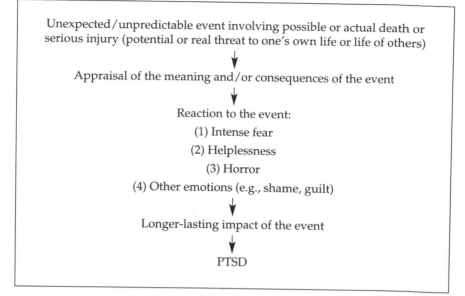

Figure 7–1. Characteristics of traumatic events and reactions to these events that may lead to posttraumatic stress disorder (modified from DSM-IV-TR).

traumatically than a situation in which no escape and no fight were possible, and the person was totally helpless, being fully exposed to the impact of the trauma. Also, traumatic events that are recurrent or happen daily, and in which the person is unable to change his or her particular circumstances (for example, the experience of being a prisoner of war or children exposed to continuous sexual and physical abuse) are likely to be experienced differently from single traumatic events, regardless of how severe the latter may be. Exposure to severe, ongoing trauma may be associated with a more severe form of PTSD than that with a single traumatic experience.

Another aspect of traumatic events is the fact that most people do not expect such events to happen to them: people do not expect to be taken hostage, witness someone's suicide, or even have a traffic accident ("Disasters happen to others"). Because traumatic events are usually unexpected and unpredicted, they can elicit different feelings and be experienced in many different ways. While some people accept the trauma as a fact of life ("That was my fate"), others are angry and may feel as if they were punished ("Why did it happen to me? Surely, I did not deserve it"). Other victims are quick to point fingers and "know" who is guilty ("The accident wouldn't have happened if the driver hadn't driven too fast"). By their very nature, traumatic events suddenly and often brutally abolish the basic notions of civilized societies—that life proceeds in some orderly fashion, that it is largely predictable, and that it is governed by law and justice. Likewise, traumatic events may suddenly invalidate any fantasy of personal invulnerability and thereby represent a deep narcissistic wound.

The DSM-IV-TR stipulation of specific emotional reactions to the trauma in the form of intense fear, sense of helplessness, and/or a feeling of horror (a complex state that combines fear, disgust, and/or disbelief) by no means represents an exhaustive list of emotions elicited by the trauma. Some traumatized people feel an overwhelming shame or even a sense of guilt, depending on the type of trauma, the nature of their participation in the event (i.e., whether their lives were threatened or whether they observed an act of crime), and personality characteristics.

Reexperiencing of the Traumatic Event

Intrusive and recurrent reexperiencing of the traumatic event is the most striking component of PTSD. Distressing dreams and nightmares involving a traumatic event are typical ways of reexperiencing the trauma. Many patients have intrusive and recurrent memories of the trauma. Others experience images or scenes of the trauma or some aspects of the trauma, with an "as-if-real," visual quality of the experience (e.g., flashbacks). These phenomena are sometimes very difficult to distinguish from visual illusions and hallucinations. The perceptual component of reexperiencing the trauma may be very prominent, with one or more senses being involved. Thus, the patient can hear, see, and/or smell the perpetrator of the crime during an episode of reliving the assault.

Reexperiencing of the trauma is an involuntary phenomenon and it is almost always distressing or painful, with patients usually feeling that they have no control over it and that they are helpless. These experiences remind patients that they cannot escape the trauma or suggest to them that trauma is like an open, bleeding wound that will never heal.

Reexperiencing of the trauma is usually brief, but may recur very often, sometimes even several times a day. This may be precipitated by certain events, situations, or perceptual stimuli that patients associate with the particular traumatic situation. For example, a patient who survived a tram crash had very vivid and frightening images of the tram turning over every time she saw the tram or heard it approaching. At the same time, she felt "paralysis" in her legs, was short of breath, and her heart was racing, so that she also reexperienced the original trauma with a physiological response.

Avoidance Behavior

Patients with PTSD commonly resort to avoidance of certain situations, places, activities, or people because they remind them of the original trauma. The avoidance can also be driven by a desire to minimize every possibility of reactivating a distressing memory of the trauma and reexperiencing it. The patient who survived a tram crash avoided not only traveling on the tram but also streets where trams were operating, because the sight or sound of a tram might provoke unpleasant images of the accident. Furthermore, this patient became afraid of all means of transportation that were not "well balanced" and that could turn over, such as trains, ships, and boats.

The avoidance may become so prominent that it accounts for most impairment in PTSD. A typical example is that of a patient who became homebound because going out might remind her of a situation in which she was raped. Many PTSD patients avoid social interactions, but this is usually a part of their pattern of general withdrawal, and is less often related to the specifically traumatic nature of some of these interactions. The pattern of avoidance in PTSD may be even more generalized in that it encompasses conversations and any internal mental activity (e.g., thinking) involving a traumatic event.

Hyperarousal Manifestations

Manifestations of hyperarousal in PTSD are related to patients' constant expectation of harm and to their consequent hypervigilance. These manifestations can become very severe over time and may dominate clinical presentation. Sometimes, hypervigilant behavior may be so prominent that patients seem paranoid. They are constantly concerned about security, extremely cautious about situations in which they find themselves (e.g., inquiring how they can escape), and checking whether all safety precautions have been taken. Symptoms of hyperarousal occur in different ways: through insomnia, exaggerated startle response, difficulties with concentration, and/or irritability.

Insomnia is a very common problem in PTSD. Sometimes it is related to distressing dreams and nightmares, and patients' overall sleep pattern is then quite disturbed. More commonly, though, insomnia is a consequence of tension, inability to relax, fear that "something bad" might happen, and the resultant need to be constantly alert. Insomnia may be particularly severe in patients whose trauma occurred at night or in darkness. It is not unusual for these patients to leave the lights or television on during the whole night.

Exaggerated startle response is another typical and common manifestation of hyperarousal. Patients with PTSD seem hypersensitive to all sudden stimuli, particularly those that are auditory and cannot be seen—hence patients' occasionally extreme reaction to any sudden, but innocuous sound (e.g., a telephone ringing or someone knocking on the door).

Difficulties with concentration in PTSD may be selective. While patients seem to have no trouble concentrating on matters related to potential or real danger, their concentration may be poor when they attempt to focus on activities they perceive as distracting; focusing on the latter might lead to their being caught off guard. For example, patients may complain of not being able to focus on reading a newspaper or watching an entertaining program on television. Difficulties with concentrating on such simple activities may make patients believe that their memory is not good, as they often have trouble remembering what they have read in the newspaper or seen on television.

Irritability, Anger, and Impulsive Behavior

Many patients with PTSD are irritable, have a "short fuse," and are prone to impulsive outbursts. These behaviors can sometimes be predicted, but they also occur without any apparent reason. The apparent lack of control that patients report with regard to their hostile impulses frightens them and often leads to feelings of remorse or guilt. Angry outbursts may be directed at anyone, including close friends and immediate family members. Such behaviors are difficult to understand, making it hard for others to empathize with patients' problems and suffering and contributing to patients' further social isolation and even rejection. As a result, patients may become even more prone to angry outbursts, thus creating a vicious circle.

In addition to being related to general hyperarousal of PTSD patients, irritability also has to do with other trauma-related feelings, thinking patterns, and experiences. For example, some patients feel almost entitled to be irritable and angry because the trauma gives them the "right" to have such feelings (e.g., "I won't be restrained after everything that I've gone through"). Other patients may be easily annoyed by what they perceive as a lack of understanding, lack of compassion, and lack of care. Irritability and anger may also be related to the sense of injustice for having been subjected to a traumatic experience, and, in such cases, patients may be preoccupied with the characteristic "Why me?" questions.

Changes in Emotional Responsiveness and Guilt Feelings

A common manifestation of PTSD is a change in emotional responsiveness, which may take many forms. For example, patients state that they have lost "all feelings," so that they are unable to feel happy, just as they cannot feel sad. Patients may report that they feel indifferent or even empty, "emotionally frozen." Sometimes it seems that their repertoire of emotional responsiveness has been reduced to fear and anger, both of which appear in response to a sense of danger associated with the trauma-related stimuli. This restricted range of emotional responsiveness is often referred to as "emotional numbness."

The emotional numbness may resemble depressive experiences. Thus, patients who are emotionally numb often report that they have lost all interest in other people, events, or activities, and that there is nothing that could make them feel happy. Other common and related experiences are loss of purpose, meaning, and goals in life. Patients' typical statements are, "Nothing seems important," "Everything is hopeless anyway," and "I see no future." To the extent that patients are painfully aware that they have changed and estranged themselves, even from their family and friends toward whom they feel "no closeness," they are likely to feel guilty about this change. That only complicates their situation, as many of them are already plagued with guilt associated with the original trauma.

Guilt feelings are commonly seen among patients with PTSD. They may feel guilty primarily because they have survived horrific traumatic experiences ("survivor guilt"), whereas their fellow soldiers, other inmates, colleagues, family members, or friends have not. In other situations, guilt feelings have a basis in reality, as some patients were directly responsible for someone's death or injury or failed to act responsibly and prevent a fatal accident. If guilt feelings are relentless and way out of proportion to the patients' real responsibility for and involvement in a traumatic event, they suggest a strong depressive component. This is particularly the case when patients vehemently accuse themselves of being "selfish" or of exhibiting "cowardice." It is important to ascertain the nature and degree of guilt feelings, as they are often associated with suicidal tendencies.

Dissociative Symptoms and Memory Problems

Dissociative phenomena are often seen as part of the trauma response. Dissociation can be conceptualized as a defense mechanism against the pain of the trauma, so that some aspects of the traumatic experience are split off, pushed away, and then forgotten. Hence, loss of memory for some aspects of the traumatic experience is a common feature of PTSD. This inability to remember certain important aspects of the trauma is in striking contrast to a vivid recollection of some other aspects of it. Some patients are quite troubled by being unable to remember what happened, and may come up with a version of the traumatic event that does not correspond to the reality. Patients then "remember" something that did not actually happen; such a recollection of the trauma may be used in the litigation process.

Dissociative mechanisms may separate memories for traumatic events (or memories for certain aspects of traumatic events) from feelings that accompanied these events. This separation can be manifested through remembering the details of the trauma, but forgetting how the patient felt at the time of the trauma. Sometimes patients seem emotionally detached and even indifferent when they talk about their traumatic experience. This may bear resemblance to the "isolation of affect" described in patients with obsessive-compulsive disorder or even to "belle indifférence" typical of those with conversion disorder (hysteria).

If the purpose of dissociation is to keep away unpleasant and painful memories of the trauma, dissociation clearly fails to do so, because memories of the trauma continue coming back to patients through dreams, nightmares, flashbacks, or intrusive recollections of the event or in some other way.

Dissociative phenomena also include various depersonalization and derealization experiences; for example, patients may describe a sense of unreality and alienation with regard to how they appear to themselves or how they perceive some aspects of their surroundings. The feeling of unreality may extend to the trauma itself, so that patients may feel that the traumatic event never occurred. Others may feel that they have been permanently changed by the trauma and have trouble recognizing themselves, others, and their physical environment. Some patients describe various "out-of-body experiences" (e.g., watching their bodies from some distance).

There may also be a marked disturbance in the integration of the perception of time and space, particularly as it relates to the trauma. Thus, patients may exhibit a marked time distortion, and the traumatic event may seem longer to them (e.g., as if it were never-ending). Sometimes they feel that the event occurred at a location different from the one where it really took place. Patients' description of the physical aspects of traumatic situation may be quite distorted.

When dissociative experiences occur immediately after the traumatic event (or as the event is still unfolding), they are usually referred to as "peritraumatic dissociation." This is often, though not invariably, considered a risk factor for the later development of PTSD (see Etiology and Pathogenesis, below).

Somatic Symptoms

Somatic symptoms can sometimes be one of the leading features of PTSD, and PTSD patients generally report somatic symptoms more often (e.g., Shalev et al., 1990). This is frequently seen in patients who were injured during the traumatic event and who have certain physical consequences as a result of such injuries. A typical example of this is chronic pain.

Some PTSD patients have somatic symptoms (e.g., headache, various gastrointestinal problems) that do not have a clear organic basis; sometimes, patients are so preoccupied with these symptoms that they attract a diagnostic label of a somatoform disorder. It appears that a response to trauma in the form of somatization is not at all rare and that it may be reinforced by cultural factors. Furthermore, somatization as part of the response to trauma may change its forms over time. Whereas cardiovascular symptoms seemed to be prominent among soldiers in the American Civil War (hence the term "soldiers' heart"), tremor was a commonly observed symptom among German soldiers in the First World War. Extreme fatigue and exhaustion were reported among soldiers who participated in more recent wars.

Posttraumatic Stress Disorder in Patients with Different Types of Traumatic Experiences

Although the patterns of response to trauma are similar, regardless of the type of trauma, the clinical presentation of PTSD may have some specific features in patients who develop the condition after different types of traumatic events.

Posttraumatic Stress Disorder in Patients Who Participated in Military Combat (Combat-Related PTSD)
Posttraumatic stress disorder in these patients may have some specific features related to the type of trauma and circumstances that led patients to find themselves in a combat situation. As the plight of the Vietnam War veterans illustrates so well, social factors play an important role in determining whether survivors of combat-related traumas develop PTSD. Participation in unpopular wars and being on the side that lost the war may suggest a higher risk of developing PTSD. Under these circumstances, soldiers are usually not welcomed back as heroes and are more likely to be regarded as

TABLE 7–1. Risk Factors That Are Relatively Specific for Developing Combat-Related Posttraumatic Stress Disorder

- Involuntary participation in war— being drafted (Kulka et al., 1990)
- Participation in a war for which public support is lacking
- Discomforts of being in a combat zone, e.g., poor accommodation conditions, sleep deprivation, poor hygiene, inadequate food, exposure to unfavorable weather conditions (King et al., 1999)
- Prolonged and more direct threats to one's life (King et al., 1999)
- Exposure to severe wounds and mutilated and/or dead bodies
- Being wounded in combat (Kulka et al., 1990)
- Poor cohesiveness within the military unit, conflicts between members of the military unit
- Participation in massacres or war crimes, or witnessing atrocities (King et al., 1999)
- Absence of enthusiastic or supportive acceptance of soldiers after the war (lack of social support)

an unpleasant reminder of the loss, shame, and national humiliation. The fact that they are directly or indirectly rejected by society, pushed into oblivion, and socially marginalized with few, if any, social supports increases the likelihood of developing PTSD. Table 7–1 lists somewhat specific risk factors for developing combat-related PTSD. (General risk factors for developing PTSD are discussed in Etiology and Pathogenesis, below.)

Features of combat-related PTSD do vary, but in this group of PTSD patients, social withdrawal, isolation, exaggerated guilt feelings, irritability, and aggressive outbursts seem to be more common. In addition, complications of PTSD such as alcoholism and drug abuse, depression, suicidality, and impaired family, occupational, and social functioning are particularly frequent. If it becomes chronic, combat-related PTSD is very difficult to treat.

Posttraumatic Stress Disorder in Former Prisoners of War and Torture and Concentration Camp Survivors

Patients with PTSD who were detained as prisoners of war or were forced to spend time in jails and concentration camps and tortured there because of belonging to a certain ethnic, religious, or political group have certain characteristics in common. This is because of the nature of the trauma to which these patients were subjected (Table 7–2).

After release from prison or liberation of a camp, many survivors have extremely strong guilt feelings. Not infrequently, suicide is the outcome of this guilt. These PTSD patients may have additional difficulties in adjusting

TABLE 7–2. Characteristics of Traumatic Experience in Patients with Posttraumatic Stress Disorder Who Were Prisoners of War or Are Survivors of Torture and Concentration Camps

• Repetitive traumatization during detention or imprisonment

• Unlimited possibilities of being physically maltreated, starved and tortured, and/or subjected to ideological or religious conversion programs ("brainwashing")

• Unpredictability of events in the person's immediate surroundings, including a possibility of being randomly selected for torture or execution

• Prominent feeling of loss of control over one's life

• Marked feelings of helplessness

• Sharing the experience of detention or imprisonment with other detainees or prisoners may be marked by competition for survival (whether real or imagined), so that opportunities for expressing adequately one's own feelings are extremely limited

to normal life circumstances; for example, they may have trouble accepting that they deserve basic human rights, which were denied to them during their detention or imprisonment. Also, patients may find that the world to which they have returned has completely changed, that they no longer recognize it as their own, or that there is no place for them in it. In these situations, patients may have to leave their country of origin and then subject themselves to another stress of adjusting to a foreign environment and culture.

Posttraumatic Stress Disorder in Victims of Rape, Physical Assault, Armed Robbery, or Other Violent Crime

Patients with PTSD who are victims of rape, physical assault, armed robbery, shooting, abduction, terrorist attack, or other violent crime often become distrustful and suspicious, particularly toward people who in some way remind them of the perpetrators of the crime. These patients may have angry outbursts and sometimes harbor strong urges to revenge. More typically, though, they present with intense fear of situations associated with the location where the crime occurred or with the person(s) who committed the crime. If this fear is accompanied by extensive avoidance, the clinical picture may be very similar to the one seen in phobias.

Posttraumatic stress disorder in victims of rape may be particularly severe, because of the nature of rape and social attitudes toward rape and its victims. First, rape is perhaps the most drastic way of violating one's physical integrity, leaving victims with a profoundly shattered sense of self-worth. As a result, the damage inflicted on self-image through rape can sometimes be irreparable. Rape may also have various symbolic meanings and corresponding consequences for its victims. Many of these pertain to the victims' sexuality and experience of intimacy, often leading to various types of sexual dysfunction and impairment of interpersonal functioning in general.

Society often expresses ambivalence in its attitude toward rape. Although rape is regarded as a crime punishable by law in most civilized countries, prejudice toward rape victims abounds. Among the latter are beliefs that victims of rape are somehow responsible for this crime, for example, by being "sexually provocative" or even by "seducing" the rapist. It does not come as a surprise, then, that rape victims often feel guilty of being raped, "dirty," disgusted with themselves, overwhelmed by a sense of self-hatred, and in need of punishment. Therefore, it is understandable that in many aspects, rape continues to be a taboo topic, with its victims often preferring to remain silent about it. If they have the strength and courage to reveal that they have been raped, victims often find that the help offered to them is inadequate, regardless of whether they are being pitied, interrogated insensitively, or treated with suspicion. The issues common to many victims of rape are summarized in Table 7–3.

TABLE 7–3. Common Issues Among Victims of Rape

Changes in Perception of Self

Shattered self-image

Poor sense of self-worth and self-esteem

Emotional Responses to Rape

Feeling of being humiliated beyond repair

Feelings of shame

Feeling guilty about rape

Behavioral Aspects

Secrecy about rape

Social withdrawal

Marked safety concerns

Extensive avoidance of places, situations, people, and other cues that remind victims of the rape

Changes Pertaining to Issues of Trust, Intimacy, and Sexuality

Profound loss of interpersonal trust

Fear of intimacy

Sexual dysfunction

Posttraumatic Stress Disorder in Victims of Traffic and Other Accidents

Patients who develop PTSD after road traffic accidents may present with a prominent phobia of driving or phobia of using certain vehicles. The functioning of these patients may be severely impaired if their job or occupation requires them to drive or use other means of transportation on a regular basis. In addition to features of PTSD, these patients may present with consequences of the injuries sustained during the accident, including pain. If permanent, as in case of the spinal cord injury or loss of a limb, such consequences are likely to have an adverse impact on the course of PTSD.

The clinical picture and prognosis of PTSD in victims of traffic accidents may be further complicated if the accident has triggered litigation, from which the patient expects compensation—hence the formerly used term "compensation neurosis." In these cases, some features of PTSD may seem exaggerated, patients are often labeled as "attention-seeking" or "difficult," they easily get angry and alienate their friends, families, and/or therapists, and they may appear unmotivated for treatment. Issues that are somewhat specific for PTSD victims of road traffic accidents are summarized in Table 7–4.

Posttraumatic Stress Disorder in Victims of Natural Disasters

Natural disasters, such as earthquakes, floods, storms, forest fires, and volcano eruptions, usually happen suddenly, with little or no forewarning. They affect a large number of people at the same time. Acute stress disorder is often seen among the survivors; if PTSD develops, it tends to have a relatively good prognosis. It may be somewhat easier to come to terms with the damage, consequences, and losses sustained as a result of natural disasters than with those caused by other people. This is partly related to the fact that losses and suffering in the former situation can be more easily shared with other survivors, as well as to the perception that natural disasters are very difficult to predict or prevent (although their consequences might be somewhat mitigated). The prognosis of PTSD associated with

Table 7–4. Issues Somewhat Specific for Victims of Road Traffic Accidents Who Have Posttraumatic Stress Disorder

- Prominent phobia of driving or phobia of using certain vehicles
- Consequences of the injuries sustained during the accident, including pain
- Litigation or compensation issues

natural disasters may be improved by massive social support, and quick repair of the damage and/or adequate compensation for the destroyed property and goods.

Varieties of Posttraumatic Stress Disorder

Partial Posttraumatic Stress Disorder

Some patients do not present with a full clinical picture of PTSD and do not meet criteria for a formal diagnosis of PTSD. In one community survey (Stein et al., 1997c), this partial, subsyndromal, or diagnostically sub-threshold form of PTSD was found in 3.4% of women and 0.3% of men. Partial PTSD exhibits longitudinal stability, as it may be present for many months and years without transformation into full-blown PTSD, but also without spontaneous resolution (Carlier and Gersons, 1995). It appears that this form of PTSD is associated with significant distress and functional impairment and it does not imply better prognosis and better response to treatment.

Complex Posttraumatic Stress Disorder

A form of PTSD with severe symptoms and permanent personality changes has been conceptualized under the terms "disorders of extreme stress not otherwise specified" (DESNOS) and "complex PTSD" (American Psychiatric Association, 1991; Herman, 1992, 1993; van der Kolk et al., 1996). In ICD-10, a similar condition was given a separate diagnostic category and called "enduring personality change after catastrophic experience." This form of PTSD is believed to be a consequence of prolonged exposure to severe and often multiple traumas (e.g., childhood abuse, torture, concentration camp) and is characterized by enduring personality characteristics that represent a clear change in comparison with the pre-trauma personality. They include profound disturbance in interpersonal relationships with estrangement from others, social withdrawal and isolation, pervasive mistrust, suspiciousness and hostility, altered perception of oneself with changes in the experience of one's own identity, feeling of emptiness, and altered sense of meaning and purpose of life. Some patients with complex PTSD may also exhibit a pattern of persistent irritability, with outbursts of anger and/or violent and destructive behavior. The concept of complex PTSD stands at the boundary of PTSD and personality disturbance and denotes effects of severe trauma and PTSD on personality. It has also generated some ongoing debate about the optimal ways of conceptualizing the relationship between severe trauma, PTSD, and severe personality disorder (e.g., borderline personality disorder).

Posttraumatic Stress Disorder with Delayed Onset

A full syndrome of PTSD may sometimes develop many months or even years after a traumatic event. DSM-IV-TR stipulates that symptoms in PTSD with delayed onset emerge at least 6 months after the trauma. Clinical practice and research (e.g., Solomon et al., 1989a) suggest that PTSD with delayed onset is relatively rare; patients who first present for treatment a long time after the occurrence of the traumatic event usually have long-standing PTSD symptoms prior to seeking help. These symptoms may not be severe enough and therefore are considered "normal" by patients; alternatively, they are overlooked or misdiagnosed by health professionals, contributing to the perception that they occurred late. Nevertheless, PTSD with delayed onset sometimes occurs as a consequence of "secondary traumatization" in patients who initially coped relatively well with the original trauma. Posttraumatic stress disorder with delayed onset may also be seen among patients who are seeking compensation.

Acute and Chronic Posttraumatic Stress Disorder

The DSM-IV-TR also makes a distinction between acute (duration of less than 3 months) and chronic (duration of more than 3 months) PTSD. Acute and chronic PTSD are clinically indistinguishable, and the cut-off of 3 months appears arbitrary. If the distinction between acute and chronic PTSD is to be retained at all, it might be more meaningful to label as chronic those patients with PTSD who have had symptoms for at least 6 months. Such a conceptualization of chronic PTSD might encompass a more homogenous group of patients and have clearer prognostic and treatment implications.

Posttraumatic Embitterment Disorder

The concept of posttraumatic embitterment disorder has recently been introduced (Linden, 2003). This condition is similar to PTSD in that both occur in the aftermath of trauma and are characterized by repetitive intrusive memories of the traumatic event. The main purported difference pertains to the pattern of emotional response to trauma: whereas there is greater variety of emotional response in PTSD with many patients exhibiting emotional blunting or numbness, emotional modulation in posttraumatic embitterment disorder is apparently intact and patients appraise traumatic event as "unjust" and respond with embitterment. Other features of posttraumatic embitterment disorder are less specific and overlap with those of PTSD, depression, anxiety and somatoform disorders. Although its validity remains to be tested, posttraumatic embitterment disorder represents an interesting attempt to conceptualize the syndrome that may be seen as a response to trauma, but is in some important aspects different from "classical" PTSD.

RELATIONSHIP BETWEEN POSTTRAUMATIC STRESS DISORDER AND OTHER DISORDERS

Patients with PTSD often have other mental disorders, and their clinical presentation may be colored by these co-occurring conditions. The overall lifetime psychiatric co-occurrence rate (at least one co-occurring mental disorder) in an epidemiological study of PTSD was 79% for women and 88% for men (Kessler et al., 1995). Indeed, it is relatively rare to find PTSD patients who do not develop any other psychiatric condition, especially with the passage of time.

Disorders that are most likely to co-occur with PTSD include depressive disorders (major depressive disorder and dysthymia), anxiety disorders, and alcohol and other substance abuse and dependence. In view of the role of trauma in the etiology of disorders other than PTSD—for example, borderline personality disorder, various dissociative disorders, and even chronic "psychogenic" pain (pain disorder)—it is not unusual to see patients whose clinical presentation is characterized by various combinations of PTSD (or PTSD-like symptoms), features of borderline personality disorder, self-harming behavior, dissociative phenomena, and pain. These patients are often given different (or multiple) diagnostic labels at different times, depending on the mode of their presentation. In many cases these labels represent different forms of expression of the same or similar underlying, trauma-related psychopathology. Some of these patients may be described as having a complex form of PTSD (see Varieties of Posttraumatic Stress Disorder, above).

Posttraumatic Stress Disorder, Major Depressive Disorder, and Dysthymia

Major depressive disorder co-occurs with PTSD in about one-half of persons with PTSD in the community (Kessler et al., 1995). Dysthymia has also been commonly found among PTSD patients, for example, in one-third of Vietnam veterans with PTSD (Kulka et al., 1990). The relationship between PTSD and depression is complex and important for several reasons. First, there is a substantial overlap in clinical manifestations (see Clinical Features, above). Sometimes PTSD is so overshadowed by the clinical features of depression (e.g., symptoms of anhedonia, prominent guilt feelings, suicidality) that PTSD is discovered only upon detailed diagnostic inquiry. Second, although there are similarities between PTSD and depression on a biological level, there also appear to be some significant differences (see Etiology and Pathogenesis, below). Third, major depressive disorder may precede the onset of PTSD by many years, it may predispose to PTSD, complicate the course of PTSD, and appear in response to trauma at approximately the same time as PTSD. The occurrence of major depressive disorder after a traumatic event may be independent from the occurrence of PTSD (Shalev et al., 1998a), or the risk for developing both is shared (Breslau et al., 2000). Finally, the presence of depression in PTSD carries an increased risk of further complications and suicide, makes the treatment more difficult, and suggests a poorer prognosis.

Posttraumatic Stress Disorder and Anxiety Disorders

Anxiety disorders are found in approximately one-third of individuals with PTSD in the community (Kessler et al., 1995). The rates with which various anxiety disorders co-occur with PTSD are similar in clinical samples. Most common among the anxiety disorders that co-occur with PTSD are generalized anxiety disorder, panic disorder and phobias, with co-occurrence rates ranging between 25% and 40% (Kulka et al., 1990; McFarlane and Papay, 1992). In some studies (Helzer et al., 1987; Breslau et al., 1991; McFarlane and Papay, 1992), obsessive-compulsive disorder was also found to accompany PTSD more often than expected. One study (Helzer et al., 1987) found that only women with PTSD (but no men) have a higher risk of panic disorder and phobias co-occurring with PTSD.

The co-occurrence of PTSD and anxiety disorders is mainly a reflection of the common features that they share and phenomenological overlap (see Differential Diagnosis, below). For example, the co-occurrence of PTSD and generalized anxiety disorder may reflect their shared clinical characteristics, such as hypervigilance, increased startle response, feelings of tension or of being on edge, restlessness, irritability, insomnia, and difficulties with concentration. There is no suggestion that co-occurrence of PTSD and anxiety disorders has etiological, prognostic, and treatment implications comparable to those of the co-occurrence of PTSD and depression.

Posttraumatic Stress Disorder and Alcohol and Other Substance Abuse or Dependence

Chronic suffering of PTSD patients may lead to their seeking some symptom alleviation by means of alcohol or other psychotropic substances.

Hence, alcohol and other substance abuse and dependence is usually a complication of PTSD, and is found in up to one-half of men with PTSD and one-third of women with PTSD (Kessler et al., 1995). The frequency of alcohol and drug abuse may be particularly high in certain populations; for example, lifetime prevalence of alcoholism in male Vietnam War veterans with PTSD was about 75% (Kulka et al., 1990). Social factors, accessibility of alcohol and other drugs, and specific effects of substances play a role in the choice of substance that is likely to be abused in any given population with PTSD. Alcohol and marijuana may be more likely to be abused because of their sedating, relaxing, and/or calming effects, whereas stimulating drugs such as amphetamine seem less likely to be abused by patients with PTSD.

ASSESSMENT

Diagnostic Issues

Although much attention has recently been paid to PTSD by mental health professionals, nonprofessional organizations, and the media, some psychiatrists are still reluctant to use the diagnosis of PTSD. This may be a result of the perception that PTSD is not a valid diagnostic concept in its own right. Traditional diagnostic labels, such as depression, anxiety, or some type of a "reactive state" are still preferred by certain psychiatrists, even when the clinical picture is consistent with the diagnosis of PTSD. Although the diagnostic concept of PTSD in its current form is not entirely satisfactory, it does provide a good descriptive framework for a multifaceted syndrome that develops in the aftermath of trauma.

The diagnosis of PTSD is based on the criteria spelled out in DSM-IV-TR and ICD-10. The diagnostic criteria in DSM-IV-TR are more detailed but also more complicated for routine use in clinical practice because of the need to memorize 17 symptoms grouped in three clusters (symptoms of reexperiencing the trauma, symptoms of avoidance and numbing of general responsiveness, and hyperarousal symptoms), with a minimum number of symptoms from each cluster required for making the diagnosis. An important advantage of the DSM-IV-TR conceptualization of PTSD is its definition of trauma that includes the event itself and reaction(s) to the event (see Clinical Features, above). In DSM-IV-TR, symptoms from all three major clusters must be present for the diagnosis of PTSD to be made.

The cluster of symptoms of reexperiencing the trauma includes vivid memories and dreams of the traumatic event, experience of the trauma as if it were occurring in the present (e.g., through flashbacks), and distress and physiological reactivity on exposure to various reminders of the trauma. The cluster of symptoms of avoidance and numbing of general responsiveness includes attempts to avoid all mental and physical activities, interpersonal interactions, people and places that are associated with or remind one of the trauma, inability to recall certain aspects of the trauma, pervasively decreased interests, feeling of detachment or estrangement from others, restricted range of feelings, and a sense that there is little, if any, future. The cluster of symptoms of hyperarousal includes insomnia, irritability and outbursts of anger, difficulties with concentration, hypervigilance, and exaggerated startle response.

The ICD-10 criteria for PTSD emphasize symptoms of reexperiencing of trauma as being most important and most specific for the diagnosis of PTSD. Indeed, a diagnosis of PTSD according to ICD-10 can be made even if avoidance behavior, numbing of general responsiveness, and symptoms of hyperarousal are not present. Making a diagnosis of PTSD according to ICD-10 is a matter of lower priority, as this diagnosis is justifiable if the criteria for diagnoses of major depressive disorder or another anxiety disorder have not been met. This approach to diagnostic conceptualization of PTSD may lead clinicians to overlook PTSD and underestimate its prevalence. It may also contribute to the erroneous notion that PTSD is a diagnosis of lesser validity than major depressive disorder and anxiety disorders.

Assessment Instruments

The gold standard for establishing the diagnosis of PTSD is the Clinician-Administered PTSD Scale (Blake et al., 1990). This instrument is based on a structured clinical interview and should be administered only by the experienced and trained clinicians. It is somewhat cumbersome and not suitable for routine use in clinical practice. Its psychometric properties are excellent, however, and it is comprehensive. In addition to being a diagnostic instrument, it can also be used for assessment of the severity of PTSD and as a measure of the changes that occur during treatment.

The Posttraumatic Stress Diagnostic Scale (Foa, 1995) is a self-report instrument, designed to assess the severity of PTSD and aid in making a diagnosis of PTSD. Because of its brevity, this instrument is relatively easy to administer and can be used as a tool for screening PTSD. It is also suitable for monitoring changes during treatment. The diagnosis of PTSD derived from the Posttraumatic Stress Diagnostic Scale should be verified by the clinician.

The Impact of Event Scale (Horowitz et al., 1979) is another self-report instrument that was originally constructed to measure the frequency of the symptoms of intrusion and avoidance associated with PTSD and other responses to trauma and stress. The modified version (Weiss and Marmar, 1996) also assesses the frequency of hyperarousal symptoms. Perhaps the greatest value of this instrument is in its use as a tool for early identification of persons who are at high risk for developing PTSD.

Differential Diagnosis

In terms of differential diagnosis of PTSD, the crucial step is to establish whether a traumatic event did occur and, if so, whether the symptoms appeared before or after the trauma. There are several conditions, mainly among the mood and anxiety disorders, that may be present before the trauma and are then exacerbated after the trauma, with or without additional PTSD-like symptoms or full-blown PTSD. Table 7–5 lists conditions that are likely to be considered in the differential diagnosis in both the acute setting (several weeks or months after the traumatic event) and the more chronic setting (several months or years after the traumatic event) The differentiation between PTSD and several disorders (e.g., depression,

TABLE 7–5. Differential Diagnosis of Posttraumatic Stress Disorder

In the More Acute Setting (several weeks or months after the traumatic event)

Acute stress disorder

Adjustment disorder

Major depressive disorder

Dissociative disorders

Panic disorder

Psychotic reactions

Malingering

In the More Chronic Setting (several months or years after the traumatic event)

Dysthymia

Major depressive disorder

Dissociative disorders

Panic disorder

Specific phobia, agoraphobia

Obsessive-compulsive disorder

Personality disorder

Malingering

dissociative disorders, panic disorder, and malingering) is important in both "acute" and "chronic" differential diagnosis of PTSD.

Acute Stress Disorder

There are many similarities between PTSD and acute stress disorder, as conceptualized by DSM-IV-TR (Table 7–6). The traumatic event that precedes both conditions is described in the same way, and the clinical picture is the same, except that acute stress disorder is also characterized by prominent dissociative symptoms (derealization, depersonalization, dissociative amnesia, reduction in awareness of one's own surroundings and/or a sense of numbing, detachment, estrangement, or absence of emotional responsiveness). Apart from this difference in clinical presentation, the main differences between PTSD and acute stress disorder (according to DSM-IV-TR) are in the course and duration of these conditions. While the symptoms of PTSD last for at least 1 month, symptoms of acute stress disorder appear and disappear within 4 weeks after the trauma. In other words, the maximum duration of acute stress disorder is about 1 month, whereas the minimum duration of PTSD is 1 month. If the symptoms of acute stress disorder continue for more than 1 month, the diagnosis is then changed to PTSD. The circumstances under which acute stress disorder leads to PTSD are not well understood and are a matter of debate (see Etiology and Pathogenesis, below).

TABLE 7–6. Similarities and Differences Between Posttraumatic Stress Disorder and Acute Stress Disorder (according to DSM-IV-TR)

Criteria for Differentiation and Similarities	Acute Stress Disorder	Posttraumatic Stress Disorder
Traumatic event that precedes the disorder	Experiencing, witnessing, or being confronted with an event that involves actual or threatened death or serious injury to oneself or others, with the person responding with intense fear, helplessness, or horror	
Clinical features	1. Prominent dissociative symptoms essential for diagnosis 2. Symptoms of reexperiencing the trauma, avoidance and hyperarousal	1. Prominent dissociative symptoms not essential for diagnosis
Onset	Within 4 weeks of traumatic event	Any time after traumatic event
Duration	Minimum 2 days, maximum 4 weeks	Minimum 1 month, no maximum duration

Adjustment Disorder

In contrast to PTSD and acute stress disorder, in which the trauma is clearly defined and always entails a direct threat to one's own life or the life of others, the nature of a traumatic event that precedes an adjustment disorder (according to DSM-IV-TR) is far less clear. Such a stressor may pertain to a traffic accident and witnessing the death of a close family member, as well as to a marital conflict, problems at work, or failure to pass a school test. Usually, however, the event that precedes an adjustment disorder is less severe in terms of the direct danger that it poses to oneself or others. Adjustment disorders are usually characterized by various symptoms of anxiety and depression and/or by disturbed behavior, and they only rarely resemble acute stress disorder and PTSD. However, if there are some clinical manifestations of acute stress disorder or PTSD following a traumatic event (as defined in DSM-IV-TR), a diagnosis of adjustment disorder can still be made. Otherwise, a diagnosis of adjustment disorder is warranted only in the absence of the full diagnostic criteria for PTSD.

Major Depressive Disorder

It is erroneous to assume that various PTSD-like symptoms that appear after trauma automatically imply that a person has developed PTSD. Some survivors of traumas may have both major depressive disorder and symptoms of PTSD, but because of the intensity, the latter may overshadow depressive symptoms. In these cases, it is particularly important to recognize the presence of depression. This may be difficult because of the significant overlap between the symptoms of these two conditions (see Clinical Features and Relationship Between Posttraumatic Stress Disorder and Other Disorders, above). Symptoms of depression, such as loss of interest, diminished emotional reactivity, anhedonia, sleep disturbance, concentration difficulties, profound guilt feelings, and inability to see future, should not be attributed to PTSD if other, more specific symptoms of PTSD are absent.

Dysthymia

Many patients with chronic PTSD have depressive symptoms that are consistent with a pattern of dysthymia or even that of "double depression" (dysthymia plus major depressive disorder). Symptoms typical of dysthymia, such as poor self-esteem, feelings of hopelessness, chronic sleep disturbance, and poor concentration, are also frequently encountered in PTSD, but as with symptoms of major depressive disorder, they should not be automatically assumed to be a part of PTSD unless other PTSD symptoms are present as well.

Dissociative Disorders

Distinguishing various dissociative disorders (e.g., dissociative amnesia, depersonalization disorder, dissociative identity disorder) from PTSD may be difficult, particularly when their onset is preceded by the trauma, as is often the case. However, the absence of other characteristics of PTSD suggests a dissociative disorder.

Personality Disorder

The relationship between PTSD and personality disturbance is complex, as already mentioned above in Clinical Features and Relationship Between Posttraumatic Stress Disorder and Other Disorders. When a significant personality dysfunction co-occurs with PTSD, it is important to ascertain whether it preceded the occurrence of trauma or developed as a complication of PTSD. There is no reason to use the diagnosis of personality disorder instead of or along with PTSD if there is no convincing evidence that personality disorder predated the traumatic event.

Psychotic Reactions

The onset of psychosis sometimes occurs after a traumatic event. According to DSM-IV-TR, brief psychotic disorder with marked stressors (brief reactive psychosis) has a maximum duration of 1 month; if psychotic features persist for more than 1 month and have some characteristics of schizophrenia, a diagnosis of schizophreniform disorder should be considered. Acute psychotic features in the context of the trauma may be related to bipolar affective disorder or be a part of delirium, substance-induced psychosis, or some other "organic" mental disorder. Hallucinatory experiences (usually visual) as part of PTSD are always related to the trauma and constitute one of the ways through which the trauma may be reexperienced. They are short-lived and often turn out to be pseudo-hallucinations rather than true hallucinations.

Malingering

Malingering should be taken into consideration in the differential diagnosis of PTSD if there is a litigation process, if criminal charges have been brought against the patient, or if political motives are implicated. The goals of malingering may be to elicit sympathy or public support, shift the blame to someone else, avoid punishment, and/or decrease the sentence. In addition, malingering may be suspected in patients who seem to exaggerate their symptoms and distress, whose clinical presentation is inconsistent or most unusual, and who exhibit significant personality disturbance.

Anxiety Disorders

Panic attacks and symptoms of panic attacks sometimes occur for the first time in the context of the trauma or shortly thereafter, and it may seem that the trauma victim suffers from panic disorder rather than PTSD. In other cases, panic disorder may be present before the onset of PTSD, with panic disorder continuing on a course of its own. Panic attacks may also become incorporated into PTSD, especially as part of the reaction to exposure to trauma reminders. As a result, symptoms of both conditions may be present at the same time and create diagnostic confusion. If panic attacks are part of panic disorder, they occur in a variety of settings and are not bound only to the situations that remind patients of their traumatic experience.

In chronic PTSD, avoidance of various cues that remind patients of the trauma may become the most prominent component of clinical presentation, resembling specific phobia (e.g., a driving phobia) or even agoraphobia (e.g., in case of the assault victims who become homebound). The distinction between phobic disorders and PTSD is based less on the presence of trauma (as the onset of both may be traced back to the specific traumatic event) and more on the reasons for avoidance behavior (which are not limited to the reminders of the trauma in phobic disorders) and presence of other characteristic symptoms of PTSD.

Intrusive and recurrent reexperiencing of the trauma may sometimes resemble obsessional phenomena seen in obsessive-compulsive disorder. However, the latter are usually experienced as alien (ego-dystonic) and are not related to any traumatic event that the patient might have experienced.

EPIDEMIOLOGY

It is not surprising that epidemiological data about the frequency of PTSD vary from one setting to another. This has resulted not only from methodological factors, such as different diagnostic criteria and different instruments used to diagnose PTSD, but also from significant differences between the settings in which epidemiological studies took place. These differences pertain to the likelihood of being traumatized, the type of trauma to which the population is likely to be exposed, and the ways in which the trauma is responded to.

For example, the general likelihood of being traumatized is lower in an affluent country with long-standing socioeconomic stability and a very low crime rate than in a developing country with political and economic instability, frequent social upheavals, and a high crime rate. The likelihood of being exposed to violent crime is higher in the impoverished, socioeconomically deprived inner-city areas than in the affluent suburbs within the same, generally affluent country. Finally, the opportunities for recovering from a traumatic event such as rape may be more limited than the opportunities for recovering from the consequences of a natural disaster.

Whatever the protective effects of living in a stable and affluent country may be, the lifetime exposure rates to traumatic events (as defined by DSM-IV) in the general adult population in Canada and the United States are staggering. These figures indicate that 74% of women and 81% of men in Canada are likely to experience at least one traumatic event during their lifetime (Stein et al., 1997c); the corresponding figures for the United States are 87% of women and 97% of men (Breslau et al., 1998). Men, extroverted persons, those with a history of childhood conduct problems and a family history of substance abuse, and persons with psychiatric disorders were found to be more likely to be exposed to trauma (Breslau et al., 1991). Data on the prevalence of PTSD in the general population should be considered on the background of these trauma exposure likelihood figures. Another factor that may affect the prevalence rates of PTSD is abuse of the diagnosis of PTSD by people who malinger and/or who are involved in the litigation process (Rosen, 2004).

In view of the differences between the various DSM editions used in different epidemiological surveys, the lifetime prevalence of PTSD in the general U.S. population ranged from 1% (Helzer et al., 1987) to 9.2% (Breslau et al., 1991). In the most recent epidemiological study in the United States, the National Comorbidity Survey, the lifetime prevalence of PTSD in the general population was estimated at 7.8% (Kessler et al., 1995).

The figures for lifetime prevalence of PTSD appear to be very different in populations exposed to different types of trauma. For example, lifetime prevalence rates of PTSD among Vietnam War veterans were 30.9% in men and 26.9% in women (Kulka et al., 1990). The lifetime prevalence rate of PTSD in women who were victims of violent acts was 25.8%, whereas the corresponding rate was 9.7% in women exposed to other types of trauma (Resnick et al., 1993).

The general risk of developing PTSD after any traumatic event, as defined according to DSM-IV, was 9.2% (Breslau et al., 1998). However, this risk varied widely, again depending on the type of trauma. The highest risk (49%) was found in victims of rape, followed by the risk in people who were "badly beaten up" (31.9%); the risk of developing PTSD was fairly low in survivors of natural disasters (3.8%) and victims of motor vehicle accidents (2.3%), while the lowest risk (0.2%) was recorded in persons who unexpectedly found a dead body (Breslau et al., 1998).

As with most other anxiety disorders and depression, epidemiological studies consistently show that there is higher prevalence of PTSD among women than among men. In the National Comorbidity Survey, women were estimated to be twice as likely as men (10.4% vs. 5%) to develop PTSD after a traumatic event (Kessler et al., 1995). The only exception to this pattern was a finding of similar prevalence of PTSD in women and men in one Australian epidemiological study (Creamer et al., 2001). The reasons for gender differences in the prevalence rates of PTSD are not clear, especially since men are generally more likely to be exposed to traumatic situations than women (Breslau et al., 1991, 1998; Kessler et al., 1995; Stein et al., 1997c). Different types of traumas that women and men are exposed to (Helzer et al., 1987; Kessler et al., 1995) may only partly account for this difference: traumas that are more often related to PTSD in men (e.g., combat) are just as likely to be associated with PTSD as are traumas that are more often related to PTSD in women (e.g., sexual assault).

The risk factors for developing PTSD are discussed in detail in Etiology and Pathogenesis (below). Table 7–7 summarizes main data about epidemiology of PTSD.

COURSE AND PROGNOSIS

Although the course of PTSD (Table 7–8) varies from one patient to another, a remarkable finding about its course is the tendency to spontaneously diminish in intensity and disappear in a substantial number of patients within a few years of its onset. For example, the duration of PTSD in one study (Breslau et al., 1998) was over 3 months in 80% of patients; at 6 months, 75% of the previously identified PTSD patients continued to have symptoms, while 2 years after its onset, PTSD continued to be present in about 50% of patients. Similarly, the proportion of the trauma survivors with PTSD in another study (Shalev et al., 1997; Freedman et al., 1999) was 39% 1 month after trauma, 17% 4 months after trauma, and 10% 1 year after trauma. More than 50% of PTSD patients 3 months following the

TABLE 7–7. Epidemiological Data for Posttraumatic Stress Disorder

- Prevalence rates of PTSD should be considered in conjunction with trauma exposure rates, as the latter vary significantly in different populations.

- Lifetime prevalence in the general population in the United States is 7.8% (National Comorbidity Survey; Kessler et al., 1995).

- Lifetime prevalence and current prevalence in victims and survivors of various traumas depend on the type of trauma (generally higher for combat-related trauma and in victims of assault and violence).

- Women appear to be two times more likely to develop PTSD than men, even when controlling for exposure to traumatic events and type of traumas.

Table 7–8. Course of Posttraumatic Stress Disorder

A. Recovery

- Tendency to spontaneously diminish in intensity and disappear in a substantial number of patients within a few years of onset

- Recovery rates decrease sharply after PTSD has become chronic and, in particular, 1–2 years after onset

- Recovery rate 5 years after onset of PTSD: 18%

B. Fluctuating course (exacerbations and partial remissions)

C. Chronic, deteriorating course, often with various complications (depression, substance abuse or dependence, enduring personality change) and lasting impairment in most areas of functioning

trauma may recover within a year. Kessler et al. (1995) also found a pattern of early disappearance of symptoms (within 1 year) in the majority of PTSD patients, with rates of recovery decreasing sharply thereafter; the overall recovery rate was 60%. Similar rates of recovery (up to 66% of patients) were reported by Blanchard et al. (1997) and Shalev et al. (1997).

It seems that a major predictor of the course of PTSD is its duration; the longer the duration of PTSD, the lower the likelihood of recovery. One study (Zlotnick et al., 1999) has found that only 18% of patients recovered 5 years after the onset of PTSD, while another (Kessler et al., 1995) reported that no recovery occurred after PTSD had lasted for 6 years. A substantial number of chronic patients have a deteriorating course, with various complications of PTSD (most commonly depression and/or substance abuse or dependence) and lasting impairments in most areas of functioning. Some patients may exhibit an enduring personality change, as described in Varieties of Posttraumatic Stress Disorder (above).

Between these extremes of complete recovery and chronic, deteriorating course are PTSD patients with a course characterized by exacerbations and incomplete remissions. About one-third of all patients with PTSD may have such a course. Exacerbations in the form of re-emergence or worsening of PTSD symptoms may be precipitated by exposure to reminders of the original trauma or by the occurrence of another traumatic event. Some patients may have a low tolerance for frustrating, tense, or stressful situations and experience difficulties in adjusting to any novelty or life change. They may react to these situations with anger or impulsive behavior, by further withdrawal, or by using alcohol, illicit drugs, and medications such as benzodiazepines. Some patients have persistent but relatively isolated symptoms of PTSD, such as nightmares and intrusive memories of the trauma, with clinical significance of these symptoms varying from one person to another.

The clinical presentation of PTSD may change over time. Symptoms of reexperiencing of the trauma are usually most prominent during the initial few months after trauma. While symptoms of reexperiencing may continue to be present long time after a traumatic event, avoidance and hyperarousal symptoms tend to be encountered later in the course of PTSD, when they also appear to be more disabling.

Table 7–9 lists prognostic factors in PTSD. Poor prognosis of PTSD is generally predicted by early appearance and long duration of symptoms. Children and the elderly seem to have poorer prognosis. The prognosis of PTSD may also be related to the type of trauma, with war-related traumas

TABLE 7–9. Poor Prognostic Factors in Posttraumatic Stress Disorder

Demographics

Female gender

Younger age (children)

Older age (elderly)

Type of Trauma

War-related traumas

Traumas related to physical or sexual assault

PTSD Symptoms

Early appearance of symptoms

Long duration of symptoms

Greater number of symptoms

Prominent numbing and hyperarousal symptoms

Co-occurring Disorders

Co-occurring medical conditions

Alcohol abuse

Pre-trauma Factors

History of childhood trauma

History of other anxiety and mood disorders

Social and Interpersonal Factors

Low level of social support

Unstable home and/or family situation

Conflicts at home or workplace

and traumas related to physical and sexual assault generally being associated with poorer prognosis than traumas related to traffic accidents and natural disasters. Low levels of social support, unstable home and family situation, and conflicts at home or at work also have a negative impact on the course and prognosis of PTSD. Additional factors that indicate poor prognosis of PTSD include female gender, childhood trauma, history of other anxiety and mood disorders, greater number of PTSD symptoms, more prominent numbing and hyperarousal symptoms, co-occurring medical conditions, and alcohol abuse (Breslau and Davis, 1992).

Patients with PTSD are impaired in all areas of functioning (marital/family, occupational, social), with a subsequently negative impact on quality of life. In this respect, PTSD has been found to have more significant consequences than other anxiety disorders (e.g., Warshaw et al., 1993). Such an impact of PTSD is more pronounced in patients with chronic symptoms and complications (e.g., depression, alcohol and other drug abuse or dependence). It also appears that chronic PTSD is associated with poorer physical health in general, deleterious health habits (e.g., smoking), higher likelihood of cardiovascular, respiratory, gastrointestinal, and neurological disease, and greater use of health-care services (e.g., Kulka et al., 1990; Kessler et al., 1995; Beckham et al., 1997).

ETIOLOGY AND PATHOGENESIS

A comprehensive conceptual model of PTSD has not been formulated yet. There are several psychological and biological models of PTSD that account to a certain extent for its etiology and pathogenesis. Before their presentation, our current knowledge of the risk factors for developing PTSD will be reviewed.

Risk Factors for Developing Posttraumatic Stress Disorder

Posttraumatic stress disorder is one of the few mental disorders in which it is known what is absolutely necessary for it to occur—a traumatic event. But even though a traumatic event is a sine qua non for the development of PTSD, it is not sufficient: only a minority of trauma victims and survivors develop PTSD, although as many as 94% have symptoms of PTSD 1 week after the trauma (Foa et al., 1991). Epidemiological and clinical research into risk factors for developing PTSD has identified numerous factors that increase vulnerability to PTSD. It is possible that a combination of all these factors, which may be unique for each individual, ultimately leads to PTSD. The risk factors are usually classified in accordance with their temporal relationship to the trauma. Some are present before the trauma, others are related to the traumatic event itself, and still a third group of risk factors includes those that manifest themselves in the period immediately after the trauma or many months and years following the trauma. Risk factors for developing PTSD that are present before the trauma and related to the trauma are listed in Table 7–10.

The research to date suggests that risk factors for developing PTSD do not affect everyone in a uniform fashion. Also, some factors appear to have a stronger predictive association with PTSD; risk factors that seem to be of greatest importance for developing PTSD are those that pertain to the trauma itself and to the clinical features appearing in the period immediately after a traumatic event. These risk factors will be examined more closely, as they also play an important role in identifying traumatized individuals who are more likely to develop PTSD and who should therefore be recipients of early treatment interventions for prevention of PTSD.

With respect to the trauma itself, there has been a suggestion that the more severe the trauma is, the greater the likelihood of developing PTSD (Foy et al., 1984; Winfield et al., 1990; Yehuda et al., 1998c). However, it is difficult to quantify the severity of traumatic experience, because its nature can be quite subjective; while some types of traumatic experiences (e.g., detention in concentration camps) would be qualified as horrific by most people, other experiences (e.g., natural disasters) may be perceived in different ways by different people and responded to accordingly. It may also be that exposure to severe trauma repeatedly or continuously over prolonged periods of time increases the risk for developing PTSD.

The occurrence of certain symptoms shortly after trauma increases the probability of the later development of PTSD (e.g., Shalev, 2002). This appears to be the case particularly with dissociative symptoms (e.g., Bremner et al., 1992; Koopman et al., 1994; Shalev et al., 1996; Ursano et al., 1999a; Holeva and Tarrier, 2001; Murray et al., 2002; Engelhard et al., 2003), depressive symptoms (e.g., Shalev et al., 1998a; Freedman et al., 1999), and increased autonomic arousal, including elevated heart rate (e.g., Shalev et al., 1998b; Yehuda et al., 1998a; Brewin et al., 1999; Bryant et al., 2000; Mellman et al., 2001). However, there are at least two problems with claims that development of PTSD can be predicted on the basis of these early symptoms. First, it is not clear under what circumstances certain early symptoms represent a risk factor for the development of PTSD; for example, opinion is divided as to whether dissociative symptoms predict PTSD, depending on whether they occur immediately after the trauma (peritraumatic dissociation) or whether they are still present several weeks after the trauma. Second, early symptoms appear to be sensitive in terms of predicting PTSD (with few false negatives), because most PTSD patients have

TABLE 7–10. Risk Factors for Developing Posttraumatic Stress Disorder That Are Present Before the Trauma and Related to the Trauma[a]

Risk Factors Present Before the Trauma

DEMOGRAPHIC FACTORS

Female gender (Breslau and Davis, 1992; Kessler et al., 1995; Breslau et al., 1997, 1999)

Lower socioeconomic status (Kessler et al., 1995)

FAMILY HISTORY

Family history of mental disorders (Davidson et al., 1985; Kulka et al., 1990)

Family or parental history of PTSD (Yehuda et al., 1998b), anxiety (Scrignar, 1984; Breslau et al., 1991), and antisocial behavior (Breslau and Davis, 1992)

CHILDHOOD-RELATED AND DEVELOPMENTAL FACTORS

Unstable family atmosphere (Kulka et al., 1990)

Disrupted parent–child attachments (Breslau et al., 1991)

Early separation from parents (McFarlane, 1988; Breslau et al., 1991)

Physical and sexual abuse in childhood (Bremner et al., 1993; Engel et al., 1993; Zaidi and Foy, 1994; Fontana et al., 1997)

Presence of mental disorders during childhood or adolescence, e.g., enuresis (Gurvits et al., 1993)

Behavioral disturbance during childhood, including conduct disorder (Helzer et al., 1987; Kulka et al., 1990)

Interference with development of the central nervous system, neurological soft signs, lower intelligence (Macklin et al., 1998; Gurvits et al., 2000)

PSYCHOPATHOLOGY

General psychological problems and psychiatric disorders (Helzer et al., 1987; McFarlane, 1989a)

Neuroticism, emotional immaturity (Kulka et al., 1990)

Personality disorders (Ursano et al., 1999b)

Past history of PTSD (Ursano et al., 1999b)

Depression and anxiety disorders (Scrignar, 1984; Breslau et al., 1991, 1997; Breslau and Davis, 1992; Kessler et al., 1995)

Risk Factors Related to the Trauma

Greater exposure to trauma or traumatic event (Shore et al., 1986; McFarlane, 1989a)

Greater severity of trauma (Foy et al., 1984; Winfield et al., 1990; Yehuda et al., 1998c)

Type of trauma and meaning of the trauma for the person (some types of trauma, such as rape, seem to be more often associated with development of PTSD than other traumas)

---

[a]In some studies these risk factors also pertain to development of chronic PTSD.

had some of these symptoms in the aftermath of the trauma (Freedman et al., 1999). However, early symptoms are nonspecific predictors (with many false positives), as the majority of traumatized individuals with these symptoms recover without developing PTSD. Therefore, the presence of identified early symptoms is *by itself* of little value for predicting PTSD.

A similar conclusion can be reached about the predictive value of acute stress disorder. If trauma victims and survivors develop acute stress disorder, there is a probability ranging from 30% (Staab et al., 1996) to 83% (Bryant and Harvey, 1998; Brewin et al., 1999) that they will later manifest PTSD. Conversely, between 10% (Schnyder et al., 2001) and 72% (Harvey and Bryant, 2000) of patients with PTSD had acute stress disorder. Across the range of studies, it appears that a majority (70%–80%) of trauma victims and survivors with acute stress disorder go on to develop PTSD, whereas about one-half (40%–60%) of PTSD patients do not have a history of acute stress disorder. These findings suggest that while the presence of acute stress disorder has a high probability of leading to PTSD, the absence of acute stress disorder is by no means a guarantee that PTSD will not occur. Therefore, the pathway leading from a traumatic event to PTSD may or may not involve acute stress disorder.

Risk factors for developing PTSD that manifest themselves in the period immediately after the trauma or many months and years following the trauma are listed in Table 7–11. These include biological and cognitive (appraisal- and memory-associated) risk factors present in the aftermath of trauma and identified by recent research.

TABLE 7–11. Posttraumatic Stress Disorder Risk Factors That Manifest Themselves After the Trauma

Clinical Factors

- Acute stress disorder (Bryant et al., 1998; 1999)
- Early development of PTSD-like symptoms (Koren et al., 1999)
- Emotional numbing early after trauma (Feinstein and Dolan, 1991; Mayou et al., 1993; Shalev et al., 1996; Epstein et al., 1998)
- Prominent avoidance and other safety-seeking behaviors (Bryant and Harvey, 1998; Ehlers et al., 1998; Dunmore et al., 2001)
- Depressive symptoms (Shalev et al., 1998a)
- Serious physical consequences of the trauma, including severe injuries, chronic pain, and other health problems (Blanchard et al., 1997; Ehlers et al., 1998)
- Great difficulty in coping with and adjusting to everyday life situations and difficulty in solving problems in various situations (Solomon et al., 1989b, 1991)

(continued)

TABLE 7–11. (*continued*)

Social and Environmental Factors

- Low levels of social and/or family support (King et al., 1998; Brewin et al., 2000)
- Unfavorable, stressful, or traumatic life events, not necessarily related to the original trauma (Blanchard et al., 1997; King et al., 1998; Brewin et al., 2000)
- Subsequent exposure to reactivating environmental factors (Kluznick et al., 1986; McFarlane, 1989a)
- Being a refugee or being separated from family, relatives, and friends

Biological Factors

- Lower cortisol levels shortly after trauma (McFarlane et al., 1997; Yehuda et al., 1998a; Delahanty et al., 2000)
- Higher heart rates in the first week after trauma (Shalev et al., 1998b; Yehuda et al., 1998a; Bryant et al., 2000)

Cognitive Factors

- Excessively negative appraisals of the trauma, its consequences, oneself, responses of other people to the trauma, and the future (Delahanty et al., 1997; Ehlers et al., 1998; Warda and Bryant, 1998a; Andrews et al., 2000; Smith and Bryant, 2000; Dunmore et al., 2001; Engelhard et al., 2002; Murray et al., 2002)

    Catastrophic appraisals of the traumatic event

    Negative appraisals of oneself

    Negative appraisals of symptoms of PTSD and other symptoms (e.g., negative appraisals of dissociative experiences)

    Negative appraisals of other people's attempts to offer support

    Exaggerated expectations of negative events in the future

    Distorted attributions (attributions of responsibility for the trauma either to oneself, with subsequent feelings of shame or guilt, or to others)

    Persistent, repetitive rumination about the traumatic event

- Memory disturbances (Harvey et al., 1998; Warda and Bryant, 1998b; Guthrie and Bryant, 2000; Moulds and Bryant, 2002)

    Difficulties in retrieving specific positive memories and positive personal information in general

    Greater likelihood of forgetting negative, trauma-related information and memories, with a tendency to avoid such information and memories

- Diminished sense of control over one's life and life events (Solomon et al., 1989b, 1991)
- Attribution of responsibility for one's own life to other people, one's environment, or circumstances beyond one's own control (Solomon et al., 1989b, 1991)

In one meta-analysis of risk factors for PTSD (Brewin et al., 2000), a lack of social support was found to have the strongest predictive power. There has been some uncertainty about the nature of social support, or lack thereof, that is so strongly associated with the development of PTSD. It appears now that a negative social environment is a better predictor of PTSD than lack of support (Zoellner et al., 1999; Ullman and Filipas, 2001). Social support and social environment issues may be particularly instrumental in the pathogenesis of PTSD in female victims of crime and sexual assault and in war veterans.

In summary, using the knowledge of various risk factors for PTSD to formulate efficacious strategies for preventing PTSD remains a challenging task.

BIOLOGICAL MODELS

Table 7–12 lists findings of biological and neuroimaginig studies that are relatively specific for PTSD.

Genetic Factors

There may be a certain genetically based predisposition for the development of PTSD. This is suggested by findings that family history of psychopathology and psychiatric disorders in general increases the risk for developing PTSD (Davidson et al., 1985; Fontana and Rosenheck, 1994).

TABLE 7–12. Findings of Biological and Neuroimaginig Studies That Are Relatively Specific for Posttraumatic Stress Disorder

Hypersensitivity of the hypothalamic-pituitary-adrenal (HPA) axis to stress
Abnormally low secretion of cortisol in response to stress, with subsequently decreased levels of cortisol
Increased negative feedback regulation of cortisol
Dysregulated mechanism of cortisol secretion
Decreased hippocampal volume on MRI scans
PET findings on exposure to stress or reminders of the trauma
Excessive activation of limbic and perilimbic structures
Activation of the visual cortex
Decreased activity of the cortical areas involved in language expression

MRI, magnetic resonance imaging; PET, positron emission tomography.

A study of male Vietnam veteran twins (True et al., 1993) reported that a significant proportion of the variance in liability for 15 PTSD symptoms—between 13% and 34%, depending on the type of PTSD symptom clusters—was accounted for by genetic factors. The study did not find evidence that shared environment experiences contributed to the development of PTSD symptoms.

Neuroendocrinology of Posttraumatic Stress Disorder

The neuroendocrinology of the normal response to stress involves the release of corticotropin-releasing hormone and arginine-vasopressin from the hypothalamus, which ultimately leads to the secretion of cortisol and catecholamines (mainly epinephrine) by the adrenal gland. As part of the hypothalamic–pituitary–adrenal (HPA) axis, cortisol in the blood then has a feedback effect on the hypothalamus and the pituitary gland, thereby controlling further release of hormones from these brain structures. Thus, with the diminution and disappearance of stress, the initially increased levels of cortisol normally decrease the secretion of corticotropin-releasing hormone and adrenocorticotropic hormone (ACTH), with the latter then bringing down cortisol levels to normal.

What happens with the HPA axis in PTSD? Although complete understanding is lacking, it appears that the HPA axis in PTSD is hypersensitive to stress. This response to stress is characterized by decreased (rather than increased) release and plasma levels of cortisol (e.g., Mason et al., 1986; Yehuda et al., 1990; Resnick et al., 1995; Goenjian et al., 1996) and increased negative feedback regulation of cortisol. The latter can be demonstrated by the dexamethasone suppression test: the suppression of cortisol following administration of dexamethasone tends to be excessive in patients with PTSD (e.g., Kudler et al., 1987; Kosten et al., 1990; Yehuda et al., 1993; Goenjian et al., 1996; Stein et al., 1997d). Low plasma cortisol level (instead of the expectedly high level) in the period immediately following the trauma may have a prognostic significance in terms of suggesting a higher likelihood for development of PTSD (McFarlane et al., 1997; Yehuda et al., 1998a; Delahanty et al., 2000; see also Table 7–10).

There are several additional findings that suggest abnormalities within the HPA axis in PTSD. First, corticotropin-releasing hormone tends to be hypersecreted in PTSD (as measured in the cerebrospinal fluid, e.g., Bremner et al., 1997a; Baker et al., 1999). Second, stimulation with corticotropin-releasing hormone does not result in markedly increased secretion of ACTH and cortisol (Smith et al., 1989). Finally, following metyrapone administration to PTSD patients, the pituitary gland was hyperresponsive, and ACTH release increased in comparison with normal controls (Yehuda et al., 1996).

These findings suggest that there are two key issues pertaining to HPA axis dysfunction in PTSD. The first is an abnormally low secretion of cortisol in response to stress, which may be related to an increased number of lymphocyte glucocorticoid receptors (Yehuda et al., 1991; 1995; Stein et al., 1997d). The second issue is a disruption in the mechanism that regulates the secretion of cortisol via corticotropin-releasing hormone and ACTH.

Although still not well understood, findings of HPA dysfunction in PTSD are also important because they seem rather unique to PTSD.

Dysfunction of Neurotransmitter Systems

Norepinephrine

Many patients with PTSD exhibit hyperarousal as a consequence of centrally increased noradrenergic stimulation and involvement of the locus coeruleus. This is similar to the changes in the norepinephrine system that may be present in panic disorder. Another similarity with panic disorder comes from studies using yohimbine, which increases noradrenergic function as an α_2 adrenergic antagonist. When yohimbine was administered to PTSD patients, a significant proportion experienced panic attacks, flashbacks, intrusive recollection of the trauma, and emotional numbing (Southwick et al., 1993; 1997). Also, noradrenergic suppressors (clonidine, propranolol) alleviate symptoms of autonomic hyperactivity (e.g., increased heart rate and blood pressure) and intrusive reexperiencing of the trauma (Kolb et al., 1984).

The potential role of norepinephrine and epinephrine in PTSD is underscored by their involvement in the normal response to stress. It has been suggested that in PTSD there may be a hyperresponsiveness of norepinephrine and epinephrine to stress (e.g., McFall et al., 1990), perhaps analogous to the hypersensitivity to stress of the HPA axis. Unlike the relative uniformity of the finding of low cortisol levels in PTSD patients, however, numerous studies in which the levels of epinephrine and/or norepinephrine were measured in blood and urine of PTSD patients produced conflicting results. This suggests that the dynamics of the norepinephrine–epinephrine system and HPA axis do not follow the same pattern in PTSD.

Serotonin

There are several findings that support the role of the serotonin system in the pathogenesis of PTSD. For example, the administration of *m*-chlorophenylpiperazine (an agonist at some serotonin receptors and antagonist at other serotonin receptors) to PTSD patients induced panic attacks and intensified symptoms of PTSD (Southwick et al., 1997). This effect was observed in one group of PTSD patients, whereas in another group, a similar effect was produced by yohimbine, which affects the norepinephrine system. This finding led to a hypothesis that there may be two subgroups of PTSD patients, one characterized by dysregulation of the serotonin system and the other characterized by dysregulation of the norepinephrine system (Southwick et al., 1997).

Serotonergic activity may be changed by corticotropin-releasing hormone, which is a part of the HPA axis and is involved in the response to stress (Kirby et al., 2000). There may also be other mechanisms through which stress affects the functioning of the serotonin system.

A heightened irritability, anger, impulsivity, aggressive behavior, and suicidality, which are often encountered in PTSD patients, have been associated with decreased functioning of the serotonin system (Evenden, 1999; Mann, 1999). Finally, the efficacy of selective serotonin reuptake inhibitors in the treatment of PTSD also suggests a role of serotonin in the pathogenesis of PTSD.

Role of Endogenous Opioid System

Largely on the basis of animal studies, it was speculated that stress might trigger release of endogenous opioids in an attempt to attenuate the unpleasant and painful effects of the experience of stress. Thus, endogenous opioids were postulated to be involved in stress-induced analgesia and, more broadly, in emotional numbing, which is one of the cardinal symptoms of PTSD (van der Kolk et al., 1984).

In the model put forward by van der Kolk and colleagues (1984), emotional numbing, analgesia, and a sense of calm occur as a result of the release of endogenous opioids upon re-exposure to stimuli that remind PTSD patients of the original trauma (see also Pitman et al., 1990). However, this probably leads to a depletion of endogenous opioids and ultimately to opioid withdrawal, which is manifested through hyperarousal symptoms. To avoid the unpleasant hyperarousal symptoms and obtain some relief, even though it results in emotional numbing and decreased motivation, PTSD patients may paradoxically seek repeated re-exposure to traumatic stimuli. This pattern has been called "trauma addiction."

Although intriguing and interesting, the trauma addiction theory of PTSD is not consistent with the clinical observation that PTSD patients are primarily trying to avoid trauma-related reexperiencing, and not necessarily the symptoms of hyperarousal.

Kindling

Kindling was originally proposed as an explanation for epilepsy, but has been considered as a mechanism that might also explain some features of PTSD. In epilepsy, kindling involves sensitization of the neurons to repeatedly administered, subthreshold electrical stimuli, so that they eventually start firing spontaneously and produce seizures, without any external stimulation (Goddard et al., 1969). In PTSD, the limbic structures become kindled, that is, sensitized to the trauma-related stimuli as a result of exposure to them, so that even in the absence of these stimuli and absence of stress, limbic structures demonstrate an exaggerated fear response, with abrupt changes in mood, anger, and impulsive and aggressive behavior. Kindling in PTSD may involve an excessive noradrenergic stimulation of the amygdala from the locus coeruleus (Post et al., 1997). The kindling theory of PTSD has served as an explanation of the efficacy of some anticonvulsants in the treatment of specific PTSD manifestations, such as mood instability and angry and impulsive outbursts.

Neuroimaging Studies

A decreased hippocampal volume in PTSD patients has been a consistent finding of magnetic resonance imagining (MRI) studies, regardless of whether PTSD was related to combat trauma (Bremner et al., 1995; Gurvits et al., 1996) or childhood abuse (Bremner et al., 1997b; Stein et al., 1997b). This finding is important for several reasons. First, as proposed by Sapolsky (1995), the necrosis of the hippocampal neurons and hippocampal atrophy may be caused by the stress-induced, persistently high levels of glucocorticoids (cortisol) in the plasma and brain. Second, the longer the exposure of the brain to high levels of cortisol, perhaps the more likely it is for the hippocampus to undergo atrophy, but this proposition is difficult to reconcile with findings of low levels of cortisol in PTSD. Finally, because the hippocampus is of crucial importance for memory, a decreased hippocampal volume may be related to memory disturbances, which are often prominent in PTSD.

Several positron emission tomography (PET) studies used PTSD symptom provocation paradigms (e.g., visualizing or viewing traumatic scenes, recalling or listening to the accounts of one's own traumatic experiences). These studies did not produce consistent findings about regional cerebral blood flow changes in PTSD patients, but some preliminary conclusions may be made on the basis of these findings. It appears that in response to traumatic stimuli, there may be decreased activity of the inferior frontal cortex (Rauch et al., 1996; Shin et al., 1999), Broca's area (Shin et al., 1997), middle temporal cortex (Rauch et al., 1996), medial prefrontal cortex, hippocampus, and visual association cortex (Bremner et al., 1999). Under the same circumstances, there was increased activity of the limbic, paralimbic, and visual cortex (Rauch et al., 1996), anterior cingulate, amygdala (Shin et al., 1997), orbitofrontal cortex, and anterior temporal pole (Shin et al., 1999). These findings suggest that PTSD may be characterized by an excessive but nonspecific response of the limbic and perilimbic structures to the trauma, in conjunction with an activation of the visual cortex and decreased response of those parts of the cortex that are pivotal for language expression. In clinical terms, this may help account for nonverbal visual reexperiencing of the trauma associated with hyperarousal, which is so common in PTSD.

PSYCHOLOGICAL MODELS

Psychological models of PTSD have grappled with more or less success to explain a condition with complex disturbances in the realms of emotion (e.g., fear, anger), cognition (e.g., memory, attention, interpretation, beliefs about trauma, oneself, and the world), and behavior (e.g., ineffective coping with stress, avoidance, impulsivity). Some models emphasize certain aspects of PTSD (e.g., memory disturbance), while others attempt to give a more comprehensive account. A review of the most prominent psychological models is presented in the text below.

Behavioral Model

This model proposes that fear in PTSD is a consequence of classical conditioning, as a learned response to a wide variety of the initially neutral stimuli that become associated with the traumatic event (Keane et al., 1985). Thus, any aspect of the traumatic situation or experience acquires the ability to elicit fear through stimulus generalization and higher-order conditioning. Analogous to the role of avoidance in phobias, PTSD is maintained through avoidance of trauma-related stimuli, because such avoidance offers "protection" against fear.

Although the behavioral model is somewhat simplistic, it has been useful in providing explanations for the seemingly inextinguishable fear of the wide variety of trauma-related stimuli and for the role of avoidance in perpetuating PTSD.

Theory of Shattered Assumptions and Beliefs

This theory highlights the impact of the trauma on PTSD patients' basic, pre-existing assumptions and beliefs (e.g., Horowitz, 1986; Janoff-Bulman, 1992; Bolton and Hill, 1996). Since the traumatic event is unpredictable and brutal, it shatters assumptions and beliefs that people may have about adherence to rules, safety, justice, fairness, reciprocity in interactions with others, and meaningfulness. Some of these assumptions and beliefs may seem naïve, but most of us live with them, without necessarily realizing that they allow normal, everyday functioning in which structure, order, stability, hope, and predictability play an important role. The traumatic event not only indicates to the person that these assumptions and beliefs are wrong, but also turns the person's whole assumptive world upside down. The person may feel confused or reacts with a sense that the trauma was unreal and never really happened. According to this model, the development of PTSD is basically a consequence of "mishandling" the basic pre-trauma assumptions and beliefs that the traumatic event abruptly transformed into illusions. In other words, PTSD is seen as a problem of poor adjustment to the trauma, with the traumatized person failing to come to terms with reality that is so incongruous with previously held illusions.

The theory of shattered assumptions and beliefs makes a lot of clinical sense, as it helps us better understand traumatized persons' attempts to reconcile previously held assumptions and beliefs with post-trauma realities. Predictions that could be made on the basis of this theory do not seem to be valid, however. For example, a lack of "illusions," perhaps as a result of previous trauma(s), should make a person less vulnerable to developing PTSD after exposure to another trauma. This is not the case, and, in fact, a history of previous trauma is one of the risk factors for developing PTSD (e.g., Bremner et al., 1993; Engel et al., 1993; Zaidi and Foy, 1994; Fontana et al., 1997).

Horowitz's Model of Alternate Reprocessing and Avoidance

Although Horowitz (1976, 1986) based his theory on psychodynamic ideas, he formulated a model of PTSD that attaches crucial importance to the traumatized person's attempts to reprocess and integrate the trauma. According to Horowitz, PTSD is characterized by alternating attempts to reprocess (work through) and avoid trauma-related information. As a result, PTSD patients oscillate between unpleasant, painful, and frightening "compulsive repetition" of the trauma (e.g., through intrusive memories and flashbacks) and temporarily comforting avoidance of all reminders of the trauma or even denial of the trauma. In this model, trauma-related information remains active and fails to be adequately reprocessed and assimilated with pre-trauma knowledge and experience.

Cognitively Based Models

Cognitively based models emphasize the central role played by specific assumptions, beliefs, and faulty information-processing and appraisals in the pathogenesis of PTSD. These models attempt to account for traumatic (or emotional) memories as the most characteristic feature of PTSD. That is, these models explicitly or implicitly conceptualize PTSD as largely being based on the failure of the trauma memories to be adequately processed. As a result, these memories appear intrusively and repeatedly, with accompanying overwhelming, negative emotions.

Information-Processing Theories

The basic tenet of information-processing theories is that PTSD results from faulty or incomplete cognitive and emotional processing of the trauma-related experience. The origin of these theories can be found in the work of Lang (1979). When his theory about emotional imagery is used in the context of PTSD, emotional or traumatic memory is conceptualized as a network that connects the following information:

- Information about the physical (perceptual) aspects of the traumatic situation
- Information about the person's reaction (emotional and physiological) to the situation
- Information about the personal meaning of the situation.

Although any of these three main components of the network can activate emotional memory, it is usually activated by stimuli that remind the person of the physical aspects of the traumatic situation. For example, exposure to the sights or sounds reminiscent of the traumatic situation automatically activates the original emotional and physiological reactions to the trauma. These reactions lead to an appraisal of the situation as currently threatening, with the consequent urge to escape. The emotional memory is strengthened by its link with the sympathetic nervous system, so that every time the person experiences autonomic arousal, the memory of the trauma reawakens.

Lang's theory served as the basis for the "network model" of PTSD postulated by Foa et al. (1989). There are several important components of this model:

1. Traumatic memory is conceived of as a network in which concepts of safety and danger play a salient role, because trauma abolishes all notions of safety.
2. Activation of the traumatic memory in PTSD is facilitated by a great variety of stimuli that are quickly associated with the notions of danger and lack of safety.
3. There is a lowered threshold for the activation of the traumatic memory network in PTSD, so that memory of the trauma is easily accessed.
4. It is difficult for PTSD patients to habituate to trauma-related stimuli because of their tendency to avoid such stimuli.

Emotional Processing Theory

The emotional processing theory brings together several aspects of the work of Foa and associates, including components of the network model (Foa and Kozak, 1986; Foa et al., 1989; Foa and Riggs, 1993; Foa and Rothbaum, 1998). In its original form, the emotional processing theory postulated a memory–fear structure in PTSD, which consists of neuronal networks that participate in selective emotional processing of trauma-related fear stimuli. This structure is maintained by avoidant behaviors, beliefs about constant external threat, perception of oneself as weak and inadequate, and appraisal of PTSD symptoms as a sign of personal failure.

In an updated version of the theory, it is proposed that cognitive rigidity makes selective emotional processing of the trauma more likely and puts the traumatized person at greater risk for developing PTSD. The cognitive rigidity pertains to inflexible pre-trauma attitudes and views about oneself (especially one's own competence) and/or the surrounding world (in terms of it being safe or dangerous), regardless of whether these attitudes and views are positive or negative. If they are excessively and rigidly optimistic, the expectations and assumptions derived from them will be contradicted by the trauma; if they are excessively and rigidly negative, the corresponding expectations and assumptions will only be confirmed by the trauma.

The emotional processing theory has served as the basis for a successful treatment approach to PTSD, which uses exposure but relies specifically on modification of the hypothesized memory–fear structure. The treatment entails adoption of positive, corrective information that is incompatible with the pathological memory–fear structure and eventually allows that structure to change. Foa and Rothbaum (1998) have given a detailed account of the mechanisms involved in exposure treatment for PTSD; some of these mechanisms (e.g., habituation) are beneficial in the same way as in the treatment of other anxiety disorders. But, more specifically, exposure modifies the memory–fear structure by "normalizing" the meaning of traumatic experience in a controlled treatment setting, making it possible for this meaning to become integrated within the memory system. Details of the exposure treatment for PTSD are presented in Psychological Treatment (below).

Dual Representation Theory
The dual representation theory of PTSD (Brewin et al., 1996) proposes that traumatic experience is represented in two different memory systems. One system is called "verbally accessible memory." Within this system, the trauma is clearly "located" in the past and memory of the trauma has been well integrated with other aspects of the personality, allowing deliberate and easy retrieval of the trauma-related information and verbal expression of this information. The other system is "situationally accessible memory," which is activated involuntarily (usually in the form of flashbacks and other intrusive memories) by the situations that remind the person of the trauma. Within situationally accessible memory, the trauma is experienced as if it were happening in the present. The memory of the trauma is represented on a perceptual level (so that the representation contains sights, sounds, and/or smells) and includes "raw," unprocessed emotions (as they were experienced at the time of the trauma) and physiological responses to the trauma (usually in the form of various symptoms of hyperarousal). This is what makes flashbacks so vivid, so detailed, and so emotionally charged.

According to the dual representation theory, PTSD may result from a disrupted balance between the two memory systems. That is, verbally accessible memory of the trauma cannot neutralize situationally accessible memory, with the latter being easily activated by numerous, unpredictable, and uncontrollable reminders of the trauma and, in that sense, enjoying a certain retrieval advantage. Therefore, when the memory of the trauma is retrieved, it is automatically experienced as if the trauma were occurring in the present, along with all the accompanying perceptual, emotional, and physiological components of such an experience.

The treatment of PTSD is initially seen as a matter of modifying the highly distressing trauma memories within situationally accessible memory so that the relatively benign trauma representations are created during exposure and cognitive restructuring. Recovery would occur after the trauma-related information contained in situationally accessible memory has been reprocessed, allowing it to be better represented in the verbally accessible memory and transferred there. Eventually, reminders of the trauma would then lead to a retrieval of the reprocessed, neutralized trauma-related information from verbally accessible memory only. In such an ideal scenario, the dissociated, automatic, uncontrollable, distressing, and largely nonverbal and incommunicable memories of the trauma are replaced by fully integrated, well-controlled, verbally expressible, and communicable memories of the trauma.

Comprehensive Cognitive Model

In a comprehensive cognitive model of PTSD, formulated by Ehlers and Clark (2000), PTSD was linked to excessively negative, specific appraisals of the trauma and its consequences, and specific memory disturbances.

Ehlers and Clark (2000) proposed that trauma victims and survivors who go on to develop PTSD process the traumatic experience and its consequences (including a variety of the ensuing symptoms) in a way that generates a sense of constant, unpredictable, and generalized threat. This threat is perceived as originating both externally (so that trauma victims and survivors expect harm and danger from others) and internally (with the correspondingly distorted, threat-laden perception of themselves and their future).

Such an appraisal of the trauma is made more likely by a specific state of mind of traumatized individuals at the time of the event. This state of mind was termed "mental defeat" (Ehlers et al., 2000), as it pertains to a sense of helplessness and loss of all control and autonomy, and readiness to give up and surrender one's own core identity. This is a profoundly disturbing experience that leads to specific trauma-related self-appraisals of weakness, loss of all confidence, inability to cope with stress, and failure to afford oneself protection from omnipresent danger. Many other factors related to negative pre-trauma experiences and specific personality characteristics also contribute to a negative appraisal of oneself, one's own future, and the surrounding world in the face of trauma.

Ehlers and Clark (2000) also suggested that there are several specific memory disturbances in PTSD that account for the corresponding clinical findings in this disorder. They proposed that memory of the trauma in PTSD is poorly integrated, poorly elaborated, and poorly contextualized. This is manifested clinically through fragmented memories of the trauma, difficulties in intentional recall of certain aspects of the trauma, and misplacing of traumatic memories as if the trauma were occurring in the present. In addition, Ehlers and Clark (2000) proposed strong associative memory in PTSD, so that memories of the trauma are firmly connected with certain cues and triggers. This explains a quick and unexpected reactivation of traumatic memories by a variety of stimuli and a disturbing lack of any control over such memories, as reported by the PTSD patients.

Another important component of the comprehensive cognitive model of PTSD is a detailed account of the processes and factors that maintain PTSD. These are of two general kinds: behavioral and cognitive. Behavioral aspects include various attempts to avoid trauma reminders and thereby prevent a return of memories of the trauma, safety behaviors designed to minimize or abolish all trauma-related threat, and use of alcohol and drugs to suppress discomfort or anxiety. The cognitive processes involved in the maintenance of PTSD include persistent, maladaptive rumination about various aspects of the trauma and its consequences and selective attention to trauma-related threat cues.

The model postulated by Ehlers and Clark (2000) has received substantial empirical support, but some aspects of the model need further testing and validation. Importantly, the model serves as the basis for cognitive therapy of PTSD, which has been efficacious in studies conducted so far (Gillespie et al., 2002; Ehlers et al., 2003).

Psychodynamic Approaches

There are several psychodynamic contributions to our understanding of PTSD. Freud speculated that "traumatic neurosis," as it was called in his time, develops when the person resorts to "repetition compulsion"; Freud believed that patients could gain control over trauma through repetitious reliving of the trauma.

Krystal (1988) proposed that the essence of PTSD is in the patients' inability to use trauma-related emotions as signals that would promptly activate adequate defense mechanisms against painful recollections of the trauma. Instead, patients perceive trauma-related emotions as a warning that the trauma will recur; in an attempt to alleviate the anticipated discomfort, avoid painful emotions, and prevent recurrence of the trauma, patients resort to somatization or use alcohol or other substances. Hence there is a relatively high frequency of psychosomatic conditions, alexithymia, and substance abuse among trauma survivors and patients with PTSD.

Regardless of the specific model, all psychodynamic approaches to PTSD emphasize importance of the personal meaning of the trauma to a patient with PTSD. This meaning is related to the personality characteristics of the patient, and its understanding is considered crucial for treatment.

The psychodynamic approach to PTSD also takes into account the specific defense mechanisms used by patients with PTSD. The purpose of these mechanisms is to alleviate the consequences of the trauma and to avoid unpleasant and painful trauma-related feelings, for example, through dissociation. Patients with PTSD often use immature defense mechanisms, such as denial and projection: patients may deny their own feelings or project anger and guilt feelings onto others. Traumatized individuals sometimes defend themselves against an unbearable feeling of helplessness through anger, revenge fantasies, or relentless pursuit of compensation.

TREATMENT

Many patients with PTSD seek professional help only reluctantly and relatively late, after a full clinical picture has emerged and even after some complications of PTSD have developed. The reasons for this situation can be found in the feelings of shame that some PTSD patients have with regard to their traumatic experience and in beliefs of other PTSD patients that they do not have a real disorder and their consequent expectations that their symptoms will go away with the passage of time. This ambivalent and sometimes quite negative attitude toward treatment can affect the treatment process adversely. The late onset of treatment of PTSD may also be a consequence of physicians' reluctance to accept PTSD as a valid psychopathological entity (see Assessment, above).

It is being increasingly recognized that the timing of therapeutic intervention in PTSD is critical, and that the best results in the treatment of PTSD may be achieved by secondary prevention. If traumatic events cannot be prevented, pathological reactions to such events can. Treatment initiated during the first few weeks after traumatic experience, at the time when there is still no diagnosis of PTSD, is more likely to be efficacious than treatment initiated later. More and more data suggest that early treatment may prevent development of the disabling features of PTSD and its complications, and it may also improve the prognosis of PTSD.

Major issues in early and preventive treatment of PTSD revolve around two questions. First, who should be treated? All victims and survivors of the trauma or only those who appear to be at risk for developing PTSD? Second, how should the early treatment be conducted? Through nonspecific or more specific psychological interventions, pharmacotherapy, or some combination of psychological and pharmacological treatment? In view of findings that most trauma victims and survivors recover without any treatment, even if they initially exhibit dramatic PTSD-like symptoms, it appears reasonable to institute early treatment to those individuals who are more likely to develop PTSD. The large body of research into risk factors for PTSD (see Etiology and Pathogenesis, above) has identified numerous risk factors, but most of them are not specific enough for PTSD and are therefore not particularly useful for identifying at-risk individuals. Clinicians are often left with their own judgment as to which combination of risk factors might be predictive of PTSD. As for the most appropriate early treatment approach, there is an increasing understanding of psychological strategies that might be useful in this phase, but very little information on efficacious pharmacotherapy. The current situation in this area will be reviewed in the text below.

When full-blown PTSD develops, it presents in different ways, with different combinations of symptoms. In view of this heterogeneity, no treatment approach is likely to be applicable to all patients, and various treatments are not likely to be efficacious for all. It follows that when making a decision about treatment of PTSD, one should take particularly into account specific characteristics of each patient. Various types of treatment, psychological and pharmacological, are usually combined in clinical practice. The severity of PTSD can serve only as a rough guide to the selection of treatment. In mild forms of PTSD, psychological treatments alone are generally recommended, whereas in the more severe forms of PTSD, a combination of psychological and pharmacological treatments is to be used (Ballenger et al., 2000).

Once the full clinical picture of PTSD has emerged, it may not be realistic to expect all of its features to completely and permanently disappear with treatment. In an effort to avoid unrealistic expectations, unfounded hopes, and disappointment, it is important to set realistic goals of treatment and for patients to understand these goals. Goals of treatment in PTSD are listed in Table 7–13.

TABLE 7–13. Goals of Treatment in Posttraumatic Stress Disorder

- Alleviation of symptoms and behavioral disturbances
- Alleviation of manifestations of any co-occurring conditions
- Better understanding of the trauma, its meanings, implications, and consequences, with sensible incorporation of the traumatic experience and traumatic memories into one's identity
- Increased resilience to stress
- Improvement in functioning
- Minimization of disability
- Prevention of complications

Pharmacological Treatment

Aspects of pharmacotherapy that are specific for PTSD are presented in Table 7–14. The role of pharmacotherapy in the treatment of PTSD is still not clear. Because PTSD is a complex and multifaceted condition, it is not likely that there will ever be a medication that will be efficacious for all of its symptoms or for their many different combinations. For that reason, several medications are often used in PTSD.

Pharmacological treatment of PTSD is used with the goals of significantly decreasing the most prominent and disabling symptoms and improving functioning. Pharmacotherapy may also be used for treatment of co-occurring psychiatric disorders. The efficacy of medications in reaching these goals depends on many factors and may vary dramatically from one patient to another. There are no clear guidelines that would help determine when pharmacotherapy is indicated. The assumption often valid for other disorders, that greater severity necessitates pharmacotherapy, may also be applicable to PTSD; patients with a more severe form of PTSD are certainly more likely to be treated with medications.

A targeted pharmacological approach to early and preventive treatment of PTSD should take into account symptoms that appear within several weeks of the traumatic event that are responsive to pharmacotherapy and highly predictive of the later development of PTSD. As already noted, several of these symptoms have been identified: depressive symptoms (e.g., Shalev et al., 1998a; Freedman et al., 1999) and symptoms of excessive

---

TABLE 7–14. Aspects of Pharmacotherapy That Are Relatively Specific for Posttraumatic Stress Disorder

- Use medications early in the aftermath of trauma, for possible prevention of full-blown PTSD.
- More classes of different medications are used in PTSD than in other anxiety disorders.
- PTSD associated with civilian trauma may be more responsive to pharmacotherapy than combat-related PTSD.
- The choice of medication(s) may be based, at least in part, on clinical features and predominant type of symptoms, but antidepressants are usually considered the treatment of choice.
- When antidepressants are used for PTSD, dropout rates are relatively high.
- When selective serotonin reuptake inhibitors (SSRIs) are used, their propensity to cause or worsen insomnia and to initially cause or worsen agitation has significant practical implications. Adding a hypnotic medication and/or initiating treatment at a very small dosage is a strategy to avoid these problems.
- Benzodiazepines have a very limited role in treatment.

autonomic arousal, including increased heart rate (e.g., Harvey and Bryant, 1998; Shalev et al., 1998b; Yehuda et al., 1998a; Brewin et al., 1999; Bryant et al., 2000; Mellman et al., 2001). In view of these findings, it is reasonable to adopt a recommendation (Ballenger et al., 2000) to start pharmacological treatment of PTSD symptoms with an antidepressant about 3 weeks after the traumatic event if the acute response to trauma has not subsided by that time. In addition, the same findings support an early, short-term use of medications that can decrease autonomic arousal, such as clonidine, propranolol, and even benzodiazepines. These medications can be used in conjunction with or instead of psychological techniques (e.g., muscle relaxation) that also aim to alleviate symptoms of hyperarousal.

It appears that certain medications work better for some symptoms of PTSD than for others, but it is still unclear to what extent medications can be combined to complement each other's modes of action. Because of the heterogeneity of the clinical picture, it is not surprising that several quite different classes of medications have been used in PTSD (Table 7–15). The choice of these medications may depend on the predominant symptomatology of

TABLE 7–15. Classes of Medications Used in Treatment of Posttraumatic Stress Disorder

---

Antidepressants

Selective serotonin reuptake inhibitors (SSRIs)

Tricyclic antidepressants (TCAs)

Nefazodone

Classical monoamine oxidase inhibitors (MAOIs)

Noradrenergic Suppressors

Clonidine

Propranolol

Mood Stabilizers and Anticonvulsants

Lithium

Anticonvulsants: carbamazepine, valproate, lamotrigine

Second-Generation Antipsychotics

Risperidone, olanzapine, quetiapine

Non-benzodiazepine Hypnotics

Zolpidem, zopiclone, zaleplon

Benzodiazepines

---

the PTSD patient (Table 7–16), although we are still far from having specific pharmacological treatments for specific clusters of PTSD symptoms.

Antidepressants in Treatment of Posttraumatic Stress Disorder

Antidepressants are the most commonly used form of pharmacotherapy for PTSD, in part because PTSD is often accompanied by depression. However, antidepressants seem to have direct and specific effects on some PTSD symptoms, regardless of the presence of depression (Kosten et al., 1991). Also, other anxiety disorders responsive to treatment with antidepressants commonly co-occur with PTSD. Several classes of antidepressants have been found to be useful in PTSD, but efficacy in controlled trials has been demonstrated only for selective serotonin reuptake inhibitors

TABLE 7–16. Aspects of Patients' Clinical Presentation That May Guide the Choice of Medication in Posttraumatic Stress Disorder

Predominant Symptomatology	Choice of Medication
Emotional numbing, social withdrawal	SSRIs
Recurrent, intrusive reexperiencing of the trauma	Phenelzine(?) SSRIs(?) Clonidine(?) Second-generation antipsychotics(?)
Trauma-related avoidance	SSRIs(?) Amitriptyline(?) Nefazodone(?)
Hyperarousal, autonomic hyperactivity	Clonidine Propranolol Benzodiazepines SSRIs(?)
Sleep disturbance	Non-benzodiazepine hypnotics Benzodiazepines Diphenhydramine TCAs Nefazodone
Restlessness, psychomotor agitation	TCAs Nefazodone(?) Second-generation antipsychotics(?)
Outbursts of anger, impulsive behavior	Lithium Carbamazepine Valproate Lamotrigine SSRIs(?)

SSRIs, selective serotonin reuptake inhibitors; TCAs, tricyclic antidepressants.

(SSRIs). In addition, there is some evidence of efficacy in PTSD for tricyclic antidepressants (TCAs), nefazodone, and phenelzine, a classical monoamine oxidase inhibitor (MAOI).

Selective Serotonin Reuptake Inhibitors
Owing to their efficacy and relatively good tolerability, SSRIs have become the first-line pharmacotherapy for PTSD. The efficacy in PTSD has been well established for sertraline (Brady et al., 2000; Davidson et al., 2001) and paroxetine (Marshall et al., 2001; Tucker et al., 2001), but some evidence of efficacy also exists for fluoxetine (Nagy et al., 1993; van der Kolk et al., 1994; Martenyi et al., 2002) and fluvoxamine (De Boer et al., 1992; Marmar et al., 1996). The PTSD symptoms that may be most responsive to SSRIs are those of emotional numbing, social withdrawal, and hyperarousal (van der Kolk et al., 1994; Brady et al., 2000; Davidson et al., 2002), but the choice of SSRIs is still not based on the most prominent PTSD symptomatology. Indeed, a response to SSRIs may be seen in various PTSD symptom clusters, and the pattern of response appears to vary from one patient to another. A study of the effects of sertraline on PTSD symptoms (Davidson et al., 2002) found an early decrease in irritability and anger, which might also partly explain the effects of sertraline on other symptoms of PTSD. Interestingly, in the same study, sertraline had more pronounced effects on the psychological than on the somatic symptoms of PTSD.

Clinical experience and at least one study (van der Kolk et al., 1994) suggest that SSRIs may be more useful for PTSD related to civilian trauma than for PTSD associated with combat trauma. There are reports of efficacy of SSRIs in combat-related PTSD (e.g., Marmar et al., 1996), but the results of some studies (e.g., Zohar et al., 2002) are conflicting. Another clinical situation in which SSRIs may be useful is when there is co-occurrence of alcohol abuse (Brady et al., 1995).

The main specific drawback of SSRIs in the treatment of PTSD is their propensity to cause or worsen insomnia, which, along with recurrent dreams of the trauma, nightmares, and other sleep disturbances, is often a prominent feature of PTSD. Thus, SSRIs are often combined with hypnotic medications (preferably non-benzodiazepine hypnotics, such as zolpidem, zopiclone, and zaleplon). Treatment with hypnotics need not begin immediately; it is recommended (Ballenger et al., 2000) that hypnotic medication be commenced after the patient has had at least four consecutive nights of disturbed sleep.

The other relatively specific feature of treatment of PTSD with SSRIs is the propensity of these medications to worsen anxiety and cause agitation during initial treatment. This effect is similar to that seen in patients with panic disorder who are treated with SSRIs. As a result, treatment with an

SSRI in PTSD should be initiated in the same way as in panic disorder—at a very small dose, which is usually one-quarter to one-half of the antidepressant dose. Depending on the side effects and treatment response, the dose of an SSRI is then gradually and very carefully increased to a level that is usually above its standard antidepressant dose. However, the range of efficacious doses of SSRIs and other medications used in the treatment of PTSD tends to be quite wide (Table 7–17).

A recent study (Vermetten et al., 2003) has suggested that long-term treatment with SSRIs (paroxetine) improves hippocampus-based verbal declarative memory and increases hippocampal volume in patients with PTSD.

Tricyclic Antidepressants

Several points need to be made about the use of TCAs (amitriptyline, imipramine) in PTSD. First, they may be helpful in PTSD, because unlike SSRIs, they have sedative properties and do not interfere with sleep. Therefore, TCAs may be useful in the treatment of PTSD patients whose sleep

TABLE 7–17. The Usual Doses of Medications Commonly Used in Treatment of Posttraumatic Stress Disorder

Medication	Dose Range
Antidepressants	
Sertraline	50–200 mg/day
Paroxetine	10–60 mg/day
Fluvoxamine	50–250 mg/day
Fluoxetine	10–80 mg/day
Amitriptyline	150–300 mg/day
Imipramine	100–250 mg/day
Nefazodone	400–600 mg/day
Phenelzine	30–90 mg/day
Noradrenergic Suppressors	
Clonidine	0.2–0.6 mg/day
Mood stabilizers and anticonvulsants	
Lithium	300–1800 mg/day
Carbamazepine	400–1200 mg/day
Valproate	250–2000 mg/day

disturbance is quite severe and/or whose agitation is a prominent component of their clinical presentation. Second, there is some suggestion that TCAs may be useful in combat-related PTSD (e.g., Bleich et al., 1986; Davidson et al., 1990), perhaps more so than other antidepressants. Finally, the specific efficacy of TCAs (amitriptyline) for PTSD symptoms may be questioned, as their efficacy in alleviating general anxiety and depressive symptoms may be more convincing (e.g., Davidson et al., 1990).

Nefazodone
Several reports (e.g., Davidson et al., 1998) have suggested that nefazodone, a serotonin antagonist and reuptake inhibitor, may be useful in the treatment of PTSD, perhaps particularly for treatment-refractory patients (Zisook et al., 2000). The advantages of nefazodone include improved sleep, mild to moderate sedation, and possible direct effects on specific PTSD symptoms.

Classical Monoamine Oxidase Inhibitors
Because of side effects and special dietary requirements, phenelzine, a classical MAOI, may be reserved for PTSD patients who have not responded to previous treatment with antidepressants. Also, the use of classical MAOIs is limited by PTSD patients' propensity to act impulsively. There is some evidence that phenelzine is efficacious in alleviating symptoms of intrusive reexperiencing of the trauma (e.g., Davidson et al., 1987; Kosten et al., 1991), and in this regard, phenelzine may be superior to imipramine (Frank et al., 1988).

Noradrenergic Suppressors

Clonidine
Clonidine, which acts as an α_2 adrenergic agonist, may be used for the specific purpose of counteracting autonomic hyperactivity. Clonidine may also alleviate various symptoms of reexperiencing trauma (e.g., nightmares, flashbacks, intrusive memories), decrease hypervigilance, and improve sleep and impulse control (Kolb et al., 1984). As already mentioned, clonidine may be suitable for initial, acute treatment of PTSD symptoms. Tolerance seems to develop to its therapeutic effects during long-term administration. It may cause severe hypotension and should therefore be used with caution.

Propranolol
Propranolol, a β-adrenergic blocker, may also be used in the treatment of PTSD, with the purpose of decreasing noradrenergic hyperactivity. As

with clonidine, propranolol may have effects on other symptoms of PTSD, but these are less clear and less convincing than in case of clonidine.

Mood Stabilizers and Anticonvulsants

Mood stabilizers and anticonvulsants—lithium, carbamazepine, valproate, and lamotrigine—may be useful in the treatment of certain features of PTSD, particularly outbursts of anger and impulsive, aggressive behavior. The rationale for using mood stabilizers and anticonvulsants is in the conceptualization of PTSD as a disorder of affective instability, based on the kindling phenomenon (see Etiology and Pathogenesis, above). The efficacy of mood stabilizers and anticonvulsants in alleviating more specific symptoms of PTSD has not been well established. These medications can be used alone or in combination with an antidepressant.

Second-Generation Antipsychotics

Second-generation antipsychotics (risperidone, olanzapine, quetiapine) are increasingly used in the treatment of PTSD, either as monotherapy or in combination with another medication, usually an antidepressant. The efficacy of these agents in PTSD and indications for their use remain to be established. In particular, it needs to be elucidated whether second-generation antipsychotics are efficacious against some of the specific PTSD symptoms (e.g., flashbacks) and quasi-hallucinatory experiences or whether they are useful only for clear-cut psychotic symptoms that sometimes co-occur with PTSD.

Benzodiazepines

Long-term treatment of PTSD with benzodiazepines is generally not recommended, particularly in patients who have poor impulse control. Benzodiazepines can sometimes disinhibit such patients and aggravate their aggressive behavior. In addition, PTSD patients seem to have more difficulty with the discontinuation of benzodiazepines and with benzodiazepine withdrawal symptoms than patients with other anxiety disorders (Risse et al., 1990). Obviously, benzodiazepines should be avoided in patients who tend to abuse alcohol and/or other substances. For all these reasons, the role of benzodiazepines in the treatment of PTSD is very limited. These medications can sometimes be used on an as-needed (prn) basis or for a relatively brief period of time, usually in conjunction with antidepressants. Benzodiazepines can be of benefit to patients who are troubled by various hyperarousal symptoms and/or insomnia, but even in this context, they should be avoided as much as possible.

Other Pharmacological Agents

Various other medications (buspirone, brofaromine, inositol, cyproheptadine, prazosin) have been used in the treatment of PTSD, some of them in an attempt to treat specific symptoms of PTSD, such as nightmares. The results of reports on these treatments are either inconsistent or suggest some efficacy in a very preliminary way.

Long-Term Pharmacological Treatment of Posttraumatic Stress Disorder

The optimal duration of pharmacological treatment of PTSD is unknown. However, for most cases of chronic PTSD, it is recommended that pharmacotherapy be continued for at least 1 year after a satisfactory response to acute treatment has been achieved (Ballenger et al., 2000). The dose administered during that time should be the same as the dose that produced the initial response.

As with other anxiety disorders, there is a risk of relapse and/or withdrawal symptoms upon discontinuation of pharmacotherapy. Therefore, if the medication is to be discontinued, it is imperative that its dose be gradually and carefully reduced (e.g., by not more than 25% every 2–3 months). In addition, psychological treatment techniques may be combined with pharmacotherapy to minimize the risk of relapse.

Pharmacotherapy of Treatment-Resistant Posttraumatic Stress Disorder

An adequate pharmacological trial for chronic PTSD consists of a minimum of 12 weeks of treatment with a first-line antidepressant (an SSRI) at the highest doses tolerated by the patient. If there is no response to an adequate trial of one antidepressant, it is reasonable to switch to another antidepressant, preferably an antidepressant from another class (Table 7–18). The usual sequence is for PTSD patients to be treated with an SSRI first; in case of treatment failure with an SSRI, nefazodone or one of the TCAs may be tried next. The last option among the antidepressants is phenelzine.

If there has been partial response to one of the antidepressants, it can be combined with a medication from another class (Table 7–18). There are no clear guidelines as to how to make these combinations, but the choice

TABLE 7–18. Choice of Medication in Treatment of Chronic Posttraumatic Stress Disorder

First-Line

SSRIs (especially sertraline and paroxetine)

Second-Line

Nefazodone or TCAs (imipramine, amitriptyline), if no response at all to an SSRI

Third-Line

A classical MAOI (phenelzine), if no response at all to an SSRI, nefazodone, or a TCA

Partial Response to First- or Second-Line Pharmacotherapy

Augmentations and combinations

1. With noradrenergic suppressors (clonidine, propranolol)
2. With mood stabilizers and anticonvulsants (lithium, carbamazepine, valproate, lamotrigine)
3. With non-benzodiazepine hypnotics
4. With benzodiazepines
5. With second-generation antipsychotics (risperidone, olanzapine, quetiapine)

Monotherapy Considerations (if no response to antidepressants or combinations of antidepressants with other medications)

1. Noradrenergic suppressors (clonidine, propranolol)
2. Mood stabilizers and anticonvulsants (lithium, carbamazepine, valproate, lamotrigine)
3. Second-generation antipsychotics (risperidone, olanzapine, quetiapine)

MAOI, monoamine oxidase inhibitor; SSRIs, selective serotonin reuptake inhibitors; TCAs, tricyclic antidepressants.

can be based in part on the symptoms that are most prominent in PTSD. Thus, patients with severe outbursts of anger and impulse control problems can be administered a mood stabilizer or an anticonvulsant, whereas patients with autonomic hyperactivity may respond well to clonidine, propranolol, or even a benzodiazepine. In case of severe insomnia, a hypnotic medication can be combined with an antidepressant. Other augmentation strategies have been tried and some reported in the literature—for example, buspirone augmentation of antidepressant treatment of PTSD. Various other pharmacological combinations and other medications as monotherapy may be used in the treatment of PTSD, particularly for patients with complex presentation or specific and incapacitating symptoms, or if they have been resistant to previous pharmacotherapy.

Psychological Treatment

General Issues in Psychological Treatment of Posttraumatic Stress Disorder

Regardless of the type of psychological treatment used for PTSD, it is likely that the nature of therapeutic relationship will play a major role in affecting the outcome of treatment. This may be obvious, but should still be emphasized because of the specific needs and characteristics of PTSD patients. Above all, PTSD patients need to feel safe in a therapeutic setting, probably more so than other patients. Indeed, the therapy can hardly proceed if patients do not feel safe enough. The sense of safety should be fostered by the therapist in multiple ways, some of which are listed below.

- The therapist should communicate an unequivocal acceptance of patients, which is possible through an understanding of the patients' traumatic experience and its impact.
- The therapist needs to be sensitive about issues that patients are preoccupied with, compassionate about their plight, and able to empathize.
- The therapist should convey a nonjudgmental attitude, which would help create an atmosphere in which patients can feel free to express their feelings and attitudes (without negative consequences to follow).
- The therapist should pay particular attention to aspects of the patients' traumatic experience that they feel guilty about, ashamed of, or embarrassed, angry, or desperate about. These aspects should be neither avoided nor excessively emphasized.
- The therapist should promote a positive attitude toward the future, while demonstrating to patients that he or she is fully aware of and understands the impact of the past trauma(s).

Because many PTSD patients have lost a sense of interpersonal trust through the traumatic experience or its consequences, it will be possible for them to restore that sense only within a safe therapeutic environment in which they are able to freely express their feelings and reactions.

There are other issues that are specific for patients with PTSD, and they often need to be addressed in the course of psychotherapy. Very broadly, these issues pertain to the different effects of the trauma on patients' sense of self-worth and their perception of other people, life, and world in general and their future in particular.

Phase-Based Approach to Psychological Treatment of Posttraumatic Stress Disorder

Posttraumatic stress disorder does not develop suddenly, and a substantial proportion of PTSD patients exhibit features of acute stress disorder following a traumatic event. Because the occurrence of trauma is a precondition for the development of PTSD and acute stress disorder is a well-known risk for developing PTSD, it appears reasonable to use psychological interventions in the period shortly after the trauma has occurred to prevent PTSD or at least alleviate its symptoms if it does develop some time after the trauma.

While the use of early psychological interventions in trauma victims and survivors is not disputable, there are controversies about most aspects of these interventions. Several questions need to be answered: which interventions should be used, for which trauma victims and survivors, at which point in time after a traumatic event, and for how long? Preliminary data suggest that only a portion of trauma victims and survivors need psychological intervention, because most manage to cope fairly well with the trauma and its consequences. Therefore, the immediate tasks following a traumatic event are to identify those victims and survivors who are at greatest risk for developing PTSD and offer specific psychological intervention to them. There has been much research into general risk factors for developing PTSD and specific risk factors present in the aftermath of a traumatic event. These risk factors are summarized in Tables 7–10 and 7–11. Another issue is the choice of early psychological intervention, which is usually psychological debriefing or cognitive-behavioral therapy (CBT), although other types of early intervention have also been used. The remaining issues about early intervention stem from the choice of intervention; these will be discussed in the text below.

After full-blown PTSD has developed (with or without other complicating psychiatric disorders or psychological issues), well-established psychological treatments can be used. These treatment approaches include several varieties of CBT, eye movement desensitization and reprocessing (EMDR), group therapy, and psychodynamic psychotherapy.

Early Psychological Interventions

Psychological Debriefing

Psychological debriefing (Mitchell, 1983; Dyregrov, 1989) was the first intervention developed specifically for use during the first several days after a traumatic event. It was designed for both group and individual format, but has increasingly been used as an individual intervention. Psychological debriefing is usually administered in a single session that takes about 2 hours. It is provided to all victims and survivors of the trauma (and even more broadly, to relatives of the victims and survivors, military personnel, emergency care workers, and others who may be in contact with the victims and survivors), regardless of the degree of their distress and presence of any symptoms of acute stress disorder.

Psychological debriefing provides victims and survivors with support and reassurance, information about normal and abnormal responses to trauma, and the opportunity to go over the event in full detail, express their feelings and thoughts associated with the event, and learn basic skills for coping with the impact of the trauma. In addition, personal meaning(s) of the trauma may be explored. The goals of psychological debriefing are to identify trauma victims and survivors who are suffering from acute stress disorder, educate them about normal and abnormal reactions to trauma and means of coping, promote normal emotional and cognitive processing of the trauma, decrease acute distress and alleviate symptoms, prevent PTSD, prepare victims and survivors for possible further symptoms and trauma-related consequences, and provide information on how to deal with them and where to seek help.

Despite the appeal of psychological debriefing as simple, based on common sense, and intuitively useful for alleviating acute distress and for preventing full-blown PTSD, long-term efficacy studies of single-session psychological debriefing have not produced generally encouraging results. Two systematic reviews and one meta-analysis (Rose and Bisson, 1998; Van Emmerick et al., 2002; Rose et al., 2003) failed to demonstrate superiority of psychological debriefing over the absence of any intervention. Two studies showed that the outcome following psychological debriefing was even worse (Bisson et al., 1997; Mayou et al., 2000). These studies have been criticized on methodological grounds, as well as on grounds of their not being representative of psychological debriefing as it is carried out in the real world and the type of victims and survivors who undergo this intervention (Deahl, 2003). There is an ongoing debate about the usefulness of psychological debriefing, with some (e.g., Wessely, 2003) arguing that it is a "waste of time," and others (e.g., Deahl, 2003) emphasizing that it is unethical "not to do anything" in the aftermath of trauma.

Resolution of this controversy does not appear to reside in either complete rejection of psychological debriefing nor in its endorsement for routine use after traumatic events. It appears that this intervention is often perceived by its recipients as having short-term benefits and that it plays an important educational role (Deahl, 2003). It is also emphasized by proponents of psychological debriefing that this is not meant to be a one-off, stand-alone intervention offered to victims and survivors of trauma, but merely the initial one, and usually as a part of a package of interventions (Mitchell and Everly, 1995; Deahl, 2003).

Because psychological debriefing is not sufficient, it may do harm by ignoring the need for additional treatment interventions and delaying their implementation (e.g., McFarlane, 1989b). Moreover, psychological debriefing should not be mandatory and should preferably not be conducted by people who are strangers to the victims and survivors, including mental health professionals (Wessely, 2003). More fundamentally, potential reasons for the lack of expected efficacy of psychological debriefing are as follows:

- Inadvertent re-traumatization of victims and survivors through their imaginal exposure to the trauma-related material too soon after the traumatic event (Rose et al., 2003)
- Emergence of the sense of shame that cannot be adequately addressed during a single session of debriefing (Rose et al., 2003)
- Interference with the natural process of post-trauma healing through medicalization of the trauma-related distress and, possibly, through an increased likelihood of PTSD symptoms actually developing instead of being prevented (Rose et al., 2003; Wessely, 2003)
- Erroneous assumptions that it is *always* salubrious for victims and survivors of the trauma to "open up," express their feelings, and give an account of what happened (Rose et al., 2003; Wessely, 2003).

Early Cognitive-Behavioral Therapy
There are relatively few reports of CBT used early after a traumatic event and/or in patients with acute stress disorder (Foa et al., 1995; Bryant et al., 1998; 1999; Gidron et al., 2001; Bryant et al., 2003). In contrast to psychological debriefing, which is administered to all trauma victims and survivors, early CBT has been used mainly in those victims and survivors who are considered to carry a high risk for developing PTSD, including victims and survivors with acute stress disorder. The two main issues concerning this version of CBT pertain to its efficacy and to its components and mode of administration (i.e., whether and how it differs from standard CBT, used for established cases of PTSD).

Studies by Bryant et al. (1998, 1999, 2003) suggest that CBT for acute stress disorder, conducted during the first month after a traumatic event, is superior to "supportive counseling," and that this difference in favor of CBT is maintained at 4-year follow-up. These studies did not make comparisons between CBT and lack of any intervention. The version of CBT used in these studies was similar to the standard CBT for PTSD, except that it was condensed, lasting 5 instead of the usual 12–16 sessions. The

comparison treatment modality, supportive counseling, specifically excluded components of CBT such as exposure, cognitive restructuring, and
anxiety management techniques, and consisted of psychoeducation, training in problem-solving skills, and support. Therefore, the superiority of
CBT could be attributed to its specific ingredients. Another potentially
important finding of these studies was a higher dropout rate among
patients treated with CBT. This suggests that use of CBT during the first
weeks after a traumatic event may not be suitable for some traumatized
patients, perhaps because of the intensity of this form of treatment and
temporal proximity to a traumatic event.

A study of four-session CBT for patients with early symptoms of
PTSD commencing 2 weeks after a traumatic event showed that it had a
better post-treatment outcome than when there was no structured treatment (Foa et al., 1995). At follow-up, however, these differences in efficacy
disappeared, suggesting that CBT might be useful in accelerating recovery
of trauma victims with PTSD symptoms.

In conclusion, there is some evidence that the use of four to five sessions of the standard CBT package for trauma victims and survivors who
are at greater risk for developing PTSD or patients with acute stress disorder during the first month following a traumatic event may bring about
relatively quick alleviation of PTSD symptoms and possibly prevent PTSD
or attenuate its manifestations if it does develop later. In addition to the
issue of patient selection on the basis of PTSD risk assessment, the possibility of dropout must be considered because of the intensive nature of
CBT administered shortly after a traumatic event. Therefore, patients
undergoing early CBT should be well prepared for it and have a good
understanding of what it entails.

Psychological Treatments for Chronic Posttraumatic Stress Disorder

Cognitive-Behavioral Therapy

There are several components of a typical CBT package for PTSD. They
include psychoeducation, exposure, cognitive restructuring, and anxiety
management techniques. In various versions of CBT these components are
used in different proportions, and different techniques are used even
within one component of CBT.

Psychoeducation. This activity is carried out at the very beginning of
treatment. Patients are informed about the nature of normal and excessive
(pathological) response to trauma. The main goals of psychoeducation are

to demystify PTSD, dispel main misconceptions about it by providing appropriate and accurate information, and agree on treatment objectives through a process of collaborative negotiation.

Exposure. This is usually considered to be the main ingredient of CBT for PTSD. The general principles of exposure therapy are the same as those for treatment of agoraphobia and other phobias (see Chapters 2 and 5). They are based on constructing hierarchies of the feared situations and stimuli to which patients are gradually being exposed, from the least fear- or discomfort-eliciting situation or stimulus to the strongest fear- or discomfort-eliciting situation or stimulus. However, there are several aspects of exposure that are relatively specific for PTSD (Table 7–19).

Most exposure-based programs for PTSD include prolonged imaginal exposure. This technique requires that patients vividly imagine the traumatic event and situation for prolonged periods of time—preferably for 1–2 hours every day, both in sessions and as homework exercises.

TABLE 7–19. Aspects of Cognitive-Behavioral Therapy That Are Relatively Specific for Posttraumatic Stress Disorder

Exposure

- Prolonged imaginal exposure is used.
- In vivo exposure usually follows imaginal exposure.
- Gradual exposure is preferable to flooding.
- Patients should be fully emotionally engaged during exposure.
- Greater flexibility may be required from the therapist for devising situations and stimuli that patients are then exposed to.
- Some improvement achieved during in-session, therapist-assisted exposure should generally precede self-exposure.

Cognitive Restructuring

Identifying, challenging, and modifying the specific trauma-related appraisals, such as

- Feeling responsible or blaming oneself for the occurrence of trauma
- Perceiving oneself as too weak
- Negative (mistrustful, hostile) attitude toward others, often because of their perceived failure to be supportive or offer help
- Perceiving symptoms of PTSD (especially reexperiencing of the trauma) as personal defeat
- Negative appraisal of one's own coping abilities

When imaginal exposure occurs in sessions, the therapist can assist with the exposure by requesting that patients provide a detailed account of their traumatic experience. To enhance this process, patients need to be emotionally engaged as much as possible. This can be achieved by asking patients to speak in the present tense and in the first person, while including in their accounts a detailed description of their emotional responses to the trauma, such as feelings of fear, helplessness, despair, disgust, shame, and/or loss of control. Patients' accounts should also include relevant trauma-related sensory cues (e.g., sounds, sights, or smells); these can subsequently be used to enhance exposure and reliving of the trauma. For example, an audiotape with a sound of a helicopter can be played to patients with combat-related PTSD.

In vivo exposure usually follows imaginal exposure and involves exposing patients to situations and stimuli that remind them of the trauma and/or that activate traumatic memories. In vivo exposure in PTSD is conducted in a way very similar to in vivo exposure in agoraphobia (see Chapter 2).

As in other anxiety disorders, exposure is beneficial in treating PTSD because it promotes habituation to patients' fears and a sense of self-mastery. In addition, there may be specific benefits of exposure in treating PTSD, as it allows patients to relive the actual traumatic experience in a controlled manner. It then becomes possible for patients to reappraise the trauma, adopt relevant corrective information (e.g., about threat and safety), and reprocess corresponding emotional reactions. Ultimately, successful exposure treatment leads to an integrated reconstruction of the trauma within the patients' memory system. This reconstruction encompasses both cognitive and emotional levels, without any component of the traumatic experience being split off. A counterconditioning model for exposure-based treatment of PTSD was recently proposed (Paunovic, 2003). The main tenet of this model is that strong-enough pleasurable emotions (e.g., learned feelings of joy or happiness) should be elicited to countercondition traumatic emotions.

Some patients are unable to complete a full exposure program because it is too unpleasant and painful. This is understandable, because exposure requires patients to face, "go over," and fully re-create a traumatic event that they are desperately trying to push aside. To minimize the risk of dropout, the therapist should carefully explain to patients the rationale and goals of exposure. The therapist also needs to be attentive to any signs that patients are becoming overwhelmed by the experience of reliving the trauma.

Cognitive restructuring. Cognitive techniques in PTSD (Table 7–19) involve identification of negative automatic thoughts and challenging of specific beliefs that patients may have about themselves, their future, the traumatic event, other people, and the world in general. In a broad sense, the goal of cognitive approaches is for patients to "normalize" the traumatic experience through reappraisal of the trauma and change in its meaning. A more balanced appraisal and understanding of the trauma would then ensue. That is, regardless of how painful the traumatic experience may be and of how incompatible it is with patients' previously held assumptions and beliefs, the goal is for patients to come to terms with it and incorporate it into their lives, so that they do not have to try to forget it, deny it, or be afraid or ashamed of it.

There are several types of cognitive distortions that are relatively specific for PTSD and, if present, should be addressed in the course of CBT. For example, patients may hold themselves responsible for the occurrence of a traumatic event when such responsibility is realistically not present. The underlying beliefs about this responsibility may drive patients to harbor an overwhelming sense of guilt. Some patients with PTSD have a particularly distorted view of others and the world, which is characterized by mistrust, suspiciousness, and hostility. Although such a view may be in the service of self-defense, it is usually based on maladaptive, exaggerated appraisals of danger that need to be modified during treatment. There may also be strong but unfounded beliefs that the trauma has permanently damaged the person and prevented accomplishment of life goals.

Anxiety management techniques. These techniques are often used as part of the CBT package, with the goals of alleviating tension, anxiety, and hyperarousal symptoms. In addition, these techniques assist PTSD patients in their struggle to regain some control over their symptoms and may help with patients' engagement with anxiety-provoking CBT procedures, particularly exposure.

Anxiety management techniques often involve use of muscle relaxation and controlled breathing, in a way similar to their use in other anxiety disorders. An intervention that is more specific for PTSD is "stress inoculation training," originally proposed by Meichenbaum (1975). In addition to muscle relaxation and/or breathing retraining, components and techniques of other versions of CBT, e.g., psychoeducation, role-playing, modeling, and some cognitive restructuring are used. A more specific component of stress inoculation training is "thought stopping" and "self-instruction" (or "self-talk"), which consists of attempts to stop or suppress intrusive thoughts. Recent research (Harvey and Bryant, 1998; Rassin et al., 2000; Wenzlaff and Wegner, 2000) suggests, however, that these attempts do not lead to a decrease or disappearance of intrusive thoughts and may even make them worse. Therefore, the original stress inoculation training program now tends to be used less often or, when used, is substantially modified.

Efficacy of cognitive-behavioral therapy. This type of treatment has been used in PTSD associated with different types of trauma. Various PTSD patients seem to require adaptations of the basic CBT techniques to address specific characteristics and needs of these patients. For example, frequent themes in the course of treatment of sexual assault victims are guilt, safety, trust, power, self-esteem, and intimacy (Resick and Schnicke, 1992; see also Table 7–3). Therefore, it is reasonable to modify CBT when treating these PTSD patients so that these themes are addressed adequately, usually through a greater emphasis on cognitive approaches. Victims of sexual assault may also be plagued by social avoidance, shame, and secrecy about their trauma (Table 7–3). Issues of pain, injury, litigation, and persistent, disabling avoidance of all trauma-related reminders are frequent during the treatment of victims and survivors of motor vehicle accidents (Table 7–4), and these should be attended to accordingly.

Studies of CBT in victims of assault and violent crime suggest that CBT is efficacious. Foa et al. (1991; 1999) found prolonged exposure (over 9 sessions) among female victims of sexual and nonsexual assault to be superior to stress inoculation training and supportive counseling, whereas stress inoculation training was more efficacious than supportive counseling. When exposure was combined with specific cognitive interventions (in "cognitive processing therapy") and compared with prolonged exposure (both conducted over 13 sessions) in the treatment of female victims of sexual assault, the two treatment modalities were approximately equally efficacious; however, patients who were treated with specific cognitive techniques improved more on measures of guilt (Resick et al., 2002).

Cognitive-behavioral therapy has also been successfully used in treatment of PTSD that results from motor vehicle accidents. Studies have demonstrated that 8–12 sessions of CBT are superior to supportive psychotherapy and no treatment (being on a waiting list for treatment) in survivors of road traffic accidents with PTSD (Fecteau and Nicki, 1999; Blanchard et al., 2003).

The results of CBT for war veterans with PTSD have been less encouraging. Possible reasons include greater severity of PTSD in many of these patients, presence of complications (e.g., alcohol and other substance abuse, enduring personality changes, and depression), and chronicity, with many patients commencing CBT years after their exposure to trauma. Nevertheless, several studies (e.g., Cooper and Clum, 1989; Keane et al., 1989; Glynn et al., 1999) suggest that CBT may be beneficial to this group of patients, even though these studies involved small samples and had other methodological shortcomings. Cognitive-behavioral therapy for combat-related PTSD may differ from CBT for PTSD related to other types of trauma in several ways. First, the course of treatment may need to be longer (14–20 sessions instead of 8–12). Second, the outcome of CBT in this patient population may crucially depend on how exposure is conducted (i.e., what proportion of exposure is imaginal and in vivo, whether exposure is gradual or performed through flooding, and how details of traumatic memories elicited by exposure and the accompanying anxiety and other emotions are dealt with).

The efficacy of a standard course of prolonged and imaginal exposure alone and cognitive therapy and restructuring alone was compared in two fairly large studies of PTSD patients with various types of traumatic experiences (Marks et al., 1998; Tarrier et al., 1999). There were no significant differences between the outcomes of the two treatment modalities, which suggests that exposure does not have to be a necessary ingredient of CBT, at least in the treatment of certain types of PTSD patients.

The formulation of a comprehensive cognitive model of PTSD (Ehlers and Clark, 2000) has led to an introduction of a cognitive therapy program, which has so far been tested in two studies. In one of these (Gillespie et al., 2002), cognitive therapy was used to treat PTSD in survivors of a terrorist attack and produced substantial improvement after an average of eight sessions. The other study (Ehlers et al., 2003), which was a randomized controlled trial, demonstrated a similarly good outcome. It should be noted that this form of cognitive therapy relies heavily on both imaginal and in vivo exposure. The emphasis, however, is on reappraisal of the trauma-related material elicited through exposure and on the elimination of avoidance, other safety behaviors, and maladaptive cognitive strategies that, according to the comprehensive cognitive model, play a crucial role in maintaining PTSD.

Eye Movement Desensitization and Reprocessing

Eye movement desensitization and reprocessing (EMDR) combines behavioral and cognitive techniques with eye movements (Shapiro, 1995). Patients are required to focus on trauma-related stimuli and memories (in a way similar to imaginal exposure), while simultaneously tracking the therapist's finger as it moves quickly across their visual field. This procedure is repeated and accompanied by cognitive techniques aimed at changing dysfunctional assumptions and beliefs about the trauma.

This technique has generated a lot of controversy, largely because its mechanism is poorly understood. The most intriguing issue, and the most controversial one, has been the role of eye movements. Numerous studies have been conducted with the aim of establishing efficacy of EMDR. Although there is no consensus on the usefulness of EMDR, it appears that it is more efficacious than nonspecific psychological interventions (e.g., supportive listening) and relaxation (Carlson et al., 1998; McNally, 1999). When EMDR was compared to CBT, it was found to be somewhat less efficacious (Devilly and Spence, 1999; Taylor et al., 2003). Moreover, initial treatment gains with EMDR do not appear to be maintained, as suggested by one 5-year follow-up study (Macklin et al., 2000). There is also a question of whether beneficial effects of EMDR may be attributed to nonspecific treatment factors (e.g., Lohr et al., 1999). Finally, it remains to be clarified whether EMDR is suitable for combat-related PTSD, and not only for PTSD associated with civilian trauma (e.g., Feske, 1998).

Group Therapy
The usefulness of group therapy in the treatment of PTSD is not clear. A group format may allow its members to share their experiences and help and support each other. It may also facilitate exposure to traumatic stimuli through encouragement from other group members and through observation of other patients' exposure during the group sessions. Many PTSD patients feel that only people who have undergone similar traumatic experiences can understand them, and are therefore keen to participate in groups composed of other PTSD patients. Others feel embarrassed or ashamed to talk about their trauma and their symptoms in front of others, and look for safety within a therapeutic relationship with their therapist. The anger and hostility of some PTSD patients are certainly destructive in the group setting and to group processes. Therefore, patients' suitability for group therapy should be assessed on a case-by-case basis. There is also an unresolved issue of how group therapy for PTSD should optimally be conducted.

The efficacy of group therapy for PTSD has not been well established, although there are many reports of its successful use within different theoretical frameworks, in a variety of contexts, and for victims and survivors of various types of traumas. One study of adult female victims of childhood sexual abuse (Zlotnick et al., 1997) found a significant decrease in PTSD symptoms following "affect management" in the course of group therapy based on CBT principles. More recently (Schnurr et al., 2003), CBT-based group therapy of Vietnam veterans with PTSD did not show better results than those of standard (supportive) group therapy.

Psychodynamic Psychotherapy

Psychodynamic psychotherapy may be suitable only for a subset of patients with PTSD. It may be indicated for patients who have a need to explore their traumatic experiences rather than suppress and merely control them. It should not be used if patients have poor impulse control, a history of aggressive outbursts, or a significant alcohol or other substance abuse problem. The goal of psychodynamic psychotherapy of PTSD is a normalizing reconstruction of the patients' traumatic experiences by means of transference. The psychotherapeutic process focuses on the understanding of the meaning of the trauma for PTSD sufferers. It may include reliving of the traumatic event, along with emotional catharsis, but only after the therapist has assessed that the patient is able to withstand strong and often overwhelming emotions likely to be aroused during such treatment.

Patients' transferrential reactions may be vehement, as much of the frustration and anger is transferred onto the therapist. The outcome of psychodynamic psychotherapy may then depend on the therapist's skillfulness in handling this transference, as well as his or her countertransference. The therapist must be careful not to succumb to feelings of helplessness that may permeate the relationship with the patient. Also, the therapist should address issues of mistrust and expectation of rejection, which PTSD patients so often bring into the therapeutic situation. Some patients test the boundaries of the therapeutic relationship by challenging the therapist's authority or by insisting that the therapist is unable to understand them. In these situations, the therapist should not respond by attempting to prove that he or she is available, compassionate, and full of acceptance and understanding. Especially in earlier phases of treatment, nonverbal communication of the unconditionally positive attitude toward patients is usually more powerful than any verbalization of this attitude. In other instances, the therapist must be careful not to plunge into a role of the patient's rescuer and should be vigilant about his or her omnipotence fantasies.

COMBINED TREATMENTS

It appears that pharmacotherapy is frequently combined with psychological treatments for PTSD, including CBT. This approach has a pragmatic rationale: since pharmacotherapy and CBT are efficacious only to a certain extent and for some domains of PTSD symptoms, combined treatment is expected to increase the overall response rate and efficacy. As yet, such expectations cannot be supported by the data, because there have been practically no studies comparing in a systematic way the efficacy of combined pharmacotherapy and CBT to that of either treatment alone.

Many of the issues identified in the combined treatment approach to panic disorder (see Chapter 2) also pertain to combined treatment of PTSD.

A recent pilot study (Otto et al., 2003) comparing combined treatment with a short course (10 sessions) of CBT and sertraline to treatment with sertraline alone in PTSD patients who had not responded to previous pharmacotherapy found advantages with the combined treatment.

References

Abraham K. 1921/1942. Contributions to the theory of the anal character. In Selected Papers of Karl Abraham, M.D. London: Hogarth Press, pp. 370–392.

Abramowitz J, Moore K, Carmin C, et al. 2001. Acute onset of obsessive-compulsive disorder in males following childbirth. Psychosomatics, 42: 429–431.

Adler CM, Craske MG, Kirshenbaum S, et al. 1989. "Fear of panic": An investigation of its role in panic occurrence, phobic avoidance, and treatment outcome. Behaviour Research and Therapy, 27: 391–396.

Adler CM, McDonough-Ryan P, Sax KW. 2000. fMRI of neuronal activation with symptom provocation in unmedicated patients with obsessive compulsive disorder. Journal of Psychiatric Research, 34: 317–324.

Agras WS, Chapin HM, Oliveau DC. 1972. The natural history of phobias: Course and prognosis. Archives of General Psychiatry, 26: 315–317.

Agras WS, Sylvester D, Oliveau D. 1969. The epidemiology of common fears and phobias. Comprehensive Psychiatry, 10: 151–156.

Akiskal HS. 1998. Toward a definition of generalized anxiety disorder as a anxious temperament type. Acta Psychiatrica Scandinavica, 98 (Suppl. 393): 66–73.

Allen AJ, Leonard HL, Swedo SE. 1995. Case study: A new infection triggered autoimmune subtype of pediatric OCD and Tourette's syndrome. Journal of the American Academy of Child and Adolescent Psychiatry, 34: 307–311.

Allgulander C. 1999. Paroxetine in social phobia: A randomized placebo-controlled study. Acta Psychiatrica Scandinavica, 100: 193–198.

Allgulander C, Hackett D, Salinas E. 2001. Venlafaxine extended release (ER) in the treatment of generalised anxiety disorder: Twenty-four week placebo-controlled dose-ranging study. British Journal of Psychiatry, 179: 15–22.

Allgulander C, Lavori PW. 1991. Excess mortality among 3302 patients with "pure" anxiety neurosis. Archives of General Psychiatry, 48: 599–602.

Alnaes R, Torgersen S. 1988. The relationship between DSM-III symptom disorders (axis I) and personality disorders (axis II) in an outpatient population. Acta Psychiatrica Scandinavica, 78: 485–492.

Altamura AC, Pioli R, Vitto M, et al. 1999. Venlafaxine in social phobia: A study in selective serotonin reuptake inhibitor non-responders. International Clinical Psychopharmacology, 14: 239–245.

American Psychiatric Association. 1980. Diagnostic and Statistical Manual of Mental Disorders, 3rd Edition (DSM-III). Washington, DC: American Psychiatric Association.

American Psychiatric Association. 1987. Diagnostic and Statistical Manual of Mental Disorders, 3rd Edition Revised (DSM-III-R). Washington, DC: American Psychiatric Association.

American Psychiatric Association. 1991. DSM-IV Draft Criteria. Washington, DC: American Psychiatric Association.

American Psychiatric Association. 1994. Diagnostic and Statistical Manual of Mental Disorders, 4th Edition (DSM-IV). Washington, DC: American Psychiatric Association.

American Psychiatric Association. 1998. Practice guidelines for the treatment of patients with panic disorder. American Journal of Psychiatry, 155 (May Supplement): 1–34.

American Psychiatric Association. 2000. Diagnostic and Statistical Manual of Mental Disorders, 4th Edition, Text Revision (DSM-IV-TR). Washington, DC: American Psychiatric Association.

Amering M, Bankier B, Berger P, et al. 1999. Panic disorder and cigarette smoking behavior. Comprehensive Psychiatry, 40: 35–38.

Amering M, Katschnig H, Berger P, et al. 1997. Embarrassment about the first panic attack predicts agoraphobia in panic disorder patients. Behaviour Research and Therapy, 35: 517–521.

Amies PL, Gelder MG, Shaw PM. 1983. Social phobia: A comparative clinical study. British Journal of Psychiatry, 142: 174–179.

Amir N, Foa EB, Coles ME. 1998. Negative interpretation bias in social phobia. Behaviour Research and Therapy, 36: 945–957.

Amir N, Foa EB, Coles ME. 2000. Implicit memory bias for threat-relevant information in individuals with generalized social phobia. Journal of Abnormal Psychology, 109: 713–720.

Ananth J, Pecknold JC, Van Den Steen N, et al. 1981. Double-blind comparative study of clomipramine and amitriptyline in obsessive neurosis. Progress in Neuropsychopharmacology and Biological Psychiatry, 5: 257–262.

Andersch S, Hetta J. 2003. A 15-year follow-up study of patients with panic disorder. European Psychiatry, 18: 401–408.

Andrade L, Eaton WW, Chilcoat H. 1994. Lifetime comorbidity of panic attacks and major depression in a population-based study: Symptom profiles. British Journal of Psychiatry, 165: 363–369.

Andrews B, Brewin CR, Rose S, et al. 2000. Predicting PTSD in victims of violent crime: The role of shame, anger and blame. Journal of Abnormal Psychology, 109: 69–73.

Andrews G, Stewart G, Allen R, et al. 1990. The genetics of six neurotic disorders: A twin study. Journal of Affective Disorders, 19: 23–29.

Antony MM, Roth D, Swinson RP, et al. 1998. Illness intrusiveness in individuals with panic disorder, obsessive-compulsive disorder, or social phobia. Journal of Nervous and Mental Disease, 186: 311–315.

Aoki Y, Fujihara S, Kitamura T. 1994. Panic attacks and panic disorder in a Japanese nonpatient population: Epidemiology and psychosocial correlates. Journal of Affective Disorders, 32: 51–59.

Apter A, Fallon TJ, King RA, et al. 1996. Obsessive-compulsive characteristics: From symptoms to syndrome. Journal of the American Academy of Child and Adolescent Psychiatry, 35: 907–912.

Arntz A. 2003. Cognitive therapy versus applied relaxation as treatment of generalized anxiety disorder. Behaviour Research and Therapy, 41: 633–646.

Aronson TA, Logue CM. 1987. On the longitudinal course of panic disorder: Developmental history and predictors of phobic complications. Comprehensive Psychiatry, 28: 344–355.

Arrindell WA, Emmelkamp PMG. 1986. Marital adjustment, intimacy and needs in female agoraphobics and their partners: A controlled study. British Journal of Psychiatry, 149: 592–602.

Arrindell WA, Emmelkamp PMG, Monsma A, et al. 1983. The role of perceived parental rearing practices in the aetiology of phobic disorders: A controlled study. British Journal of Psychiatry, 143: 183–187.

Asmundson G, Larsen D, Stein M. 1998. Panic disorder and vestibular disturbance: An overview of empirical findings and clinical evaluations. Journal of Psychosomatic Research, 44: 107–120.

Aston-Jones G, Foote SL, Bloom FE. 1984. Anatomy and physiology of locus coeruleus neurons: Functional implications. In Ziegler M, Lake CR, editors: Norepinephrine (Frontiers of Clinical Neuroscience), Volume 2. Baltimore: Williams & Wilkins, pp. 92–116.

Avery DH, Osgodd TB, Ishiki DM, et al. 1985. The DST in psychiatric outpatients with generalized anxiety disorder, panic disorder, or primary affective disorder. American Journal of Psychiatry, 142: 844–848.

Baer L, Jenike MA, Black DW, et al. 1992. Effect of axis II diagnoses on treatment outcome with clomipramine in 55 patients with obsessive-compulsive disorder. Archives of General Psychiatry, 49: 862–866.

Baer L, Jenike MA, Ricciardi JN, et al. 1990. Standardized assessment of personality disorders in obsessive-compulsive disorder. Archives of General Psychiatry, 47: 826–830.

Baer L, Rauch SL, Ballantine HT, et al. 1995. Cingulotomy for intractable obsessive-compulsive disorder: Prospective long-term follow-up of 18 patients. Archives of General Psychiatry, 52: 384–392.

Baetz M, Bowen R. 1998. Efficacy of divalproex sodium in patients with panic disorder and mood instability who have not responded to conventional therapy. Canadian Journal of Psychiatry, 43: 73–77.

Bajwa WK, Asnis GM, Sanderson WC, et al. 1992. High cholesterol levels in patients with panic disorder. American Journal of Psychiatry, 149: 376–378.

Baker DG, West SA, Nicholson WE, et al. 1999. Serial CSF corticotropin-releasing hormone levels and adrenocortical activity in combat veterans with posttraumatic stress disorder. American Journal of Psychiatry, 156: 585–588.

Bakker A, Spinhoven P, van Balkom AJLM, et al. 2002a. Relevance of assessment of cognitions during panic attacks in the treatment of panic disorder. Psychotherapy and Psychosomatics, 71: 158–161.

Bakker A, van Balkom AJLM, Spinhoven P. 2002b. SSRIs vs. TCAs in the treatment of panic disorder: A meta-analysis. Acta Psychiatrica Scandinavica, 106: 163–167.

Baldwin D, Bobes J, Stein DJ, et al. 1999. Paroxetine in the treatment of social phobia/social phobia: Randomized, double-blind, placebo-controlled study. British Journal of Psychiatry, 175: 120–126.

Ball SG, Otto MW, Pollack MH, et al. 1994. Predicting prospective episodes of depression in patients with panic disorder: A longitudinal study. Journal of Consulting and Clinical Psychology, 62: 359–365.

Ballenger JC, Burrows GD, DuPont RL, et al. 1988. Alprazolam in panic disorder and agoraphobia: Results from a multicenter trial: I. Efficacy in short-term treatment. Archives of General Psychiatry, 45: 413–422.

Ballenger JC, Davidson JRT, Lecrubier Y, et al. 2000. Consensus statement on post-traumatic stress disorder from the International Consensus Group on Depression and Anxiety. Journal of Clinical Psychiatry, 61 (Suppl. 5): 60–66.

Ballenger JC, Lydiard RB. 1997. Panic disorder: Results of a patient survey. Human Psychopharmacology, 12: S27–S33.

Ballenger JC, Wheadon DE, Steiner M, et al. 1998. Double-blind, fixed-dose, placebo-controlled study of paroxetine in the treatment of panic disorder. American Journal of Psychiatry, 155: 36–42.

Bandelow B. 1995. Assessing the efficacy of treatment for panic disorder and agoraphobia. II. The Panic and Agoraphobia Scale. International Clinical Psychopharmacology, 10: 73–81.

Bandelow B. 1999. Panic and Agoraphobia Scale (PAS). Seattle: Hogrefe & Huber Publishers.

Bandura A. 1977. Social Learning Theory. Englewood Cliffs, NJ: Prentice-Hall.

Barlow DH. 1988. Anxiety and Its Disorders: The Nature and Treatment of Anxiety and Panic. New York: Guilford Press.

Barlow DH, Craske MG, Cerny JA, et al. 1989. Behavioral treatment of panic disorder. Behavior Therapy, 20: 261–282.

Barlow DH, Gorman JM, Shear MK, et al. 2000. Cognitive-behavioral therapy, imipramine, or their combination for panic disorder: A randomised controlled trial. Journal of the American Medical Association: 283: 2529–2536.

Barlow DH, Rapee RM, Brown TA. 1992. Behavioral treatment of generalized anxiety disorder. Behavior Therapy, 23: 551–570.

Barsky AJ, Delamater BA, Clancy SA, et al. 1996. Somatized psychiatric disorder presenting as palpitations. Archives of Internal Medicine, 156: 1102–1108.

Basoglu M, Lax T, Kasvikis Y, et al. 1988. Predictors of improvement in obsessive-compulsive disorder. Journal of Anxiety Disorders, 2: 299–317.

Basoglu M, Marks IM, Kilic K, et al. 1994. Alprazolam and exposure for panic disorder with agoraphobia: Attribution of improvement to medication predicts subsequent relapse. British Journal of Psychiatry, 164: 652–659.

Baxter LR, Phelps ME, Mazziotta JC, et al. 1987. Local cerebral glucose metabolic rates in obsessive-compulsive disorder: A comparison with rates in unipolar depression and in normal controls. Archives of General Psychiatry, 44: 211–218.

Baxter LR, Schwartz JM, Bergman KS, et al. 1992. Caudate glucose metabolic rate changes with both drug and behavior therapy for obsessive-compulsive disorder. Archives of General Psychiatry, 49: 681–689.

Beck AT, Emery G, Greenberg RI. 1985. Anxiety Disorders and Phobias: A Cognitive Perspective. New York: Basic Books.

Beck AT, Epstein N, Brown G, et al. 1988. An inventory for measuring clinical anxiety: Psychometric properties. Journal of Consulting and Clinical Psychology, 56: 893–897.

Beckham J, Kirby AC, Feldman ME, et al. 1997. Prevalence and correlates of heavy smoking in Vietnam veterans with chronic posttraumatic stress disorder. Addictive Behaviors, 22: 637–647.

Beidel DC, Turner SM. 1999. The natural course of shyness and related syndromes. In Schmidt LA, Schulkin JS, editors: Extreme Fear, Shyness, and Social Phobia: Origins, Biological Mechanisms, and Clinical Outcomes. New York: Oxford University Press, pp. 203–223.

Beitman BD, Basha IM, Flaker G, et al. 1987. Major depression in cardiology chest pain patients without coronary artery disease and with panic disorder. Journal of Affective Disorders, 13: 51–59.

Bejerot S. 2003. Psychosurgery for obsessive-compulsive disorders—concerns remain. Acta Psychiatrica Scandinavica, 107: 241–243.

Bellodi L, Scuito G, Diafera G, et al. 1992. Psychiatric disorders in the families of patients with obsessive compulsive disorder. Psychiatry Research, 42: 111–120.

Benedetti A, Perugi G, Toni C, et al. 1997. Hypochondriasis and illness phobia in panic-agoraphobic patients. Comprehensive Psychiatry, 38: 124–131.

Benkelfat C, Nordahl TE, Semple WE, et al. 1990. Local cerebral glucose metabolic rates in obsessive-compulsive disorder: Patients treated with clomipramine. Archives of General Psychiatry, 47: 840–848.

Berman I, Kalinowski A, Berman SM, et al. 1995. Obsessive and compulsive symptoms in chronic schizophrenia. Comprehensive Psychiatry, 36: 6–10.

Bernstein DA, Borkovec TD. 1973. Progressive Relaxation Training. Champaign, IL: Research Press.

Biber B, Alkin T. 1999. Panic disorder subtypes: Differential response to CO_2 challenge. American Journal of Psychiatry, 156: 739–744.

Bienvenu OJ, Nestadt G, Eaton WW. 1998. Characterizing generalized anxiety: Temporal and symptomatic thresholds. Journal of Nervous and Mental Disease, 186: 51–56.

Bienvenu OJ, Samuels JF, Riddle MA, et al. 2000. The relationship of obsessive-compulsive disorder to possible spectrum disorders: Results from a family study. Biological Psychiatry, 48: 287–293.

Biondi M, Picardi A. 2003. Increased probability of remaining in remission from panic disorder with agoraphobia after drug treatment in patients who received concurrent cognitive-behavioural therapy: A follow-up study. Psychotherapy and Psychosomatics, 72: 34–42.

Birbaumer N, Grodd W, Diedrich O, et al. 1998. fMRI reveals amygdala activation to human faces in social phobics. Neuroreport, 9: 1223–1226.

Bisserbe JC, Lane RM, Flament MF. 1997. A double-blind comparison of sertraline and clomipramine in outpatients with obsessive-compulsive disorder. European Psychiatry, 12: 82–93.

Bisson JI, Jenkins PL, Alexander J, et al. 1997. Randomised controlled trial of psychological debriefing for victims of acute burn trauma. British Journal of Psychiatry, 171: 78–81.

Black A. 1974. The natural history of obsessional neurosis. In Beech HR, editor: Obsessional States. London: Methuen Press, pp. 1–23.

Black DW, Monahan P, Gable J, et al. 1998. Hoarding and treatment response in 38 non-depressed subjects with obsessive-compulsive disorder. Journal of Clinical Psychiatry, 59: 420–425.

Black DW, Wesner R, Bowers W, et al. 1993. A comparison of fluvoxamine, cognitive therapy, and placebo in the treatment of panic disorder. Archives of General Psychiatry, 50: 44–50.

Blake DD, Weathers FW, Nagy LN, et al. 1990. A clinician rating scale for assessing current and lifetime PTSD: The CAPS-1. Behavior Therapist, 18: 187–188.

Blanchard EB, Hickling EJ, Devineni T, et al. 2003. A controlled evaluation of cognitive behavioral therapy for posttraumatic stress in motor vehicle accident survivors. Behaviour Research and Therapy, 41: 79–96.

Blanchard EB, Hickling EJ, Forneris CA, et al. 1997. Prediction of remission of acute posttraumatic stress disorder in motor vehicle accident victims. Journal of Traumatic Stress, 10: 215–234.

Bland RC, Newman SC, Orn H. 1988a. Age of onset of psychiatric disorders. Acta Psychiatrica Scandinavica, 77 (Suppl. 338): 43–49.

Bland RC, Orn H, Newman SC. 1988b. Lifetime prevalence of psychiatric disorders in Edmonton. Acta Psychiatrica Scandinavica, 77 (Suppl. 338): 24–32.

Blashfield R, Noyes R, Reich J, et al. 1994. Personality disorder traits in generalized anxiety and panic disorder patients. Comprehensive Psychiatry, 35: 329–334.

Blazer D, George LK, Hughes D. 1991a. The epidemiology of anxiety disorders: An age comparison. In Salzman C, Lebowitz BD, editors: Anxiety in the Elderly: Treatment and Research. New York: Springer-Verlag, pp. 17–30.

Blazer DG, Hughes D, George LK, et al. 1991b. Generalized anxiety disorder. In Robins LN, Regier DA, editors: Psychiatric Disorders in America: The Epidemiologic Catchment Area Study. New York: Free Press, pp. 180–203.

Bleich A, Siegel B, Garb R, et al. 1986. Post-traumatic stress disorder following combat exposure: Clinical features and psychopharmacological treatment. British Journal of Psychiatry, 149: 365–369.

Blomhoff S, Haug TT, Hellstrom K, et al. 2001. Randomised controlled general practice trial of sertraline, exposure therapy and combined treatment in generalised social phobia. British Journal of Psychiatry, 179: 23–30.

Boersma K, Den Hengst S, Dekker J, et al. 1976. Exposure and response prevention in the natural environment: A comparison with obsessive-compulsive patients. Behaviour Research and Therapy, 14: 19–24.

Bolton D, Hill J. 1996. Mind, Meaning, and Mental Disorder. Oxford: Oxford University Press.

Borkovec TD, Costello E. 1993. Efficacy of applied relaxation and cognitive-behavioral therapy in the treatment of generalized anxiety disorder. Journal of Consulting and Clinical Psychology, 61: 611–619.

Borkovec TD, Inz J. 1990. The nature of worry in generalized anxiety disorder: A predominance of thought activity. Behaviour Research and Therapy, 28: 153–158.

Borkovec TD, Ray WJ, Stoeber J. 1998. Worry: A cognitive phenomenon intimately linked to affective, physiological, and interpersonal behavioral processes. Cognitive Therapy and Research, 22: 561–576.

Borkovec TD, Shadick RN, Hopkins M. 1991. The nature of normal and pathological worry. In Rapee RM, Barlow DH, editors: Chronic Anxiety: Generalized Anxiety Disorder and Mixed Anxiety-Depression. New York: Guilford, pp. 29–51.

Bourdon KH, Boyd JH, Rae DS, et al. 1988. Gender differences in phobias: Results of the ECA community survey. Journal of Anxiety Disorders, 2: 227–241.

Bourque P, Ladouceur R. 1980. An investigation of various performance-based treatments with acrophobics. Behaviour Research and Therapy, 18: 161–170.

Bowen RC, Offord DR, Boyle MH. 1990. The prevalence of overanxious disorder and separation anxiety disorder: Results from the Ontario Child Health Study. Journal of the American Academy of Child and Adolescent Psychiatry, 29: 753–758.

Bowlby J. 1973. Separation: Anxiety and Anger, Vol. 2. New York: Basic Books.

Boyd JH, Rae DS, Thompson JW, et al. 1990. Social phobia: Prevalence and risk factors. Social Psychiatry and Psychiatric Epidemiology, 25: 314–323.

Brady K, Pearlstein T, Asnis GM, et al. 2000. Efficacy and safety of sertraline treatment of posttraumatic stress disorder: A randomized controlled trial. Journal of the American Medical Association, 283: 1837–1844.

Brady KT, Sonne SC, Roberts JM. 1995. Sertraline treatment of comorbid posttraumatic stress disorder and alcohol dependence. Journal of Clinical Psychiatry, 56: 502–505.

Brantigan CO, Brantigan TA, Joseph N. 1982. Effect of beta blockade and beta stimulation on stage fright. American Journal of Medicine, 72: 88–94.

Brantley PJ, Mehan DJ, Ames SC, et al. 1999. Minor stressors and generalized anxiety disorder among low-income patients attending primary care clinics. Journal of Nervous and Mental Disease, 187: 435–440.

Brawman-Mintzer O, Lydiard RB. 1996. Generalized anxiety disorder: Issues in epidemiology. Journal of Clinical Psychiatry, 57 (Suppl. 7): 3–8.

Brawman-Mintzer O, Lydiard RB. 1997. Biological basis of generalized anxiety disorder. Journal of Clinical Psychiatry, 58 (Suppl. 3): 16–25.

Brawman-Mintzer O, Lydiard RB, Emmanuel N, et al. 1993. Psychiatric comorbidity in patients with generalized anxiety disorder. American Journal of Psychiatry, 150: 1216–1218.

Breier A, Charney DS, Heninger GR. 1984. Major depression in patients with agoraphobia and panic disorder. Archives of General Psychiatry, 41: 1129–1135.

Breier A, Charney DS, Heninger GR. 1985. The diagnostic validity of anxiety disorders and their relationship to depressive illness. American Journal of Psychiatry, 142: 787–797.

Breier A, Charney DS, Heninger GR. 1986. Agoraphobia with panic attacks: Development, diagnostic stability, and course of illness. Archives of General Psychiatry, 43: 1029–1036.

Breiter HC, Rauch SL, Kwong KK, et al. 1996. Functional magnetic resonance imaging of symptom provocation in obsessive-compulsive disorder. Archives of General Psychiatry, 53: 595–606.

Bremner JD, Innis RB, White T, et al. 2000. SPECT [I-123]iomazenil measurement of the benzodiazepine receptor in panic disorder. Biological Psychiatry, 47: 96–106.

Bremner JD, Licinio J, Darnell A, et al. 1997a. Elevated CSF corticotropin-releasing factor concentrations in posttraumatic stress disorder. American Journal of Psychiatry, 154: 624–629.

Bremner JD, Narayan M, Staib LH, et al. 1999. Neural correlates of memories of childhood sexual abuse in women with and without posttraumatic stress disorder. American Journal of Psychiatry, 156: 1787–1795.

Bremner JD, Randall P, Scott, TM, et al. 1995. MRI-based measurement of hippocampal volume in patients with combat-related posttraumatic stress disorder. American Journal of Psychiatry, 152: 973–981.

Bremner JD, Randall P, Vermetten E, et al. 1997b. Magnetic resonance imaging–based measurement of hippocampal volume in posttraumatic stress disorder related to childhood physical and sexual abuse: A preliminary report. Biological Psychiatry, 41: 23–32.

Bremner JD, Southwick SM, Brett E, et al. 1992. Dissociation and posttraumatic stress disorder in Vietnam combat veterans. American Journal of Psychiatry, 149: 328–332.

Bremner JD, Southwick SM, Johnson DR, et al. 1993. Childhood physical abuse and combat-related posttraumatic stress disorder in Vietnam veterans. American Journal of Psychiatry, 150: 235–239.

Breslau N, Chilcoat HD, Kessler RC, et al. 1999. Vulnerability to assaultive violence: Further specification of the sex difference in post-traumatic stress disorder. Psychological Medicine, 29: 813–821.

Breslau N, Davis GC. 1992. Posttraumatic stress disorder in an urban population of young adults: Risk factors for chronicity. American Journal of Psychiatry, 149: 671–675.

Breslau N, Davis GC, Andreski P, et al. 1991. Traumatic events and posttraumatic stress disorder in an urban population of young adults. Archives of General Psychiatry, 48: 216–222.

Breslau N, Davis GC, Andreski P, et al. 1997. Sex differences in posttraumatic stress disorder. Archives of General Psychiatry, 54: 1044–1048.

Breslau N, Davis GC, Peterson EL, et al. 2000. A second look at comorbidity in victims of trauma: The posttraumatic stress disorder–major depression connection. Biological Psychiatry, 48: 902–909.

Breslau N, Kessler RC, Chilcoat HD, et al. 1998. Trauma and posttraumatic stress disorder in the community: The 1996 Detroit Area Survey of Trauma. Archives of General Psychiatry, 55: 626–632.

Breslau N, Klein D. 1999. Smoking and panic attacks. Archives of General Psychiatry, 56: 1141–1147.

Brewin CR, Andrews B, Rose S, et al. 1999. Acute stress disorder and posttraumatic stress disorder in victims of violent crime. American Journal of Psychiatry, 156: 360–365.

Brewin CR, Andrews B, Valentine JD. 2000. Meta-analysis of risk factors for posttraumatic stress disorder in trauma-exposed adults. Journal of Consulting and Clinical Psychology, 68: 748–766.

Brewin CR, Dalgleish T, Joseph S. 1996. A dual representation theory of post-traumatic stress disorder. Psychological Review, 103: 670–686.

Briggs A, Stretch D, Brandon S. 1993. Subtyping of panic disorder by symptom profile. British Journal of Psychiatry, 163: 201–209.

Brooks RB, Baltazar PL, Munjack DJ. 1989. Co-occurrence of personality disorders with panic disorder, social phobia, and generalized anxiety disorder: A review of the literature. Journal of Anxiety Disorders, 3: 259–285.

Brown EJ, Heimberg RG, Juster HR. 1995. Social phobia subtype and avoidant personality disorder: Effect on severity of social phobia, impairment, and outcome of cognitive-behavioral treatment. Behavior Therapy, 26: 467–486.

Brown TA. 1997. The nature of generalized anxiety disorder and pathological worry: Current evidence and conceptual models. Canadian Journal of Psychiatry, 42: 817–825.

Brown TA, Barlow DH, Liebowitz MR. 1994. The empirical basis of generalized anxiety disorder. American Journal of Psychiatry, 151: 1272–1280.

Brown TA, O'Leary TA, Barlow DH. 1993. Generalized anxiety disorder. In Barlow DH, editor: Clinical Handbook of Psychological Disorders, 2nd Edition. New York: Guilford Press, pp. 137–188.

Bruce SE, Vasile RG, Goisman RM, et al. 2003. Are benzodiazepines still the medication of choice for patients with panic disorder with or without agoraphobia? American Journal of Psychiatry, 160: 1432–1438.

Bryant RA, Harvey AG. 1998. Relationship of acute stress disorder and posttraumatic stress disorder following mild traumatic brain injury. American Journal of Psychiatry, 155: 625–629.

Bryant RA, Harvey AG, Dang ST, et al. 1998. Treatment of acute stress disorder: A comparison of cognitive-behavioral therapy and supportive counseling. Journal of Consulting and Clinical Psychology, 66: 862–866.

Bryant RA, Harvey AG, Guthrie RM, et al. 2000. A prospective study of psychophysiological arousal, acute stress disorder and posttraumatic stress disorder. Journal of Abnormal Psychology, 109: 341–344.

Bryant RA, Moulds ML, Nixon RVD. 2003. Cognitive behaviour therapy of acute stress disorder: A four-year follow-up. Behaviour Research and Therapy, 41: 489–494.

Bryant RA, Sackville T, Dang ST, et al. 1999. Treating acute stress disorder: An evaluation of cognitive behavior therapy and supportive counseling techniques. American Journal of Psychiatry, 156: 1780–1786.

Buchanan AW, Meng KS, Marks IM. 1996. What predicts improvement and compliance during the behavioral treatment of obsessive compulsive disorder? Anxiety, 2: 22–27.

Buglass D, Clarke J, Henderson A, et al. 1977. A study of agoraphobic housewives. Psychological Medicine, 7: 73–86.

Burns LE, Thorpe GL, Cavallaro LA. 1986. Agoraphobia eight years after behavioral treatment: A follow-up study with interview, self-report, and behavioral data. Behavior Therapy, 17: 580–591.

Butler G, Cullington A, Munby M, et al. 1984. Exposure and anxiety management in the treatment of social phobia. Journal of Consulting and Clinical Psychology, 52: 642–650.

Butler G, Fennell M, Robson P, et al. 1991. A comparison of behavior therapy and cognitive-behavior therapy in the treatment of generalized anxiety disorder. Journal of Consulting and Clinical Psychology, 59: 167–175.

Butler G, Mathews A. 1983. Cognitive processes in anxiety. Advances in Behaviour Research and Therapy, 5: 51–62.

Butler G, Wells A. 1995. Cognitive-behavioral treatments: Clinical applications. In Heimberg RG, Liebowitz MR, Hope DA, Schneier FR, editors: Social Phobia: Diagnosis, Assessment, and Treatment. New York: Guilford Press, pp. 310–333.

Candilis PJ, McLean RY, Otto MW, et al. 1999. Quality of life in patients with panic disorder. Journal of Nervous and Mental Disease, 187: 429–434.

Carlier IV, Gersons BPR. 1995. Partial posttraumatic stress disorder (PTSD): The issue of psychological scars and the occurrence of PTSD symptoms. Journal of Nervous and Mental Disease, 183: 107–109.

Carlson JG, Chemtob CM, Rusnak K, et al. 1998. Eye movement desensitization and reprocessing (EMDR) treatment for combat-related posttraumatic stress disorder. Journal of Traumatic Stress, 11: 3–24.

Cassano GB, Petracca A, Perugi G. 1988. Clomipramine for panic disorder: I. The first 10 weeks of a long-term comparison with imipramine. Journal of Affective Disorders, 14: 123–127.

Castle DJ, Deale A, Marks IM, et al. 1994. Obsessive-compulsive disorder: Prediction of outcome from behavioral psychotherapy. Acta Psychiatrica Scandinavica, 89: 393–398.

Chambers J, Yeragani VK, Keshavan MS. 1986. Phobias in India and the United Kingdom: A trans-cultural study. Acta Psychiatrica Scandinavica, 74: 388–391.

Chambless DL, Caputo GC, Bright P, et al. 1984. Assessment of fear in agoraphobics: The Body Sensations Questionnaire and the Agoraphobic Cognitions Questionnaire. Journal of Consulting and Clinical Psychology, 52: 1090–1097.

Chambless DL, Caputo GC, Jasin SE, et al. 1985. The Mobility Inventory for Agoraphobia. Behaviour Research and Therapy, 23: 35–44.

Chambless DL, Mason J. 1986. Sex, sex role stereotyping, and agoraphobia. Behaviour Research and Therapy, 24: 231–235.

Chambless DL, Renneberg B, Goldstein A, et al. 1992. MCMI-diagnosed personality disorders among agoraphobic outpatients: Prevalence and relationship to severity and treatment outcome. Journal of Anxiety Disorders, 6: 193–211.

Charney DS, Heninger GR. 1986. Abnormal regulation of noradrenergic function in panic disorders: Effects of clonidine in healthy subjects and patients with agoraphobia and panic disorder. Archives of General Psychiatry, 43: 1042–1054.

Charney DS, Heninger GR, Breier A. 1984. Noradrenergic function in panic anxiety: Effects of yohimbine in healthy subjects and patients with agoraphobia and panic disorder. Archives of General Psychiatry, 41: 751–763.

Chartier MJ, Hazen AL, Stein MB. 1998. Lifetime patterns of social phobia: A retrospective study of the course of social phobia in a nonclinical population. Depression and Anxiety, 7: 113–121.

Chavira DA, Stein MB, Malcarne VL. 2002. Scrutinizing the relationship between shyness and social phobia. Journal of Anxiety Disorders, 16: 585–598.

Chen YW, Dilsaver SC. 1995. Comorbidity of panic disorder in bipolar illness: Evidence from the Epidemiologic Catchment Area survey. American Journal of Psychiatry, 152: 280–282.

Chen YP, Ehlers A, Clark DM, et al. 2002. Patients with generalized social phobia direct their attention away from faces. Behaviour Research and Therapy, 40: 677–687.

Chignon JM, Lepine JP, Ades J. 1993. Panic disorder in cardiac outpatients. American Journal of Psychiatry, 150: 780–785.

Clark DA, Steer RA, Beck AT. 1994a. Common and specific dimensions of self-reported anxiety and depression: Implications for the cognitive and tripartite models. Journal of Abnormal Psychology, 103: 645–654.

Clark DM. 1986. A cognitive approach to panic. Behaviour Research and Therapy, 24: 461–470.

Clark DM. 1988. A cognitive model of panic attacks. In Rachman S, Maser JD, editors: Panic: Psychological Perspectives. Hillsdale, NJ: Erlbaum, pp. 71–89.

Clark DM, Beck AT. 1988. Cognitive approaches. In Last CG, Hersen M, editors: Handbook of Anxiety Disorders. New York: Pergamon Press, pp. 362–385.

Clark DM, Salkovskis PM, Hackmann A, et al. 1994b. A comparison of cognitive therapy, applied relaxation and imipramine in the treatment of panic disorder. British Journal of Psychiatry, 164: 759–769.

Clark DM, Wells A. 1995. A cognitive model of social phobia. In Heimberg R, Liebowitz M, Hope DA, Schneier FR, editors: Social Phobia: Diagnosis, Assessment and Treatment. New York: Guilford Press, pp. 69–93.

Clark LA, Watson D. 1991. Tripartite model of anxiety and depression: Psychometric evidence and taxonomic implications. Journal of Abnormal Psychology, 100: 316–336.

Clayton IC, Richards JC, Edwards CJ. 1999. Selective attention in obsessive-compulsive disorder. Journal of Abnormal Psychology, 108: 171–175.

Cloitre M, Shear MK. 1995. Psychodynamic perspectives. In Stein MB, Editor: Social Phobia: Clinical and Research Perspectives. Washington, DC: American Psychiatric Press, pp. 163–187.

Clomipramine Collaborative Study Group. 1991. Clomipramine in the treatment of patients with obsessive-compulsive disorder. Archives of General Psychiatry, 48: 730–738.

Clum GA, Knowles SL. 1991. Why do some people with panic disorders become avoidant? A review. Clinical Psychology Review, 11: 295–313.

Cooper NA, Clum GA. 1989. Imaginal flooding as a supplementary treatment for PTSD in combat veterans: A controlled study. Behavior Therapy, 20: 381–391.

Cooper PJ, Eke M. 1999. Childhood shyness and maternal social phobia: A community study. British Journal of Psychiatry, 174: 439–443.

Coryell W, Noyes R, Clancy J. 1982. Excess mortality in panic disorder: A comparison with primary unipolar depression. Archives of General Psychiatry, 39: 701–703.

Coryell W, Noyes R, House JD. 1986. Mortality among outpatients with anxiety disorders. American Journal of Psychiatry, 143: 508–510.

Cottraux J, Messy P, Marks IM, et al. 1993. Predictive factors in the treatment of obsessive-compulsive disorders with fluvoxamine and/or behaviour therapy. Behavioural Psychotherapy, 21: 45–50.

Cottraux J, Mollard E, Bouvard M, et al. 1990. A controlled study of fluvoxamine and exposure in obsessive-compulsive disorder. International Clinical Psychopharmacology, 5: 17–30.

Cowley DS, Arana GW. 1990. The diagnostic utility of lactate sensitivity in panic disorder. Archives of General Psychiatry, 47: 277–284.

Cowley DS, Dager SR, McClellan J, et al. 1988. Response to lactate infusion in generalized anxiety disorder. Biological Psychiatry, 24: 409–414.

Cowley DS, Ha EH, Roy-Byrne PP. 1997. Determinants of pharmacologic treatment failure in panic disorder. Journal of Clinical Psychiatry, 58: 555–561.

Cox BJ, Direnfeld DM, Swinson RP, et al. 1994a. Suicidal ideation and suicide attempts in panic disorder and social phobia. American Journal of Psychiatry, 151: 882–887.

Cox BJ, Endler NS, Swinson RP, et al. 1992. Situations and specific coping strategies associated with clinical and nonclinical panic attacks. Behaviour Research and Therapy, 30: 67–69.

Cox BJ, Swinson RP, Endler NS, et al. 1994b. The symptom structure of panic attacks. Comprehensive Psychiatry, 35: 349–353.

Craske MG. 1996. An integrated approach to panic disorder. Bulletin of the Menninger Clinic, 60 (Suppl.): A87–A104.

Craske MG, Barlow DH, O'Leary TA. 1992. Mastery of Your Anxiety and Worry. Albany, NY: Graywind.

Craske MG, Brown TA, Barlow DH. 1991. Behavioral treatment of panic disorder: A two-year follow-up. Behavior Therapy, 22: 289–304.

Craske MG, Lang AJ, Mystkowski JL, et al. 2002. Does nocturnal panic represent a more severe form of panic disorder? Journal of Nervous and Mental Disease, 190: 611–618.

Craske MG, Rapee RM, Barlow DH. 1988. The significance of panic-expectancy for individual patterns of avoidance. Behavior Therapy, 19: 577–592.

Craske MG, Sipsas A. 1992. Animal phobias vs. claustrophobias: Exteroceptive vs. interoceptive cues. Behaviour Research and Therapy, 30: 569–581.

Creamer M, Burgess P, McFarlane AC. 2001. Post-traumatic stress disorder: Findings from the Australian National Survey of Mental Health and Well-Being. Psychological Medicine, 31: 1237–1247.

Crino RD. 1999. Obsessive-compulsive spectrum disorders. Current Opinion in Psychiatry, 12: 151–155.

Crits-Christoph PC, Connolly MB, Azarian K, et al. 1996. An open trial of brief supportive-expressive psychotherapy in the treatment of generalized anxiety disorder. Psychotherapy, 33: 418–430.

Cross-National Collaborative Panic Study, Second Phase Investigators. 1992. Drug treatment of panic disorder: Comparative efficacy of alprazolam, imipramine, and placebo. British Journal of Psychiatry, 160: 191–202.

Crowe RR, Noyes R, Pauls DL, et al. 1983. A family study of panic disorder. Archives of General Psychiatry, 40: 1065–1069.

Curtis GC, Magee WJ, Eaton WW, et al. 1998. Specific fears and phobias: Epidemiology and classification. British Journal of Psychiatry, 173: 212–217.

Dannon PN, Sasson Y, Hirschmann S, et al. 2000. Pindolol augmentation in treatment-resistant obsessive-compulsive disorder: A double-blind placebo-controlled trial. European Neuropsychopharmacology, 10: 165–169.

Darcis T, Ferreri M, Natens J, et al. 1995. A multicentre double-blind, placebo-controlled study investigating the anxiolytic efficacy of hydroxyzine in patients with generalized anxiety. Human Psychopharmacology, 10: 181–187.

Davey GCL, Levy S. 1998. Catastrophic worrying: Personal inadequacy and a perseverative iterative style as features of the catastrophizing process. Journal of Abnormal Psychology, 107: 576–586.

Davey GCL, McDonald AS, Hirisave U, et al. 1998. A cross-cultural study of animal fears. Behaviour Research and Therapy, 36: 735–750.

Davidson J, Kudler H, Smith R, et al. 1990. Treatment of posttraumatic stress disorder with amitriptyline and placebo. Archives of General Psychiatry, 47: 259–266.

Davidson J, Swartz M, Storck M, et al. 1985. A diagnostic and family study of posttraumatic stress disorder. American Journal of Psychiatry, 142: 90–93.

Davidson JR, Landerman LR, Farfel GM, et al. 2002. Characterizing the effects of sertraline in post-traumatic stress disorder. Psychological Medicine, 32: 661–670.

Davidson JRT, DuPont RL, Hedges D, et al. 1999. Efficacy, safety and tolerability of venlafaxine extended release and buspirone in outpatients with generalized anxiety disorder. Journal of Clinical Psychiatry, 60: 528–535.

Davidson JRT, Hughes DL, George LK, et al. 1993a. The epidemiology of social phobia: Findings from the Duke Epidemiological Catchment Area Study. Psychological Medicine, 23: 709–718.

Davidson JRT, Petts N, Richichi E, et al. 1993b. Treatment of social phobia with clonazepam and placebo. Journal of Clinical Psychopharmacology, 13: 423–428.

Davidson JRT, Rothbaum BO, van der Kolk BA, et al. 2001. Multicenter, double-blind comparison of sertraline and placebo in the treatment of posttraumatic stress disorder. Archives of General Psychiatry, 58: 485–492.

Davidson JRT, Walker JI, Kilts C. 1987. A pilot study of phenelzine in the treatment of post-traumatic stress disorder. British Journal of Psychiatry, 150: 252–255.

Davidson JRT, Weisler RH, Malik ML, et al. 1998. Treatment of posttraumatic stress disorder with nefazodone. International Clinical Psychopharmacology, 13: 111–113.

Davies SJ, Ghahramani P, Jackson PR, et al. 1999. Association of panic disorder and panic attacks with hypertension. American Journal of Medicine, 107: 310–316.

Deahl M. 2003. In debate: Psychological debriefing is a waste of time. Against. British Journal of Psychiatry, 183: 13–14.

de Araujo LA, Ito LM, Marks IM. 1996. Early compliance and other factors predicting outcome of exposure for obsessive-compulsive disorder. British Journal of Psychiatry, 169: 747–752.

DeBellis MD, Casey BJ, Dahl RE, et al. 2000. A pilot study of amygdala volumes in pediatric generalized anxiety disorder. Biological Psychiatry, 48: 51–57.

de Beurs E, van Balkom AJ, Lange A, et al. 1995. Treatment of panic disorder with agoraphobia: Comparison of fluvoxamine, placebo, and psychological panic management combined with exposure and of exposure in vivo alone. American Journal of Psychiatry, 152: 683–691.

De Boer M, Op den Velde W, Falger PJR, et al. 1992. Fluvoxamine treatment for chronic PTSD: A pilot study. Psychotherapy and Psychosomatics, 57: 158–163.

Degonda M, Angst J. 1993. The Zurich Study, XX: Social phobia and agoraphobia. European Archives of Psychiatry and Clinical Neuroscience, 243: 95–102.

Degonda M, Wyss M, Angst J. 1993. The Zurich Study, XVIII. Obsessive-compulsive disorders and syndromes in the general population. European Archives of Psychiatry and Clinical Neuroscience, 243: 16–22.

de Haan HE, van Oppen P, van Balkom AJLM, et al. 1997. Prediction of outcome and early vs. late improvement in OCD patients treated with cognitive behavior therapy and pharmacotherapy. Acta Psychiatrica Scandinavica, 96: 354–361.

De Jongh A, Muris P, Ter Horst G, et al. 1995. One-session cognitive treatment of dental phobia: Preparing dental phobics for treatment by restructuring negative cognitions. Behaviour Research and Therapy, 33: 947–954.

Delahanty DL, Herberman HB, Craig KJ, et al. 1997. Acute and chronic distress and posttraumatic stress disorder as a function of responsibility for serious motor vehicle accidents. Journal of Consulting and Clinical Psychology, 65: 560–567.

Delahanty DL, Raimonde AJ, Spoonster E. 2000. Initial posttraumatic urinary cortisol levels predict subsequent PTSD symptoms in motor vehicle accident victims. Biological Psychiatry, 48: 940–947.

Delle Chiaie R, Pancheri P, Casacchia M, et al. 1995. Assessment of the efficacy of buspirone in patients affected by generalized anxiety disorder, shifting to buspirone from prior treatment with lorazepam: A placebo-controlled, double-blind study. Journal of Clinical Psychopharmacology, 15: 12–19.

Demal U, Gerhardt L, Mayrhofer A, et al. 1993. Obsessive compulsive disorder and depression. Psychopathology, 26: 145–150.

DeMartinis N, Rynn M, Rickels K, et al. 2000. Prior benzodiazepine use and buspirone response in the treatment of generalized anxiety disorder. Journal of Clinical Psychiatry, 61: 91–94.

Demartino R, Mollica RF, Wilk V. 1995. Monoamine oxidase inhibitors in posttraumatic stress disorder. Journal of Nervous and Mental Disease, 183: 510–515.

den Boer JA, Westenberg HGM, Kamerbeek WDJ. 1987. Effect of serotonin uptake inhibitors in anxiety disorders: A double-blind comparison of clomipramine and fluvoxamine. International Clinical Psychopharmacology, 2: 21–32.

Denney DR, Sullivan BJ, Thiry MR. 1977. Participant modeling and self-verbalization training in the reduction of spider fears. Journal of Behavior Therapy and Experimental Psychiatry, 8: 247–253.

deRuiter C, Rijken H, Garssen B, et al. 1989. Comorbidity among the anxiety disorders. Journal of Anxiety Disorders, 3: 57–68.

Devilly GJ, Spence SH. 1999. The relative efficacy and treatment distress of EMDR and a cognitive-behavior trauma treatment protocol in the amelioration of posttraumatic stress disorder. Journal of Anxiety Disorders, 13: 131–157.

DeWit DJ, Ogborne A, Offord DR, et al. 1999. Antecedents of the risk of recovery from DSM-III social phobia. Psychological Medicine, 29: 569–582.

Diaferia G, Sciuto G, Perna G, et al. 1993. DSM-III-R personality disorders in panic disorder. Journal of Anxiety Disorders, 7: 153–161.

Diamond DB. 1985. Panic attacks, hypochondriasis, and agoraphobia: A self-psychology formulation. American Journal of Psychotherapy, 39: 114–125.

Diamond DB. 1987. Psychotherapeutic approaches to the treatment of panic attacks, hypochondriasis and agoraphobia. British Journal of Medical Psychology, 60: 79–84.

DiNardo PA, Guzy LT, Jenkins JA, et al. 1988. Etiology and maintenance of dog fears. Behaviour Research and Therapy, 26: 241–244.

Dougherty DD, Baer L, Cosgrove GR, et al. 2002. Prospective long-term follow-up of 44 patients who received cingulotomy for treatment-refractory obsessive-compulsive disorder. American Journal of Psychiatry, 159: 269–275.

Dreessen L, Arntz A, Luttels C, et al. 1994. Personality disorders do not influence the results of cognitive behavior therapies for anxiety disorders. Comprehensive Psychiatry, 35: 265–274.

Dreessen L, Hoekstra R, Arntz A. 1997. Personality disorders do not influence the results of cognitive and behavior therapy for obsessive compulsive disorder. Journal of Anxiety Disorders, 11: 503–521.

Dugas MJ, Freeston MH, Ladouceur R, et al. 1998a. Worry themes in primary GAD, secondary GAD, and other anxiety disorders. Journal of Anxiety Disorders, 12: 253–261.

Dugas MJ, Gagnon F, Ladouceur R, et al. 1998b. Generalized anxiety disorder: A preliminary test of a conceptual model. Behaviour Research and Therapy, 36: 215–226.

Dugas MJ, Ladouceur R, Leger E, et al. 2003. Group cognitive-behavioral therapy for generalized anxiety disorder: Treatment outcome and long-term follow-up. Journal of Consulting and Clinical Psychology, 71: 821–825.

Dunmore E, Clark DM, Ehlers A. 2001. A prospective investigation of the role of cognitive factors in persistent posttraumatic stress disorder (PTSD) after physical or sexual assault. Behaviour Research and Therapy, 39: 1063–1084.

Durham RC, Murphy T, Allan T, et al. 1994. Cognitive therapy, analytic psychotherapy and anxiety management training for generalised anxiety disorder. British Journal of Psychiatry, 165: 315–323.

Dyregrov A. 1989. Caring for helpers in disaster situations: Psychological debriefing. Disaster Management, 2: 25–30.

Eaton WW, Dryman A, Weissman MM. 1991. Panic and phobias. In Robins LN, Regier DA, editors: Psychiatric Disorders in America: The Epidemiologic Catchment Area Study. New York: Free Press, pp. 155–179.

Eaton WW, Kessler RC, Wittchen HU, et al. 1994. Panic and panic disorder in the United States. American Journal of Psychiatry, 151: 413–420.

Echeburua E, De Corral P, Bajos EG, et al. 1993. Interactions between self-exposure and alprazolam in the treatment of agoraphobia without current panic: An exploratory study. Behavioural and Cognitive Psychotherapy 21: 219–238.

Ehlers A, Clark DM. 2000. A cognitive model of posttraumatic stress disorder. Behaviour Research and Therapy, 38: 319–345.

Ehlers A, Clark DM, Hackmann A, et al. 2003. A randomized controlled trial of cognitive therapy, a self-help booklet, and repeated assessments as early interventions for posttraumatic stress disorder. Archives of General Psychiatry, 60: 1024–1032.

Ehlers A, Hofmann SG, Herda CA, et al. 1994. Clinical characteristics of driving phobia. Journal of Anxiety Disorders, 8: 323–339.

Ehlers A, Maercker A, Boos A. 2000. Posttraumatic stress disorder following political imprisonment: The role of mental defeat, alienation, and perceived permanent change. Journal of Abnormal Psychology, 109: 45–55.

Ehlers A, Mayou RA, Bryant RA. 1998. Psychological predictors of chronic PTSD after motor vehicle accidents. Journal of Abnormal Psychology, 107: 508–519.

Eisen JL, Beer DA, Pato MT, et al. 1997. Obsessive-compulsive disorder in patients with schizophrenia or schizoaffective disorder. American Journal of Psychiatry, 154: 271–273.

Eisen JL, Rasmussen SA. 1993. Obsessive-compulsive disorder with psychotic features. Journal of Clinical Psychiatry, 54: 373–379.

Eisen JL, Rasmussen SA, Phillips KA, et al. 2001. Insight and treatment outcome in obsessive-compulsive disorder. Comprehensive Psychiatry, 42: 494–497.

Emmelkamp PMG, Gerlsma C. 1994. Marital functioning and the anxiety disorders. Behavior Therapy, 25: 407–429.

Emmelkamp PMG, van den Heuvell C, van Linden RM, et al. 1989. Home-based treatment of obsessive-compulsive patients: Intersession interval and therapist involvement. Behaviour Research and Therapy, 27: 89–93.

Engel CC, Engel AL, Campbell SJ, et al. 1993. Posttraumatic stress disorder symptoms and precombat sexual and physical abuse in Desert Storm veterans. Journal of Nervous and Mental Disease, 181: 683–688.

Engelhard IM, van den Hout MA, Arntz A. 2002. A longitudinal study of "intrusion-based reasoning" and posttraumatic stress disorder after exposure to a train disaster. Behaviour Research and Therapy, 40: 1415–1425.

Engelhard IM, van den Hout MA, Kindt M, et al. 2003. Peritraumatic dissociation and posttraumatic stress after pregnancy loss: A prospective study. Behaviour Research and Therapy, 41; 67–78.

Epstein RS, Fullerton CS, Ursano RJ. 1998. Posttraumatic stress disorder following an air disaster: A prospective study. American Journal of Psychiatry, 155: 934–938.

Evenden J. 1999. Impulsivity: A discussion of clinical and experimental findings. Journal of Psychopharmacology, 13: 180–192.

Fahy TJ, O'Rourke DO, Bropky J, et al. 1992. The Galway study of panic disorder. I. Clomipramine and lofepramine in DSM-III-R panic disorder: A placebo-controlled trial. Journal of Affective Disorders, 25: 63–76.

Fallon BA, Liebowitz MR, Campeas R, et al. 1998. Intravenous clomipramine for obsessive-compulsive disorder refractory to oral clomipramine: A placebo-controlled study. Archives of General Psychiatry, 55: 918–924.

Faravelli C, Degl'Innocenti BG, Giardinelli L. 1989. Epidemiology of anxiety disorders in Florence. Acta Psychiatrica Scandinavica, 79: 308–312.

Faravelli C, Pallanti S. 1989. Recent life events and panic disorder. American Journal of Psychiatry, 146: 622–626.

Faravelli C, Panichi C, Pallanti S, et al. 1991. Perception of early parenting in panic and agoraphobia. Acta Psychiatrica Scandinavica, 84: 6–8.

Faravelli C, Paterniti S, Scarpato MA. 1995. A 5-year prospective, naturalistic follow-up study of panic disorder. Comprehensive Psychiatry, 36: 271–277.

Faravelli C, Webb T, Ambonetti A, et al. 1985. Prevalence of traumatic early life events in 31 agoraphobic patients with panic attacks. American Journal of Psychiatry, 142: 1493–1494.

Fava GA, Grandi S, Canestrari R. 1988. Prodromal symptoms in panic disorder with agoraphobia. American Journal of Psychiatry, 145: 1564–1567.

Fava GA, Grandi S, Rafanelli C, et al. 1992. Prodromal symptoms in panic disorder with agoraphobia: A replication study. Journal of Affective Disorders, 25: 85–88.

Fava GA, Grandi S, Saviotti FM, et al. 1990. Hypochondriasis with panic attacks. Psychosomatics, 31: 351–353.

Fava GA, Zielezny M, Savron G, et al. 1995. Long-term effects of behavioural treatment for panic disorder with agoraphobia. British Journal of Psychiatry, 166: 87–92.

Fecteau G, Nicki R. 1999. Cognitive behavioural treatment of posttraumatic stress disorder after motor vehicle accident. Behavioural and Cognitive Psychotherapy, 27: 201–215.

Feinstein A, Dolan R. 1991. Predictors of post-traumatic stress disorder following physical trauma: An examination of the stressor criterion. Psychological Medicine, 21: 85–91.

Fenichel O. 1945. The Psychoanalytic Theory of Neurosis. New York: W.W. Norton.

Fenigstein F, Scheier MF, Buss AK. 1975. Public and private self-consciousness: Assessment and theory. Journal of Consulting and Clinical Psychology, 43: 522–527.

Fenton WS, McGlashan TH. 1986. The prognostic significance of obsessive-compulsive symptoms in schizophrenia. American Journal of Psychiatry, 143: 437–441.

Feske U. 1998. Eye movement desensitization and reprocessing treatment for post-traumatic stress disorder. Clinical Psychology: Science and Practice, 5: 171–181.

Feske U, Chambless DL. 1995. Cognitive-behavioral versus exposure only treatment for social phobia: A meta-analysis. Behavior Therapy, 26: 695–720.

Fifer SK, Mathias SD, Patrick DL, et al. 1994. Untreated anxiety among adult primary care patients in a health maintenance organization. Archives of General Psychiatry, 51: 740–750.

Fineberg N. 1999. Evidence-based pharmacotherapy for obsessive-compulsive disorder. Advances in Psychiatric Treatment, 5: 357–365.

Fineberg NA, O'Doherty C, Rajagopal S, et al. 2003. How common is obsessive-compulsive disorder in a dermatology outpatient clinic? Journal of Clinical Psychiatry, 64: 152–155.

Fireman B, Koran LM, Leventhal JL, et al. 2001. The prevalence of clinically recognized obsessive-compulsive disorder in a large health maintenance organization. American Journal of Psychiatry, 158: 1904–1910.

Fishbein M, Middlestadt SE, Ottati V, et al. 1988. Medical problems among ICSOM musicians: Overview of a national survey. Medical Problems of Performing Artists, 3: 1–8.

Fisher PL, Durham RC. 1999. Recovery rates in generalized anxiety disorder following psychological therapy: An analysis of clinically significant change in the STAI-T across outcome studies since 1990. Psychological Medicine, 29: 1425–1434.

Flament MF, Rapoport JL, Berg CJ, et al. 1985. Clomipramine treatment of childhood obsessive-compulsive disorder. A double-blind controlled study. Archives of General Psychiatry, 42: 977–983.

Flament MF, Whitaker A, Rapoport JL, et al. 1988. Obsessive compulsive disorder in adolescence: An epidemiological study. Journal of the American Academy of Child and Adolescent Psychiatry, 27: 764–771.

Fleet RP, Dupuis G, Marchand A, et al. 1996. Panic disorder in emergency department chest pain patients: Prevalence, comorbidity, suicidal ideation, and physician recognition. American Journal of Medicine, 101: 371–380.

Fleet RP, Lavoie K, Beitman BD. 2000a. Is panic disorder associated with coronary artery disease? A critical review of the literature. Journal of Psychosomatic Research, 48: 347–356.

Fleet RP, Martel J-P, Lavoie KL, et al. 2000b. Non-fearful panic disorder: A variant of panic in medical patients? Psychosomatics, 41: 311–320.

Fleming B, Faulk A. 1989. Discriminating factors in panic disorder with and without agoraphobia. Journal of Anxiety Disorders, 3: 209–219.

Foa EB. 1979. Failure in treating obsessive compulsives. Behaviour Research and Therapy, 17: 169–179.

Foa EB. 1995. Posttraumatic Stress Diagnostic Scale Manual. Minneapolis: National Computer Systems.

Foa EB, Dancu CV, Hembree EA, et al. 1999. A comparison of exposure therapy, stress inoculation training, and their combination for reducing posttraumatic stress disorder in female assault victims. Journal of Consulting and Clinical Psychology, 67: 194–200.

Foa EB, Goldstein A. 1978. Continuous exposure and complete response prevention of obsessive-compulsive disorder. Behavior Therapy, 9: 821–829.

Foa EB, Grayson JB, Steketee G, et al. 1983. Success and failure in behavioral treatment of obsessive compulsives. Journal of Consulting and Clinical Psychology, 51: 287–297.

Foa EB, Hearst-Ikeda D, Perry KJ. 1995. Evaluation of a brief cognitive-behavioral program for the prevention of chronic PTSD in recent assault victims. Journal of Consulting and Clinical Psychology, 63: 948–955.

Foa EB, Kozak MJ. 1986. Emotional processing of fear: Exposure to corrective information. Psychological Bulletin, 99: 20–35.

Foa EB, Kozak MJ. 1995. DSM-IV field trial: Obsessive-compulsive disorder. American Journal of Psychiatry, 152: 90–96.

Foa EB, Kozak MJ. 1996. Psychological treatment for obsessive-compulsive disorder. In Mavissakalian MR, Prien RF, editors: Long-Term Treatments of Anxiety Disorders. Washington, DC: American Psychiatric Press, pp. 285–309.

Foa EB, McNally RJ. 1996. Mechanisms of change in exposure therapy. In Rapee RM, editor: Current Controversies in the Anxiety Disorders. New York: Guilford Press, pp. 329–343.

Foa EB, Riggs DS. 1993. Post-traumatic stress disorder in rape victims. In Oldham J, Riba MB, Tasman A, editors: American Psychiatric Press Review of Psychiatry, Volume 12. Washington, DC: American Psychiatric Press, pp. 273–303.

Foa EB, Rothbaum BO. 1998. Treating the Trauma of Rape: Cognitive-Behavioral Therapy for PTSD. New York: Guilford Press.

Foa EB, Rothbaum BO, Riggs DS, et al. 1991. Treatment of posttraumatic stress disorder in rape victims: A comparison between cognitive-behavioral procedures and counseling. Journal of Consulting and Clinical Psychology, 59: 715–723.

Foa EB, Steketee GS, Grayson JB. 1981. Success and failure in treating obsessive-compulsives. Biological Psychiatry, 5: 1099–1102.

Foa EB, Steketee GS, Grayson JB, et al. 1984. Deliberate exposure and blocking of obsessive-compulsive rituals: Immediate and long-term effects. Behavior Therapy, 15: 450–472.

Foa EB, Steketee GS, Ozarow BJ. 1985. Behavior therapy with obsessive compulsives: From theory to treatment. In Mavissakalian M, Turner SM, Michelson L, editors: Obsessive Compulsive Disorder: Psychological and Pharmacological Treatments. New York: Plenum Press, pp. 49–129.

Foa EB, Steketee G, Rothbaum BO. 1989. Behavioral/cognitive conceptualization of post-traumatic stress disorder. Behavior Therapy, 20: 155–176.

Fodor IG. 1974. The phobic syndrome in women: Implications for treatment. In Franks V, Burtle V, editors: Women in Therapy. New York: Brunner/Mazel, pp. 132–168.

Fontana A, Rosenheck R. 1994. Posttraumatic stress disorder among Vietnam theater veterans: A causal model of etiology in a community sample. Journal of Nervous and Mental Disease, 182: 677–684.

Fontana A, Schwartz LS, Rosenheck R. 1997. Posttraumatic stress disorder among female Vietnam veterans: A causal model of etiology. American Journal of Public Health, 87: 169–175.

Foy DW, Sipprelle RC, Rueger DB, et al. 1984. Etiology of posttraumatic stress disorder in Vietnam veterans. Journal of Consulting and Clinical Psychology, 40: 1323–1328.

Frances A, Dunn P. 1975. The attachment–autonomy conflict in agoraphobia. International Journal of Psychoanalysis, 56: 435–439.

Frank E, Cyranowski JM, Rucci P, et al. 2002. Clinical significance of lifetime panic spectrum symptoms in the treatment of patients with bipolar I disorder. Archives of General Psychiatry, 59: 905–911.

Frank JB, Kosten TR, Giller EL, et al. 1988. A randomized clinical trial of phenelzine and imipramine for posttraumatic stress disorder. American Journal of Psychiatry, 145: 1289–1291.

Franklin JA. 1987. The changing nature of agoraphobic fears. British Journal of Clinical Psychology, 26: 127–133.

Fredrikson M, Annas P, Fischer H, et al. 1996. Gender and age differences in the prevalence of specific fears and phobias. Behaviour Research and Therapy, 34: 33–39.

Freedman SA, Peri T, Brandes D, et al. 1999. Predictors of chronic PTSD—A prospective study. British Journal of Psychiatry, 174: 353–359.

Freeman CPL, Trimble MR, Deakin JFW, et al. 1994. Fluvoxamine versus clomipramine in the treatment of obsessive compulsive disorder: A multicenter, randomized, double-blind, parallel group comparison. Journal of Clinical Psychiatry, 55: 301–305.

Freeston MH, Rhéaume JL, Dugas MJ, et al. 1994. Why do people worry? Personality and Individual Differences, 17: 791–802.

Freeston MH, Rhéaume J, Ladouceur R. 1996. Correcting faulty appraisals of obsessional thoughts. Behaviour Research and Therapy, 34: 433–446.

Freud S. 1908/1959. Character and anal erotism. In Strachey J, editor: The Standard Edition of the Complete Psychological Works of Sigmund Freud, Vol. 9. London: Hogarth Press, pp. 167–175.

Freud S. 1909/1955a. Analysis of a phobia in a five-year-old boy. In Strachey J, editor: The Standard Edition of the Complete Psychological Works of Sigmund Freud, Vol. 10. London: Hogarth Press, pp. 3–149.

Freud S. 1909/1955b. Notes upon a case of obsessional neurosis. In Strachey J, editor: The Standard Edition of the Complete Psychological Works of Sigmund Freud, Vol. 10. London: Hogarth Press, pp. 151–318.

Freud S. 1913/1958. The disposition to obsessional neurosis. In Strachey J, editor: The Standard Edition of the Complete Psychological Works of Sigmund Freud, Vol. 12. London: Hogarth Press, pp. 317–326.

Freud S. 1926/1959. Inhibitions, symptoms and anxiety. In Strachey J, editor: The Standard Edition of the Complete Psychological Works of Sigmund Freud, Vol. 20. London: Hogarth Press, pp. 77–175.

Frost RO, Krause MS, Steketee G. 1996. Hoarding and obsessive-compulsive symptoms. Behavior Modification, 20: 116–132.

Furer P, Walker JR, Chartier MJ, et al. 1997. Hypochondriacal concerns and somatization in panic disorder. Depression and Anxiety, 6: 78–85.

Furmark T, Tillfors M, Stattin H, et al. 2000. Social phobia subtypes in the general population revealed by cluster analysis. Psychological Medicine, 30: 1335–1344.

Fyer AJ, Mannuzza S, Chapman TF, et al. 1993. A direct interview family study of social phobia. Archives of General Psychiatry, 50: 286–293.

Fyer AJ, Mannuzza S, Chapman TF, et al. 1995. Specificity in familial aggregation of phobic disorders. Archives of General Psychiatry, 52: 564–573.

Fyer AJ, Mannuzza S, Gallops MS, et al. 1990. Familial transmission of simple phobias and fears. Archives of General Psychiatry, 47: 252–256.

Gabbard GO. 1992. Psychodynamics of panic disorder and social phobia. Bulletin of the Menninger Clinic, 56 (Suppl. A): A3–A13.

Garvey MJ, Cook B, Noyes R. 1988. The occurrence of a prodrome of generalized anxiety in panic disorder. Comprehensive Psychiatry, 29: 445–449.

Gelenberg AJ, Lydiard RB, Rudolph RL, et al. 2000. Efficacy of venlafaxine extended-release capsules in nondepressed outpatients with generalized anxiety disorder: A 6-month randomized controlled trial. Journal of the American Medical Association, 283: 3082–3088.

Gelernter CS, Uhde TW, Cimbolic P, et al. 1991. Cognitive-behavioral and pharmacological treatments of social phobia: A controlled study. Archives of General Psychiatry, 48: 938–945.

Gentil V, Lotufoo-Neto F, Andrade L, et al. 1993. Clomipramine, a better reference drug for panic/agoraphobia. I. Effectiveness comparison with imipramine. Journal of Psychopharmacology, 7: 316–324.

Gidron Y, Gal R, Freedman S, et al. 2001. Translating research findings to PTSD prevention: Results of a randomized controlled trial. Journal of Traumatic Stress, 14: 773–780.

Giedd JN, Rapoport JL, Garvey MA, et al. 2000. MRI assessment of children with obsessive-compulsive disorder or tics associated with streptococcal infection. American Journal of Psychiatry, 157: 281–283.

Gilbert AR, Moore GJ, Keshavan MS, et al. 2000. Decrease in thalamic volumes of pediatric patients with obsessive-compulsive disorder who are taking paroxetine. Archives of General Psychiatry, 57: 449–456.

Gillespie K, Duffy M, Hackmann A, et al. 2002. Community-based cognitive therapy in the treatment of post-traumatic stress disorder following the Omagh bomb. Behaviour Research and Therapy, 40: 345–357.

Gittelman R, Klein DF. 1984. Relationship between separation anxiety and agoraphobic disorders. Psychopathology, 17 (Suppl. 1): 56–65.

Glynn SM, Eth S, Randolph ET, et al. 1999. A test of behavioral family therapy to augment exposure for combat-related posttraumatic stress disorder. Journal of Consulting and Clinical Psychology, 67: 243–251.

Goddard AW, Brouette T, Almai A, et al. 2001a. Early coadministration of clonazepam with sertraline for panic disorder. Archives of General Psychiatry, 58: 681–686.

Goddard AW, Mason GF, Almai A, et al. 2001b. Reductions in occipital cortex GABA levels in panic disorder detected with ^{1}H-magnetic resonance spectroscopy. Archives of General Psychiatry, 58: 556–561.

Goddard GV, McIntyre DC, Leech CK. 1969. A permanent change in brain function resulting from daily electrical stimulation. Experimental Neurology, 25: 295–330.

Goenjian AK, Yehuda R, Pynoos RS, et al. 1996. Basal cortisol, dexamethasone suppression of cortisol, and MHPG in adolescents after the 1988 earthquake in Armenia. American Journal of Psychiatry, 153: 929–934.

Goisman RM, Warshaw MG, Steketee GS, et al. 1995. DSM-IV and the disappearance of agoraphobia without a history of panic disorder: New data on a controversial diagnosis. American Journal of Psychiatry, 152: 1438–1443.

Goldberg DP, Lecrubier Y. 1995. Form and frequency of mental disorders across centres. In Ustun TB, Sartorius N, editors: Mental Illness in General Health Care: An International Study. New York: Wiley, pp. 323–334.

Goldstein AJ, Chambless DL. 1978. A reanalysis of agoraphobia. Behavior Therapy, 9: 47–59.

Goldstein RB, Weissman MM, Adams PB, et al. 1994. Psychiatric disorders in relatives of probands with panic disorder and/or major depression. Archives of General Psychiatry, 51: 383–394.

Goldstein RB, Wickramaratne PJ, Horwath E, et al. 1997. Familial aggregation and phenomenology of 'early'-onset (at or before age 20 years) panic disorder. Archives of General Psychiatry, 54: 271–278.

Goodman WK, McDougle CJ, Price LH, et al. 1990a. Beyond the serotonin hypothesis: A role for dopamine in some forms of obsessive compulsive disorder? Journal of Clinical Psychiatry, 51 (Suppl. 8): 36–43.

Goodman WK, Price LH, Delgado PL, et al. 1990b. Specificity of serotonin reuptake inhibitors in the treatment of obsessive-compulsive disorder: Comparison of fluvoxamine and desipramine. Archives of General Psychiatry, 47: 577–585.

Goodman WK, Price LH, Rasmussen SA, et al. 1989a. The Yale-Brown Obsessive Compulsive Scale: I. Development, use, and reliability. Archives of General Psychiatry, 46: 1006–1011.

Goodman WK, Price LH, Rasmussen SA, et al. 1989b. Efficacy of fluvoxamine in obsessive-compulsive disorder: A double-blind comparison with placebo. Archives of General Psychiatry, 46: 36–44.

Goodwin DW, Guze SB, Robbins E. 1969. Follow-up studies in obsessional neurosis. Archives of General Psychiatry, 20: 182–187.

Gorman JM, Askanazi J, Liebowitz MR, et al. 1984. Response to hyperventilation in a group of patients with panic disorder. American Journal of Psychiatry, 141: 857–861.

Gorman JM, Fyer MR, Goetz R, et al. 1988. Ventilatory physiology of patients with panic disorder. Archives of General Psychiatry, 45: 31–39.

Gorman JM, Kent JM, Sullivan GM, et al. 2000. Neuroanatomical hypothesis of panic disorder, revised. American Journal of Psychiatry, 157: 493–505.

Gorman JM, Liebowitz MR, Fyer AJ, et al. 1989. A neuroanatomical hypothesis for panic disorder. American Journal of Psychiatry, 146: 148–161.

Gorman JM, Papp LA. 1990. Respiratory physiology of panic. In Ballenger JC, editor: Neurobiology of Panic Disorder. New York: Wiley-Liss, pp. 187–203.

Gorman JM, Sloan RP. 2000. Heart rate variability in depressive and anxiety disorders. American Heart Journal, 140 (Suppl. 4): 77–83.

Green MA, Curtis GC. 1988. Personality disorders in panic patients: Response to termination of antipanic medication. Journal of Personality Disorders, 2: 303–314.

Greenberg PE, Sisitsky T, Kessler RC, et al. 1999. The economic burden of anxiety disorders in the 1990s. Journal of Clinical Psychiatry, 60: 427–435.

Greist J, Chouinard G, DuBoff E, et al. 1995a. Double-blind parallel comparison of three dosages of sertraline and placebo in outpatients with obsessive-compulsive disorder. Archives of General Psychiatry, 52: 289–295.

Greist JH, Jefferson JW, Kobak KA, et al. 1995b. A 1-year double-blind placebo-controlled fixed dose study of sertraline in the treatment of obsessive-compulsive disorder. International Clinical Psychopharmacology, 10: 57–65.

Grunhaus L, Pande AC, Brown MB, et al. 1994. Clinical characteristics of patients with concurrent major depressive disorder and panic disorder. American Journal of Psychiatry, 151: 541–546.

Gurvits TV, Gilbertson MW, Lasko NB, et al. 2000. Neurologic soft signs in chronic posttraumatic stress disorder. Archives of General Psychiatry, 57: 181–186.

Gurvits TV, Lasko NB, Schachter SC, et al. 1993. Neurological status of Vietnam veterans with chronic posttraumatic stress disorder. Journal of Neuropsychiatry and Clinical Neurosciences, 150: 183–188.

Gurvits TV, Shenton ME, Hokama H, et al. 1996. Magnetic resonance imaging study of hippocampal volume in chronic, combat-related posttraumatic stress disorder. Biological Psychiatry, 40: 1091–1099.

Guthrie R, Bryant RA. 2000. Attempting suppression of traumatic memories over extended periods in acute stress disorder. Behaviour Research and Therapy, 38: 899–907.

Hackmann A, Surawy C, Clark DM. 1998. Seeing yourself through others' eyes: A study of spontaneously occurring images in social phobia. Behavioural and Cognitive Psychotherapy, 26: 3–12.

Hafner RJ. 1977. The husbands of agoraphobic women and their influence on treatment outcome. British Journal of Psychiatry, 131: 289–294.

Hallam RS. 1978. Agoraphobia: A critical review of the concept. British Journal of Psychiatry, 133: 314–319.

Hallam RS, Hafner J. 1978. Fears of phobic patients: Factor analyses of self-report data. Behaviour Research and Therapy, 16: 1–6.

Hamilton M. 1959. The assessment of anxiety states by rating. British Journal of Medical Psychology, 32: 50–55.

Hartley LR, Ungapen S, Davie I, et al. 1983. The effect of beta-adrenergic blocking drugs on speakers' performance and memory. British Journal of Psychiatry, 142: 512–517.

Harvey AG, Bryant RA. 1998. The effect of attempted thought suppression in acute stress disorder. Behaviour Research and Therapy, 36: 583–590.

Harvey AG, Bryant RA. 2000. Two-year prospective evaluation of the relationship between acute stress disorder and posttraumatic stress disorder following mild traumatic brain injury. American Journal of Psychiatry, 157: 626–628.

Harvey AG, Bryant RA, Dang S. 1998. Autobiographical memory in acute stress disorder. Journal of Consulting and Clinical Psychology, 66: 500–506.

Haug TT, Blomhoff S, Hellstrom K, et al. 2003. Exposure therapy and sertraline in social phobia: 1-year follow-up of a randomised controlled trial. British Journal of Psychiatry, 182: 312–318.

Hay P, Sachdev P, Cumming S, et al. 1993. Treatment of obsessive-compulsive disorder by psychosurgery. Acta Psychiatrica Scandinavica, 87: 197–207.

Heimberg RG, Dodge CS, Hope DA, et al. 1990a. Cognitive-behavioral treatment of social phobia: Comparison to a credible placebo control. Cognitive Therapy and Research, 14: 1–23.

Heimberg RG, Hope DA, Dodge CS, et al. 1990b. DSM-III-R subtypes of social phobia: Comparison of generalized social phobics and public speaking phobics. Journal of Nervous and Mental Disease, 178: 172–179.

Heimberg RG, Liebowitz MR, Hope DA, et al. 1998. Cognitive-behavioral group therapy versus phenelzine in social phobia: 12-week outcome. Archives of General Psychiatry, 55: 1133–1141.

Heimberg RG, Salzman DG, Holt CS, et al. 1993. Cognitive-behavioral group treatment for social phobia: Effectiveness at five-year follow-up. Cognitive Therapy and Research, 17: 325–339.

Heiser NA, Turner SM, Beidel DC. 2003. Shyness: Relationship to social phobia and other psychiatric disorders. Behaviour Research and Therapy, 41: 209–221.

Hellström K, Öst L-G. 1995. One-session therapist-directed exposure vs. two forms of manual-directed self-exposure in the treatment of spider phobia. Behaviour Research and Therapy, 33: 959–965.

Helzer JE, Robins LN, McEvoy L. 1987. Post-traumatic stress disorder in the general population: Findings of the Epidemiologic Catchment Area survey. New England Journal of Medicine, 317: 1630–1634.

Herbert JD, Hope DA, Bellack AS. 1992. Validity of the distinction between generalized social phobia and avoidant personality disorder. Journal of Abnormal Psychology, 101: 332–339.

Herman JL. 1992. Trauma and Recovery. New York: Basic Books.

Herman JL. 1993. Sequelae of prolonged and repeated trauma: Evidence for a complex posttraumatic syndrome (DESNOS). In Davidson JRT, Foa EB, editors: Posttraumatic Stress Disorder: DSM-IV and Beyond. Washington, DC: American Psychiatric Press, pp. 213–228.

Hewlett WA, Vinogradov S, Agras WS. 1992. Clomipramine, clonazepam, and clonidine treatment of obsessive-compulsive disorder. Journal of Clinical Psychopharmacology, 12: 420–430.

Himle JA, McPhee K, Cameron OG, et al. 1989. Simple phobia: Evidence for heterogeneity. Psychiatry Research, 28: 25–30.

Hirschmann S, Dannon PN, Iancu I, et al. 2000. Pindolol augmentation in patients with treatment-resistant panic disorder: A double-blind, placebo-controlled trial. Journal of Clinical Psychopharmacology, 20: 556–559.

Hodgson RJ, Rachman S. 1977. Obsessional compulsive complaints. Behaviour Research and Therapy, 15: 389–395.

Hoehn-Saric R, Hazlett RL, McLeod DR. 1993a. Generalized anxiety disorder with early and late onset of anxiety symptoms. Comprehensive Psychiatry, 34: 291–298.

Hoehn-Saric R, McLeod DR, Hipsley PA. 1993b. Effect of fluvoxamine on panic disorder. Journal of Clinical Psychopharmacology, 13: 321–326.

Hoehn-Saric R, McLeod DR, Zimmerli WD. 1988. Differential effects of alprazolam and imipramine in generalized anxiety disorder: Somatic versus psychic symptoms. Journal of Clinical Psychiatry, 49: 293–301.

Hoehn-Saric R, McLeod DR, Zimmerli WD. 1989. Somatic manifestations in women with generalized anxiety disorder: Psychophysiological responses to psychological stress. Archives of General Psychiatry, 46: 1113–1119.

Hoehn-Saric R, Merchant AF, Keyser ML, et al. 1981. Effects of clonidine on anxiety disorders. Archives of General Psychiatry, 38: 1278–1282.

Hoffart A, Martinsen E. 1993. The effects of personality disorders and anxious-depressive comorbidity on outcome of patients with unipolar depression and with panic disorder and agoraphobia. Journal of Personality Disorders, 7: 304–311.

Hofmann SG, Lehman CL, Barlow DH. 1997. How specific are specific phobias? Journal of Behavior Therapy and Experimental Psychiatry, 28: 233–240.

Hohagen F, Winkelmann G, Rasche-Rauchle H, et al. 1998. Combination of behaviour therapy with fluvoxamine in comparison with behaviour therapy and placebo: Results of a multicentre study. British Journal of Psychiatry, 173: 71–78.

Holeva V, Tarrier N. 2001. Personality and peritraumatic dissociation in the prediction of PTSD in victims of road traffic accidents. Journal of Psychosomatic Research, 51: 687–692.

Hollander E. 1993. Obsessive-Compulsive Related Disorders. Washington, DC: American Psychiatric Press.

Hollander E, Allen A, Steiner M, et al. 2003. Acute and long-term treatment and prevention of relapse of obsessive-compulsive disorder with paroxetine. Journal of Clinical Psychiatry, 64: 1113–1121.

Hollander E, Bienstock C, Pallanti S, et al. 2002. Refractory obsessive-compulsive disorder: State-of-the-art treatment. Journal of Clinical Psychiatry, 63 (Suppl. 6): 20–29.

Hollander E, Fay M, Cohen B, et al. 1988. Serotonergic and noradrenergic sensitivity in obsessive-compulsive disorder: Behavioral findings. Archives of General Psychiatry, 45: 1015–1023.

Hollander E, Kwon J, Stein D, et al. 1996. Obsessive-compulsive and spectrum disorders: Overview and quality of life issues. Journal of Clinical Psychiatry, 57 (Suppl. 8): 3–6.

Hollander E, Wong CM. 1995. Obsessive-compulsive spectrum disorders. Journal of Clinical Psychiatry, 56 (Suppl. 4): 3–6.

Hollander E, Wong CM. 1998. Psychosocial functions and economic costs of obsessive compulsive disorder. CNS Spectrums, 3 (Suppl. 1): 48–58.

Hollingsworth CE, Tanguay PE, Grossman L, et al. 1980. Long-term outcome of obsessive-compulsive disorder in childhood. Journal of the American Academy of Child and Adolescent Psychiatry, 19: 134–144.

Holt CS, Heimberg RG, Hope DA. 1992. Avoidant personality disorder and the generalized subtype of social phobia. Journal of Abnormal Psychology, 101: 318–325.

Holt PE, Andrews G. 1989. Provocation of panic: Three elements of the panic reaction in four anxiety disorders. Behaviour Research and Therapy, 27: 253–261.

Hoogduin CAL, Duivenvoorden JH. 1988. A decision model in the treatment of obsessive-compulsive disorder. Behaviour Research and Therapy, 22: 455–459.

Hope DA, Heimberg RG. 1988. Public and private self-consciousness and social phobia. Journal of Personality Assessment, 52: 626–639.

Hope DA, Heimberg RG, Klein JF. 1990. Social anxiety and the recall of interpersonal information. Journal of Cognitive Psychotherapy, 4: 185–195.

Hornig CD, McNally RJ. 1995. Panic disorder and suicide attempt: A reanalysis of data from the Epidemiologic Catchment Area study. British Journal of Psychiatry, 167: 76–79.

Horowitz MJ. 1976. Stress Response Syndromes. New York: Aronson.

Horowitz MJ. 1986. Stress Response Syndromes, 2nd Edition. Northvale, NJ: Jason Aronson.

Horowitz MJ, Wilner N, Alvarez W. 1979. Impact of Event Scale: A measure of subjective distress. Psychosomatic Medicine, 41: 209–218.

Horwath E, Lish JD, Johnson J, et al. 1993. Agoraphobia without panic: Clinical reappraisal of an epidemiological finding. American Journal of Psychiatry, 150: 1496–1501.

Hubbard J, Realmuto GM, Northwood AK, et al. 1995. Comorbidity of psychiatric diagnoses with posttraumatic stress disorder in survivors of childhood trauma. Journal of the American Academy of Child and Adolescent Psychiatry, 34: 1167–1173.

Hwu HG, Yeh EK, Chang LY. 1989. Prevalence of psychiatric disorders in Taiwan defined by the Chinese Diagnostic Interview Schedule. Acta Psychiatrica Scandinavica, 79: 136–147.

Ingram IM. 1961. The obsessional personality and obsessional illness. American Journal of Psychiatry, 117: 1016–1019.

Insel TR. 1992. Toward a neuroanatomy of obsessive-compulsive disorder. Archives of General Psychiatry, 49: 739–744.

Insel TR, Akiskal HS. 1986. Obsessive-compulsive disorder with psychotic features: A phenomenological analysis. American Journal of Psychiatry, 143: 1527–1533.

Insel TR, Murphy DL, Cohen RM, et al. 1983. Obsessive-compulsive disorder: A double-blind trial of clomipramine and clorgyline. Archives of General Psychiatry, 40: 605–612.

Irle E, Exner C, Thielen K, et al. 1998. Obsessive-compulsive disorder and ventromedial frontal lesions: Clinical and neuropsychological findings. American Journal of Psychiatry, 155: 255–263.

Jacob RG, Furman JM, Durrant JD, et al. 1996. Panic, agoraphobia, and vestibular dysfunction. American Journal of Psychiatry, 153: 503–512.

Jacobson E. 1938. Progressive Relaxation. Chicago: University of Chicago Press.

Jacobson NS, Wilson L, Tupper C. 1988. The clinical significance of treatment gains resulting from exposure-based interventions for agoraphobia: A re-analysis of outcome data. Behavior Therapy, 19: 539–554.

Jaisoorya TS, Reddy YCJ, Srinath S. 2003. The relationship of obsessive-compulsive disorder to putative spectrum disorders: Results from an Indian study. Comprehensive Psychiatry, 44: 317–323.

James IA, Blackburn IM. 1995. Cognitive therapy with obsessive-compulsive disorder. British Journal of Psychiatry, 166: 444–450.

Janoff-Bulman R. 1992. Shattered Assumptions: Towards a New Psychology of Trauma. New York: Free Press.

Jansson L, Jerremalm A, Öst L-G. 1986. Follow-up of agoraphobic patients treated with exposure in vivo or applied relaxation. British Journal of Psychiatry, 149: 486–490.

Jansson L, Öst L-G. 1982. Behavioral treatments for agoraphobia: An evaluative review. Clinical Psychology Review, 2: 311–336.

Jenike MA. 1998. Neurosurgical treatment of obsessive-compulsive disorder. British Journal of Psychiatry, 173 (Suppl. 35): 79–90.

Jenike MA, Baer L, Ballantine T, et al. 1991. Cingulotomy for refractory obsessive-compulsive disorder: A long-term follow-up of 33 patients. Archives of General Psychiatry, 48: 548–555.

Jenike MA, Baer L, Minichiello WE, et al. 1986. Concomitant obsessive-compulsive disorder and schizotypal personality disorder. American Journal of Psychiatry, 143: 530–532.

Jenike MA, Baer L, Minichiello WE, et al. 1997. Placebo-controlled trial of fluoxetine and phenelzine for obsessive-compulsive disorder. American Journal of Psychiatry, 154: 1261–1264.

Johnson J, Weissman MM, Klerman GL. 1990. Panic disorder, comorbidity, and suicide attempts. Archives of General Psychiatry, 47: 805–808.

Johnston DG, Troyer IE, Whitsett SF. 1988. Clomipramine treatment of agoraphobic women: An 8-week controlled trial. Archives of General Psychiatry, 45: 453–459.

Kagan J, Reznick JS, Clarke C, et al. 1984. Behavioral inhibition to the unfamiliar. Child Development, 55: 2212–2225.

Kagan J, Reznick JS, Snidman N. 1987. The physiology and psychology of behavioral inhibition in children. Child Development, 58: 1459–1473.

Kagan J, Reznick JS, Snidman N. 1988. Biological basis of childhood shyness. Science, 240: 167–171.

Kahn RJ, McNair DM, Lipman RS, et al. 1986. Imipramine and chlordiazepoxide in depressive and anxiety disorders: II. Efficacy in anxious outpatients. Archives of General Psychiatry, 43: 79–85.

Kampman M, Keijsers GPJ, Hoogduin CAL, et al. 2002. Addition of cognitive-behaviour therapy for obsessive-compulsive disorder patients non-responding to fluoxetine. Acta Psychiatrica Scandinavica, 106: 314–319.

Kaplan D, Masand P, Gupta S. 1996. The relationship between irritable bowel syndrome and panic disorder. Annals of Clinical Psychiatry, 8: 81–88.

Karasu TB. 1994. A developmental metatheory of psychopathology. American Journal of Psychotherapy, 48: 581–599.

Karno M, Golding JM, Sorenson SB, et al. 1988. The epidemiology of obsessive-compulsive disorder in five US communities. Archives of General Psychiatry, 45: 1094–1099.

Katerndahl DA. 1990. Infrequent and limited-symptom panic attacks. Journal of Nervous and Mental Disease, 178: 313–317.

Katerndahl DA. 1993. Panic and prolapse: Meta-analysis. Journal of Nervous and Mental Disease, 181: 539–544.

Katerndahl DA, Realini JP. 1993. Lifetime prevalence of panic states. American Journal of Psychiatry, 150: 246–249.

Katon W. 1990. Chest pain, cardiac disease and panic disorder. Journal of Clinical Psychiatry, 51: 27–30.

Katon W. 1996. Panic disorder: Relationship to high medical utilization, unexplained physical symptoms, and medical costs. Journal of Clinical Psychiatry, 57 (Suppl. 10): 11–18.

Katon W, Vitaliano PP, Russo J, et al. 1986. Panic disorder: Epidemiology in primary care. Journal of Family Practice, 23: 233–239.

Katschnig H, Amering M, Stolk JM, et al. 1995. Long-term follow-up after a drug trial for panic disorder. British Journal of Psychiatry, 167: 487–494.

Katschnig H, Stein MB, Buller R. 1997. Moclobemide in social phobia: A double-blind, placebo-controlled clinical study. European Archives of Psychiatry and Clinical Neurosciences, 247: 71–80.

Katzelnick DJ, Kobak KA, Greist JH, et al. 1995. Sertraline for social phobia: A double-blind, placebo-controlled crossover study. American Journal of Psychiatry, 152: 1368–1371.

Kawachi I, Golditz GA, Ascherio A, et al. 1994. Prospective study of phobic anxiety and risk of coronary heart disease in men. Circulation, 89: 1992–1997.

Kawachi I, Sparrow D, Vokonas PS, et al. 1995. Decreased heart rate variability in men with phobic anxiety: Data from the Normative Aging Study. American Journal of Cardiology, 75: 882–885.

Keane TM, Fairbank JA, Caddell JM, et al. 1989. Implosive (flooding) therapy reduced symptoms of PTSD in Vietnam combat veterans. Behavior Therapy, 20: 245–260.

Keane TM, Zimering RT, Caddell RT. 1985. A behavioral formulation of PTSD in Vietnam veterans. Behavior Therapist, 8: 9–12.

Keijsers GPJ, Hoogduin CAL, Schaap CPDR. 1994. Predictors of treatment outcome in the behavioural treatment of obsessive-compulsive disorder. British Journal of Psychiatry, 165: 781–786.

Kelly CB, Cooper SJ. 1998. Differences in variability in plasma noradrenaline between depressive and anxiety disorders. Journal of Psychopharmacology, 12: 161–167.

Kendler KS. 1996. Major depression and generalised anxiety disorder: Same genes, (partly) different environments—revisited. British Journal of Psychiatry, 168: 68–75.

Kendler KS, Karkowski LM, Prescott CA. 1999. Fears and phobias: Reliability and heritability. Psychological Medicine, 29: 539–553.

Kendler KS, Neale MC, Kessler RC, et al. 1992a. Generalized anxiety disorder in women: A population-based twin study. Archives of General Psychiatry, 49: 267–272.

Kendler KS, Neale MC, Kessler RC, et al. 1992b. Major depression and generalized anxiety disorder: Same genes, (partly) different environments? Archives of General Psychiatry, 49: 716–722.

Kendler KS, Neale MC, Kessler RC, et al. 1992c. The genetic epidemiology of phobias in women: The interrelationship of agoraphobia, social phobia, situational phobia, and simple phobia. Archives of General Psychiatry, 49: 273–281.

Kendler KS, Neale MC, Kessler RC, et al. 1993. Panic disorder in women: A population-based twin study. Psychological Medicine, 23: 397–406.

Kennedy BL, Schwab JJ. 1997. Utilization of medical specialists by anxiety disorder patients. Psychosomatics, 38: 109–112.

Kent G, Gibbons R. 1987. Self-efficacy and the control of anxious cognitions. Journal of Behavior Therapy and Experimental Psychiatry, 18: 33–40.

Kessler RC, Crum RM, Warner LA, et al. 1997. Lifetime co-occurrence of DSM-III-R alcohol abuse and dependence with other psychiatric disorders in the National Comorbidity Survey. Archives of General Psychiatry, 54: 313–321.

Kessler RC, DuPont RL, Berglund P, et al. 1999a. Impairment in pure and comorbid generalized anxiety disorder and major depression at 12 months in two national surveys. American Journal of Psychiatry, 156: 1915–1923.

Kessler RC, McGonagle KA, Zhao S, et al. 1994. Lifetime and 12-month prevalence of DSM-III-R psychiatric disorders in the United States: Results from the National Comorbidity Survey. Archives of General Psychiatry, 51: 8–19.

Kessler RC, Sonnega A, Bromet E, et al. 1995. Posttraumatic stress disorder in the National Comorbidity Survey. Archives of General Psychiatry, 52: 1048–1060.

Kessler RC, Stang P, Wittchen HU, et al. 1999b. Lifetime co-morbidities between social phobia and mood disorders in the US National Comorbidity Survey. Psychological Medicine, 29: 555–567.

Kessler RC, Stein MB, Berglund P. 1998. Social phobia subtypes in the National Comorbidity Survey. American Journal of Psychiatry, 155: 613–619.

Kimble CE, Zehr HD. 1982. Self-consciousness, information load, self-presentation, and memory in a social situation. Journal of Social Psychology, 118: 39–46.

King DW, King LA, Foy DW, et al. 1999. Posttraumatic stress disorder in a national sample of female and male Vietnam veterans: Risk factors, war-zone stressors, and resilience-recovery variables. Journal of Abnormal Psychology, 108: 164–170.

King LA, King DW, Fairbank JA. 1998. Resilience-recovery factors in post-traumatic stress disorder among female and male Vietnam veterans: Hardiness, postwar social support, and additional stressful life events. Journal of Personality and Social Psychology: Personality Processes and Individual Differences, 74: 420–434.

Kirby L, Rice K, Valentino R. 2000. Effects of corticotropin-releasing factor on neuronal activity in the serotonergic dorsal raphe nucleus. Neuropsychopharmacology, 22: 148–162.

Klein DF. 1981. Anxiety reconceptualized. In Klein DF, Rabkin JG, editors: Anxiety: New Research and Changing Concepts. New York: Raven Press, pp. 235–264.

Klein DF. 1993. False suffocation alarms, spontaneous panics, and related conditions: An integrative hypothesis. Archives of General Psychiatry, 50: 306–317.

Klein DF, Klein HM. 1989. The definition and psychopharmacology of spontaneous panic and phobia. In Tyrer P, editor: Psychopharmacology of Anxiety. New York: Oxford University Press, pp. 135–162.

Kleiner L, Marshall WL. 1987. The role of interpersonal problems in the development of agoraphobia with panic attacks. Journal of Anxiety Disorders, 1: 313–323.

Klerman GL, Weissman MM, Ouellette R, et al. 1991. Panic attacks in the community: Social morbidity and health care utilization. Journal of the American Medical Association: 265: 742–746.

Klosko JS, Barlow DH, Tassinari R, et al. 1990. A comparison of alprazolam and behavior therapy in the treatment of panic disorder. Journal of Consulting and Clinical Psychology, 58: 77–84.

Kluznick JC, Speed N, Van Valkenburg C, et al. 1986. Forty-year follow-up of United States prisoners of war. American Journal of Psychiatry, 143: 1443–1446.

Kobak KA, Greist JH, Jefferson JW, et al. 1998. Behavioral versus pharmacological treatments of obsessive-compulsive disorder: A meta-analysis. Psychopharmacology (Berlin), 136: 205–216.

Kohut H. 1971. The Analysis of the Self. New York: International Universities Press.

Kohut H. 1977. The Restoration of the Self. New York: International Universities Press.

Kolb LC, Burris BC, Griffiths S. 1984. Propranolol and clonidine in treatment of the chronic post-traumatic stress disorder of war. In van der Kolk BA, editor: Post-Traumatic Stress Disorder: Psychological and Biological Sequelae. Washington, DC: American Psychiatric Press, pp. 97–105.

Koopman C, Classen C, Spiegel D. 1994. Predictors of posttraumatic stress symptoms among survivors of the Oakland/Berkeley, California firestorm. American Journal of Psychiatry, 151: 888–894.

Koran LM, McElroy SL, Davidson JRT, et al. 1996. Fluvoxamine versus clomipramine for obsessive-compulsive disorder: A double-blind comparison. Journal of Clinical Psychopharmacology, 16: 121–129.

Koran LM, Sallee FR, Pallanti S. 1997. Rapid benefit of intravenous pulse loading of clomipramine in obsessive-compulsive disorder. American Journal of Psychiatry, 154: 396–401.

Koren D, Arnon I, Klein E. 1999. Acute stress response and posttraumatic stress disorder in traffic accident victims: A one-year prospective, follow-up study. American Journal of Psychiatry, 156: 367–373.

Kosten TR, Frank JB, Dan E, et al. 1991. Pharmacotherapy for posttraumatic stress disorder using phenelzine or imipramine. Journal of Nervous and Mental Disease, 179: 366–370.

Kosten TR, Wahby V, Giller E, et al. 1990. The dexamethasone suppression test and thyrotropin-releasing hormone stimulation test in posttraumatic stress disorder. Biological Psychiatry, 28: 657–664.

Kozak MJ, Foa EB. 1994. Obsessions, overvalued ideas, and delusions in obsessive-compulsive disorder. Behaviour Research and Therapy, 32: 343–353.

Kringlen E. 1965. Obsessional neurotics: A long term follow-up. British Journal of Psychiatry, 111: 709–722.

Kronig MH, Apter J, Asnis G, et al. 1999. Placebo-controlled, multicenter study of sertraline treatment for obsessive-compulsive disorder. Journal of Clinical Psychopharmacology, 19: 172–176.

Krystal H. 1988. Integration and Self-Healing: Affect, Trauma, Alexithymia. Hillsdale, NJ: Analytic Press.

Kudler H, Davidson J, Meador K, et al. 1987. The DST and posttraumatic stress disorder. American Journal of Psychiatry, 144: 1068–1071.

Kulka RA, Schlenger WE, Fairbank JA, et al. 1990. Trauma and the Vietnam War Generation: Report of Findings from the National Vietnam Veterans Readjustment Study. New York: Brunner/Mazel.

Kushner MG, Beitman BD. 1990. Panic attacks without fear: An overview. Behaviour Research and Therapy, 28: 469–479.

Labbate LA, Pollack MH, Otto MW, et al. 1994. Sleep panic attacks: An association with childhood anxiety and adult psychopathology. Biological Psychiatry, 36: 57–60.

Lader M, Scotto JC. 1998. A multicentre double-blind comparison of hydroxyzine, buspirone and placebo in patients with generalized anxiety disorder. Psychopharmacology, 139: 402–406.

Ladouceur R, Blais F, Freeston MH, et al. 1998. Problem solving and problem orientation in generalized anxiety disorder. Journal of Anxiety Disorders, 12: 139–152.

Ladouceur R, Dugas MJ, Freeston MH, et al. 2000. Efficacy of a cognitive-behavioral treatment for generalized anxiety disorder: Evaluation in a controlled clinical trial. Journal of Clinical and Consulting Psychology, 68: 957–964.

Ladouceur R, Freeston MH, Dugas MJ. 1993. L'intolérance à l'incertitude et les raisons pour s'inquiéter dans le trouble d'anxiété généralisée. Presented at the Annual Convention of the Quebec Society for Research in Psychology, Quebec City, Quebec, Canada.

Ladouceur R, Talbot F, Dugas MJ. 1997. Behavioral expressions of intolerance of uncertainty in worry: Experimental findings. Behavior Modification, 21: 355–371.

Lampe L, Slade T, Issakidis C, et al. 2003. Social phobia in the Australian National Survey of Mental Health and Well-Being (NSMHWB). Psychological Medicine, 33: 637–646.

Lang PJ. 1979. A bio-informational theory of emotional imagery. Journal of Psychophysiology, 16: 495–512.

Lange A, van Dyck R. 1992. The function of agoraphobia in the marital relationship. Acta Psychiatrica Scandinavica, 85: 89–93.

Leckman JF, Walker DE, Cohen DJ. 1993. Premonitory urges in Tourette's syndrome. American Journal of Psychiatry, 150: 98–102.

Leckman JF, Walker DE, Goodman WK, et al., 1994. "Just right" perceptions associated with compulsive behavior in Tourette's syndrome. American Journal of Psychiatry, 151: 675–680.

Lecrubier Y. 1998. Comorbidity in social anxiety disorder: Impact on disease burden and management. Journal of Clinical Psychiatry, 59: 33–37.

Lecrubier Y, Bakker A, Judge R. 1997. A comparison of paroxetine, clomipramine, and placebo in the treatment of panic disorder. Acta Psychiatrica Scandinavica, 95: 145–152.

Lecrubier Y, Judge R. 1997. Long-term evaluation of paroxetine, clomipramine and placebo in panic disorder. Acta PsychiatricaScandinavica, 95: 153–160.

Lecrubier Y, Weiller E. 1997. Comorbidities in social phobia. International Clinical Psychopharmacology, 12 (Suppl. 6): 17–21.

Lee CK, Kwak YS, Yamamoto J, et al. 1990a. Psychiatric epidemiology in Korea. Part I: Gender and age differences in Seoul. Journal of Nervous and Mental Disease, 178: 242–246.

Lee CK, Kwak YS, Yamamoto J, et al. 1990b. Psychiatric epidemiology in Korea. Part II: Urban and rural differences. Journal of Nervous and Mental Disease, 178: 247–252.

Lelliott P, Marks I, McNamee G, et al. 1989. Onset of panic disorder with agoraphobia: Toward an integrated model. Archives of General Psychiatry, 46: 1000–1004.

Lelliott PT, Noshirvani HF, Basoglu M, et al. 1988. Obsessive-compulsive beliefs and treatment outcome. Psychological Medicine, 18: 697–702.

Lenane MC, Swedo SE, Leonardo H, et al. 1990. Psychiatric disorders in first degree relatives of children and adolescents with obsessive compulsive disorder. Journal of the American Academy of Child and Adolescent Psychiatry, 29: 407–412.

Lensi P, Cassano GB, Correddu G, et al. 1996. Obsessive-compulsive disorder: Familial-developmental history, symptomatology, comorbidity and course with special reference to gender-related differences. British Journal of Psychiatry, 169: 101–107.

Leon AC, Porter AL, Weissman MM. 1995. The social costs of anxiety disorders. British Journal of Psychiatry, 166 (Suppl. 27): 19–22.

Leon CA, Leon A. 1990. Panic disorder and parental bonding. Psychiatric Annals, 20: 503–508.

Leonard HL, Swedo SE. 2001. Paediatric autoimmune neuropsychiatric disorders associated with streptococcal infection (PANDAS). International Journal of Neuropsychopharmacology, 4: 191–198.

Leonard HL, Swedo SE, Lenane MC, et al. 1991. A double-blind desipramine substitution during long-term clomipramine treatment in children and adolescents with obsessive-compulsive disorder. Archives of General Psychiatry, 48: 922–927.

Leonard HL, Swedo SE, Rapoport JL, et al. 1989. Treatment of obsessive-compulsive disorder with clomipramine and desipramine in children and adolescents: A double-blind crossover comparison. Archives of General Psychiatry, 46: 1088–1092.

Lepine JP, Chignon JM, Teherani M. 1993. Suicide attempts in patients with panic disorder. Archives of General Psychiatry, 50: 144–149.

Lepine JP, Lellouch J. 1994. Classification and epidemiology of anxiety disorders. In Darcourt G, Mendlewicz J, Racagni G, Brunello N, editors: Current Therapeutic Approaches to Panic and Other Anxiety Disorders. Basel: Karger, pp. 1–14.

Lepola UM, Wade AG, Leinonen EV, et al. 1998. A controlled, prospective, 1-year trial of citalopram in the treatment of panic disorder. Journal of Clinical Psychiatry, 59: 528–534.

Lesch KP, Wiesmann M, Hoh A, et al. 1992. 5-HT1A receptor-effector system responsivity in panic disorder. Psychopharmacology, 106: 111–117.

Lesser IM, Rubin RT, Pecknold JC, et al. 1988. Secondary depression in panic disorder and agoraphobia: I. Frequency, severity, and response to treatment. Archives of General Psychiatry, 45: 437–443.

Lieb R, Wittchen H-U, Hoefler M, et al. 2000. Parental psychopathology, parenting styles, and the risk of social phobia in offspring: A prospective-longitudinal community study. Archives of General Psychiatry, 57: 859–866.

Liebowitz MR. 1987. Social phobia. Modern Problems in Pharmacopsychiatry, 22: 141–173.

Liebowitz MR, Campeas R, Hollander E. 1987. Possible dopamine dysregulation in social phobia and atypical depression. Psychiatry Research, 22: 89–90.

Liebowitz MR, DeMartinis NA, Weihs K, et al. 2003. Efficacy of sertraline in severe generalized social phobia: Results of a double-blind, placebo-controlled study. Journal of Clinical Psychiatry, 64: 785–792.

Liebowitz MR, Gorman JM, Fyer AJ, et al. 1985. Lactate provocation of panic attacks: II. Biochemical and physiological findings. Archives of General Psychiatry, 42: 709–719.

Liebowitz MR, Heimberg RG, Fresco DM, et al. 2000. Social phobia or social anxiety disorder: What's in a name? Archives of General Psychiatry, 57: 191–192.

Liebowitz MR, Quitkin FM, Stewart JW, et al. 1988. Antidepressant specificity in atypical depression. Archives of General Psychiatry, 45: 129–137.

Liebowitz MR, Schneier F, Campeas R, et al. 1992. Phenelzine vs. atenolol in social phobia: A placebo-controlled comparison. Archives of General Psychiatry, 49: 290–300.

Lilienfeld SO, Turner SM, Jacob RG. 1993. Anxiety sensitivity: An examination of theoretical and methodological issues. Advances in Behaviour Research and Therapy, 15: 147–183.

Lindemann CG, Zitrin CM, Klein DF. 1984. Thyroid dysfunction in phobic patients. Psychosomatics, 25: 603–606.

Linden M. 2003. Posttraumatic embitterment disorder. Psychotherapy and Psychosomatics, 72: 195–202.

Lipsitz, JD, Barlow DH, Mannuzza S, et al. 2002. Clinical features of four DSM-IV-specific phobia subtypes. Journal of Nervous and Mental Disease, 190: 471–478.

Llorca PM, Spadone C, Sol O, et al. 2002. Efficacy and safety of hydroxyzine in the treatment of generalized anxiety disorder: A 3-month double-blind study. Journal of Clinical Psychiatry, 63: 1020–1027.

Logue MB, Thomas AM, Barbee JG, et al. 1993. Generalized anxiety disorder patients seek evaluation for cardiological symptoms at the same frequency as patients with panic disorder. Journal of Psychiatric Research, 27: 55–59.

Lohr JM, Lilienfeld SO, Tolin DF, et al. 1999. Eye movement desensitisation and reprocessing: An analysis of specific versus nonspecific treatment factors. Journal of Anxiety Disorders, 13: 185–207.

Londborg PD, Wolkow R, Smith WT. 1998. Sertraline in the treatment of panic disorder: A multi-site, double-blind, placebo-controlled, fixed-dose investigation. British Journal of Psychiatry, 173: 54–60.

Lteif GN, Mavissakalian MR. 1995. Life events and panic disorder/agoraphobia. Comprehensive Psychiatry, 36: 118–122.

Lucock MP, Salkovskis PM. 1988. Cognitive factors in social anxiety and its treatment. Behaviour Research and Therapy, 26: 297–302.

Lydiard RB. 1997. Anxiety and the irritable bowel syndrome: Psychiatric, medical, or both? Journal of Clinical Psychiatry, 58 (Suppl. 3): 51–58.

Lydiard RB, Fosser MD, Marsh W, et al. 1993. Prevalence of psychiatric disorders in patients with irritable bowel syndrome. Psychosomatics, 34: 229–234.

Lydiard RB, Greenwald S, Weissman MM, et al. 1994. Panic disorder and gastrointestinal symptoms: Findings from the National Institute of Mental Health Epidemiologic Catchment Area project. American Journal of Psychiatry, 151: 64–70.

Macdonald PA, Antony MM, Macleod CM, et al. 1997. Memory and confidence in memory judgments among individuals with obsessive compulsive disorder and non-clinical controls. Behaviour Research and Therapy, 35: 497–505.

Mackinnon D, Xu J, McMahon F, et al. 1997. Panic disorder with familial bipolar disorder. Biological Psychiatry, 42: 90–95.

Macklin ML, Metzger LJ, Lasko NB, et al. 2000. Five-year follow-up study of eye movement desensitization and reprocessing therapy for combat-related posttraumatic stress disorder. Comprehensive Psychiatry, 41: 24–27.

Macklin ML, Metzger LJ, Litz BT, et al. 1998. Lower precombat intelligence is a risk factor for posttraumatic stress disorder. Journal of Consulting and Clinical Psychology, 66: 323–326.

MacLeod C, Mathews A, Tata P. 1986. Attentional bias in emotional disorders. Journal of Abnormal Psychology, 95: 15–20.

Magee WJ, Eaton WW, Wittchen HU, et al. 1996. Agoraphobia, simple phobia, and social phobia in the National Comorbidity Survey. Archives of General Psychiatry, 53: 159–168.

Maier W, Gaensicke M, Freyberger HJ, et al. 2000. Generalized anxiety disorder (ICD-10) in primary care from a cross-cultural perspective: A valid diagnostic entity? Acta Psychiatrica Scandinavica, 101: 29–36.

Maier W, Minges J, Lichtermann D. 1995. The familial relationship between panic disorder and unipolar depression. Journal of Psychiatric Research, 29: 375–388.

Malizia AL, Cunningham VJ, Bell CJ, et al. 1998. Decreased brain GABA$_A$-benzodiazepine receptor binding in panic disorder: Preliminary results from a quantitative PET study. Archives of General Psychiatry, 55: 715–720.

Mancuso DM, Townsend MH, Mercante DE. 1993. Long-term follow-up of generalized anxiety disorder. Comprehensive Psychiatry, 34: 441–446.

Mann JJ. 1999. Role of the serotonergic system in the pathogenesis of major depression and suicidal behavior. Neuropsychopharmacology, 21: 99S–105S.

Mannuzza S, Schneier FR, Chapman TF, et al. 1995. Generalized social phobia: Reliability and validity. Archives of General Psychiatry, 52: 230–237.

Mansell W, Clark DM. 1999. How do I appear to others? Social anxiety and processing of the observable self. Behaviour Research and Therapy, 37: 419–434.

Marazziti D, Dell'Osso L, Di Nasso E, et al. 2002. Insight in obsessive-compulsive disorder: A study of an Italian sample. European Psychiatry, 17: 407–410.

Marcaurelle R, Belanger C, Marchand A. 2003. Marital relationship and the treatment of panic disorder with agoraphobia: A critical review. Clinical Psychology Review, 23: 247–276.

Margraf J, Barlow DH, Clark DM, et al. 1993. Psychological treatment of panic: Work in progress in outcome, active ingredients, and follow-up. Behaviour Research and Therapy, 31: 1–8.

Margraf J, Ehlers A, Roth WT. 1986. Sodium lactate infusions and panic attacks: A review and critique. Psychosomatic Medicine, 48: 23–51.

Margraf J, Ehlers A, Roth WT. 1988. Mitral valve prolapse and panic disorder: A review of their relationship. Psychosomatic Medicine, 50: 93–113.

Markowitz JS, Weissman MM, Ouellette R, et al. 1989. Quality of life in panic disorder. Archives of General Psychiatry, 46: 984–992.

Marks IM. 1988. Blood-injury phobia: A review. American Journal of Psychiatry, 145: 1207–1213.

Marks IM, Boulogouris JC, Marcet P. 1971. Flooding versus desensitization in the treatment of phobic patients: A cross-over study. British Journal of Psychiatry, 119: 353–375.

Marks IM, Gray S, Cohen D, et al. 1983. Imipramine and brief therapist-aided exposure in agoraphobics having self-exposure homework. Archives of General Psychiatry, 40: 153–162.

Marks IM, Hodgson R, Rachman S. 1975. Treatment of chronic obsessive-compulsive neurosis by in vivo exposure: A 2-year follow-up and issues in treatment. British Journal of Psychiatry, 127: 349–364.

Marks IM, Lelliott P, Basoglu M, et al. 1988. Clomipramine, self-exposure and therapist-aided exposure for obsessive compulsive rituals. British Journal of Psychiatry, 152: 522–534.

Marks IM, Lovell K, Noshirvani H, et al. 1998. Treatment of posttraumatic stress disorder by exposure and/or cognitive restructuring: A controlled study. Archives of General Psychiatry, 55: 317–325.

Marks IM, Mathews AM. 1979. Brief standard self-rating scale for phobic patients. Behaviour Research and Therapy, 17: 263–267.

Marks IM, Stern RS, Mawson D, et al. 1980. Clomipramine and exposure for obsessive-compulsive rituals. British Journal of Psychiatry, 136: 1–25.

Marks IM, Swinson RP, Basoglu M, et al. 1993. Alprazolam and exposure alone and combined in panic disorder with agoraphobia: A controlled study in London and Toronto. British Journal of Psychiatry, 162: 776–787.

Marmar CR, Schoenfeld F, Weiss DS, et al. 1996. Open trial of fluvoxamine treatment for combat-related posttraumatic stress disorder. Journal of Clinical Psychiatry, 57 (Suppl. 8): 66–72.

Marshall RD, Beebe KL, Oldham M, et al. 2001. Efficacy and safety of paroxetine treatment for chronic PTSD: A fixed-dose, placebo-controlled study. American Journal of Psychiatry, 158: 1982–1988.

Martenyi F, Brown EB, Zhang H, et al. 2002. Fluoxetine versus placebo in posttraumatic stress disorder. Journal of Clinical Psychiatry, 63: 199–206.

Marzillier JS, Lambert C, Kellett J. 1976. A controlled evaluation of systematic desensitization and social skills training for socially inadequate psychiatric patients. Behaviour Research and Therapy, 14: 225–238.

Mason JW, Giller EL, Kosten TR, et al. 1986. Urinary free-cortisol levels in posttraumatic stress disorder patients. Journal of Nervous and Mental Disease, 174: 145–149.

Massion AO, Dyck IR, Shea MT, et al. 2002. Personality disorders and time to remission in generalized anxiety disorder, social phobia, and panic disorder.
— Archives of General Psychiatry, 59: 434–440.

Massion AO, Warshaw MG, Keller MB. 1993. Quality of life and psychiatric morbidity in panic disorder and generalized anxiety disorder. American Journal of Psychiatry, 150: 600–607.

Mataix-Cols D, Rauch SL, Baer L, et al. 2002. Symptom stability in adult obsessive-compulsive disorder: Data from a naturalistic two-year follow-up study. American Journal of Psychiatry, 159: 263–268.

Mataix-Cols D, Rauch SL, Manzo PA, et al. 1999. Use of factor-analyzed symptom dimensions to predict outcome with serotonin reuptake inhibitors and placebo in the treatment of obsessive-compulsive disorder. American Journal of Psychiatry, 156: 1409–1416.

Mathews A, Mogg K, May J, et al. 1989. Implicit and explicit memory bias in anxiety. Journal of Abnormal Psychology, 98: 236–240.

Mattick RP, Peters L. 1988. Treatment of severe social phobia: Effects of guided exposure with and without cognitive restructuring. Journal of Consulting and Clinical Psychology, 56: 251–260.

Mattick RP, Peters L, Clarke JC. 1989. Exposure and cognitive restructuring for social phobia: A controlled study. Behavior Therapy, 20: 3–23.

Mavissakalian M. 1988. The relationship between panic, phobic and anticipatory anxiety in agoraphobia. Behaviour Research and Therapy, 26: 235–240.

Mavissakalian M, Hamman MS. 1987. DSM-III personality disorders in agoraphobia: II. Changes with treatment. Comprehensive Psychiatry, 28: 356–361.

Mavissakalian M, Hamman MS, Haidar SA, et al. 1993. DSM-III personality disorders in generalized anxiety, panic/agoraphobia, and obsessive-compulsive disorders. Comprehensive Psychiatry, 34: 243–248.

Mavissakalian M, Michelson L. 1986a. Two year follow-up of exposure and imipramine treatment of agoraphobia. American Journal of Psychiatry 143: 1106–1112.

Mavissakalian M, Michelson L. 1986b. Agoraphobia: Relative and combined effectiveness of therapist-assisted in vivo exposure and imipramine. Journal of Clinical Psychiatry, 47: 117–122.

Mavissakalian M, Perel JM. 1989. Imipramine dose-response relationship in panic disorder with agoraphobia: Preliminary findings. Archives of General Psychiatry, 46: 127–131.

Mavissakalian M, Perel JM. 1992. Protective effects of imipramine maintenance treatment in panic disorder with agoraphobia. American Journal of Psychiatry, 149: 1053–1057.

Mavissakalian M, Perel JM. 1995. Imipramine treatment of panic disorder with agoraphobia: Dose ranging and plasma level–response relationships. American Journal of Psychiatry, 152: 673–682.

Mavissakalian MR, Perel JM. 2002. Duration of imipramine therapy and relapse in panic disorder with agoraphobia. Journal of Clinical Psychopharmacology, 22: 294–299.

Mayou R, Bryant B, Duthie R. 1993. Psychiatric consequences of road traffic accidents. British Medical Journal, 307: 647–651.

Mayou R, Ehlers A, Hobbs M. 2000. Psychological debriefing for road traffic accident victims: Three-year follow-up of a randomised controlled trial. British Journal of Psychiatry, 176: 589–593.

McDougle CJ, Barr LC, Goodman WK, et al. 1995. Lack of efficacy of clozapine monotherapy in refractory obsessive compulsive disorder. American Journal of Psychiatry, 152: 1812–1814.

McDougle CJ, Epperson CN, Pelton GH, et al. 2000. A double-blind, placebo-controlled study of risperidone addition in serotonin reuptake inhibitor–refractory obsessive-compulsive disorder. Archives of General Psychiatry, 57: 794–801.

McDougle CJ, Goodman WK, Leckman JF, et al. 1994. Haloperidol addition in fluvoxamine-refractory obsessive-compulsive disorder: A double-blind, placebo-controlled study in patients with and without tics. Archives of General Psychiatry, 51: 302–308.

McElroy SL, Altshuler LL, Suppes T, et al. 2001. Axis I psychiatric comorbidity and its relationship to historical illness variables in 288 patients with bipolar disorder. American Journal of Psychiatry, 158: 420–426.

McEwan KL, Devins GM. 1983. Is increased arousal in social anxiety noticed by others? Journal of Abnormal Psychology, 92: 417–421.

McFall M, Murburg M, Ko G, et al. 1990. Autonomic response to stress in Vietnam combat veterans with post-traumatic stress disorder. Biological Psychiatry, 27: 1165–1175.

McFall ME, Wollersheim JP. 1979. Obsessive-compulsive neurosis: A cognitive-behavioral formulation and approach to treatment. Cognitive Therapy and Research, 3: 333–348.

McFarlane AC. 1988. The longitudinal course of posttraumatic morbidity: The range of outcomes and their predictors. Journal of Nervous and Mental Disease, 176: 30–39.

McFarlane AC. 1989a. The etiology of post-traumatic morbidity: Predisposing, precipitating and perpetuating factors. British Journal of Psychiatry, 154: 221–228.

McFarlane AC. 1989b. The treatment of post-traumatic stress disorder. British Journal of Medical Psychology, 62: 81–90.

McFarlane AC, Atchison M, Yehuda R. 1997. The acute stress response following motor vehicle accidents and its relation to PTSD. Annals of the New York Academy of Sciences, 821: 437–441.

McFarlane AC, Papay P. 1992. Multiple diagnoses in posttraumatic stress disorder in the victims of a natural disaster. Journal of Nervous and Mental Disease, 180: 498–504.

McGee R, Feehan M, Williams S, et al. 1990. DSM-III disorders in a large sample of adolescents. Journal of the American Academy of Child and Adolescent Psychiatry, 29: 611–619.

McKay D. 1997. A maintenance program for obsessive-compulsive disorder using exposure with response prevention: 2-year follow-up. Behaviour Research and Therapy, 35: 367–369.

McKay D, Neziroglu F, Todaro J, et al. 1996. Changes in personality disorders following behavior therapy for obsessive-compulsive disorder. Journal of Anxiety Disorders, 10: 47–57.

McLeod JD. 1994. Anxiety disorders and marital quality. Journal of Abnormal Psychology, 103: 767–776.

McNally RJ. 1987. Preparedness and phobias: A review. Psychological Bulletin, 101: 283–303.

McNally RJ. 1999. Research on eye movement desensitization and reprocessing as a treatment for PTSD. PTSD Research Quarterly, 10: 1–7.

McNally RJ. 2002. Disgust has arrived. Journal of Anxiety Disorders, 16: 561–566.

McPherson FM, Brougham L, McLaren S. 1980. Maintenance of improvement in agoraphobic patients treated by behavioural methods: A four-year follow-up. Behaviour Research and Therapy, 18: 150–152.

Meichenbaum D. 1975. Self-instructional methods. In Kanfer FH, Goldstein AP, editors: Helping People Change. New York: Pergamon Press, pp. 357–391.

Mellings TMB, Alden LE. 2000. Cognitive processes in social anxiety: The effects of self-focus, rumination and anticipatory processing. Behaviour Research and Therapy, 38: 243–257.

Mellman TA, David D, Bustamante V, et al. 2001. Predictors of post-traumatic stress disorder following severe injury. Depression and Anxiety, 14: 226–231.

Mendlewicz J, Papadimitriou G, Wilmotte J. 1993. Family study of panic disorder: Comparison with generalized anxiety disorder, major depression, and normal subjects. Psychiatric Genetics, 3: 73–78.

Mennin DS, Heimberg RG, Jack MS. 2000. Comorbid generalized anxiety disorder in primary social phobia: Symptom severity, functional impairment, and treatment response. Journal of Anxiety Disorders, 14: 325–343.

Menzies RG, Clarke JC. 1993a. The etiology of childhood water phobia. Behaviour Research and Therapy, 31: 499–501.

Menzies RG, Clarke JC. 1993b. The etiology of fear of heights and its relationship to severity and individual response patterns. Behaviour Research and Therapy, 31: 355–365.

Menzies RG, Clarke JC. 1995. The etiology of phobias: A nonassociative account. Clinical Psychology Review, 15: 23–48.

Meyer TJ, Miller RL, Metzger R, et al. 1990. Development and validation of the Penn State Worry Questionnaire. Behaviour Research and Therapy, 28: 487–495.

Michelson D, Allgulander C, Dantendorfer K, et al. 2001. Efficacy of usual antidepressant dosing regimens of fluoxetine in panic disorder: Randomised, placebo-controlled trial. British Journal of Psychiatry, 179: 514–518.

Michelson D, Lydiard RB, Pollack MH, et al. 1998. Outcome assessment and clinical improvement in panic disorder: Evidence from a randomized controlled trial of fluoxetine and placebo. American Journal of Psychiatry, 155: 1570–1577.

Michelson D, Pollack M, Lydiard RB. 1999. Continuing treatment of panic disorder after acute response: Randomised, placebo-controlled trial with fluoxetine. British Journal of Psychiatry, 172: 213–218.

Mick MA, Telch MJ. 1998. Social anxiety and history of behavioral inhibition in young adults. Journal of Anxiety Disorders, 12: 1–20.

Miguel EC, Coffey BJ, Baer L, et al. 1995. Phenomenology of intentional repetitive behaviors in obsessive-compulsive disorder and Tourette's disorder. Journal of Clinical Psychiatry, 56: 246–255.

Mikkelson EJ, Deltor J, Cohen DJ. 1981. School avoidance and social phobia triggered by haloperidol in patients with Tourette's syndrome. American Journal of Psychiatry, 138: 1572–1576.

Miller ML. 1953. On street fear. International Journal of Psychoanalysis, 34: 232–252.

Milrod B, Busch F, Cooper A, Shapiro T. 1997. Manual of Panic-Focused Psychodynamic Psychotherapy. Washington, DC: American Psychiatric Press.

Mineka S, Watson D, Clark LA. 1998. Comorbidity of anxiety and unipolar mood disorders. Annual Review of Psychology, 49: 377–412.

Minichiello WE, Baer L, Jenike MA. 1987. Schizotypal personality disorder: A poor prognostic indicator for behavior therapy in the treatment of obsessive-compulsive disorder. Journal of Anxiety Disorders, 1: 273–276.

Mitchell JT. 1983. When disaster strikes . . . the critical incident stress debriefing process. Journal of Emergency Medical Services, 8: 36–39.

Mitchell JT, Everly GS. 1995. Critical Incident Stress Debriefing: An Operation Manual for the Prevention of Traumatic Stress among Emergency Services and Disaster Workers. Elliott City, MD: Chevron Publishing.

Modigh K, Westberg P, Eriksson E. 1992. Superiority of clomipramine over imipramine in the treatment of panic disorder: A placebo-controlled trial. Journal of Clinical Psychopharmacology, 12: 251–261.

Mogg K, Bradley BP, Miller T, et al. 1994. Interpretation of homophones related to threat: Anxiety or response bias effects? Cognitive Therapy and Research, 18: 461–477.

Montgomery SA, McIntyre A, Osterheider M, et al. 1993. A double-blind, placebo-controlled study of fluoxetine in patients with DSM-III-R obsessive-compulsive disorder. European Neuropsychopharmacology, 3: 143–152.

Morgenstern J, Langenbucher J, Labouvie E, et al. 1997. The comorbidity of alcoholism and personality disorders in a clinical population: Prevalence rates and relation to alcohol typology. Journal of Abnormal Psychology, 106: 74–84.

Moritz, S, Fricke S, Jacobsen D, et al. 2004. Positive schizotypal symptoms predict treatment outcome in obsessive-compulsive disorder. Behaviour Research and Therapy, 42: 217–227.

Moulds ML, Bryant RA. 2002. Directed forgetting in acute stress disorder. Journal of Abnormal Psychology, 111: 175–179.

Mowrer O. 1960. Learning Theory and Behavior. New York: Wiley.

Mulkens S, de Jong PJ, Dobbelaar A, et al. 1999. Fear of blushing: Fearful preoccupation irrespective of facial coloration. Behaviour Research and Therapy, 37: 1119–1128.

Mullaney JA, Trippett CJ. 1979. Alcohol dependence and phobias: Clinical description and relevance. British Journal of Psychiatry, 135: 565–573.

Munby J, Johnston DW. 1980. Agoraphobia: The long-term follow-up of behavioral treatment. British Journal of Psychiatry, 137: 418–427.

Mundo E, Mainia G, Uslenghi C. 2000. Multicentre, double-blind comparison of fluvoxamine and clomipramine in the treatment of obsessive-compulsive disorder. International Clinical Psychopharmacology, 15: 69–76.

Muris P, Merckelbach H, Van Haaften H, et al. 1997. Eye movement desensitisation and reprocessing versus exposure in vivo. A single-session crossover study of spider-phobic children. British Journal of Psychiatry, 171: 82–86.

Murphy TK, Goodman WK, Fudge MW, et al. 1997. Lymphocyte antigen D8/17: A peripheral marker for childhood-onset obsessive-compulsive disorder and Tourette's syndrome? American Journal of Psychiatry, 154: 402–407.

Murray J, Ehlers A, Mayou RA. 2002. Dissociation and post-traumatic stress disorder: Two prospective studies of road traffic accident survivors. British Journal of Psychiatry, 180: 363–368.

Nagy LM, Krystal JH, Woods SW, et al. 1989. Clinical and medication outcome after short-term alprazolam and behavioral group treatment in panic disorder: 2.5 year naturalistic follow-up study. Archives of General Psychiatry, 46: 993–999.

Nagy LM, Morgan CA, Southwick SM, et al. 1993. Open prospective trial of fluoxetine for posttraumatic stress disorder. Journal of Clinical Psychopharmacology, 13: 107–113.

Nardi AE, Nascimento I, Valenca AM, et al. 2003. Respiratory panic disorder subtype: Acute and long-term response to nortriptyline, a noradrenergic tricyclic antidepressant. Psychiatry Research, 120: 283–293.

Narrow WE, Rae DS, Robins LN, et al. 2002. Revised prevalence estimates of mental disorders in the United States: Using a clinical significance criterion to reconcile 2 surveys' estimates. Archives of General Psychiatry, 59: 115–123.

Neftel KA, Adler RH, Kappell K, et al. 1982. Stage fright in musicians: A model illustrating the effect of beta-blockers. Psychosomatic Medicine, 44: 461–469.

Nelson E, Rice J. 1997. Stability of diagnosis of obsessive-compulsive disorder in the Epidemiological Catchment Area Study. American Journal of Psychiatry, 154: 826–831.

Nelson EC, Grant JD, Bucholz KK, et al. 2000. Social phobia in a population-based female adolescent twin sample: Co-morbidity and associated suicide-related symptoms. Psychological Medicine, 30: 797–804.

Nemiah JC. 1988. Psychoneurotic disorders. In Nicholi AM, editor: The New Harvard Guide to Psychiatry. Cambridge, MA: Belknap Press of Harvard University Press, pp. 234–258.

Nestadt G, Samuels J, Riddle M, et al. 2000. A family study of obsessive-compulsive disorder. Archives of General Psychiatry, 57: 358–363.

Newman MG, Hofmann SG, Trabert W, et al. 1994. Does behavioural treatment of social phobia lead to cognitive changes? Behavior Therapy, 25: 503–517.

Neziroglu F, Anemone R, Yaryura-Tobias JA. 1992. Onset of obsessive-compulsive disorder in pregnancy. American Journal of Psychiatry, 149: 947–950.

Nisita C, Petracca A, Akiskal HS, et al. 1990. Delimitation of generalized anxiety disorder: Clinical comparisons with panic and major depressive disorders. Comprehensive Psychiatry, 31: 409–415.

Norton GR, Dorward J, Cox BJ. 1986. Factors associated with panic attacks in non-clinical subjects. Behavior Therapy, 17: 239–252.

Noshirvani HF, Kasvikis YG, Marks IM, et al. 1991. Gender divergent aetiological factors in obsessive-compulsive disorder. British Journal of Psychiatry, 158: 260–263.

Noyes R. 1999. The relationship of hypochondriasis to anxiety disorders. General Hospital Psychiatry, 21: 8–17.

Noyes R, Clancy J, Garvey MJ, Anderson DJ. 1987a. Is agoraphobia a variant of panic disorder or a separate illness? Journal of Anxiety Disorders, 1: 3–13.

Noyes R, Clancy J, Woodman C, et al. 1993. Environmental factors related to the outcome of panic disorder: A seven-year follow-up study. Journal of Nervous and Mental Disease, 181: 529–538.

Noyes R, Clarkson C, Crowe RR, et al. 1987b. A family study of generalized anxiety disorder. American Journal of Psychiatry, 144: 1019–1024.

Noyes R, Crowe RR, Harris EL, et al. 1986. Relationship between panic disorder and agoraphobia: A family study. Archives of General Psychiatry, 43:227–232.

Noyes R, Garvey MJ, Cook B. 1991. Controlled discontinuation of benzodiazepine treatment for patients with panic disorder. American Journal of Psychiatry, 148: 517–523.

Noyes R, Moroz G, Davidson JTR, et al. 1997. Moclobemide in social phobia: A controlled dose–response trial. Journal of Clinical Psychopharmacology, 17: 247–254.

Nutt DJ, Glue P, Lawson C, et al. 1990. Flumazenil provocation of panic attacks: Evidence for altered benzodiazepine receptor sensitivity in panic disorder. Archives of General Psychiatry, 47: 917–925.

Obsessive Compulsive Cognitions Working Group. 1997. Cognitive assessment of obsessive-compulsive disorder. Behaviour Research and Therapy, 35: 667–681.

Oehrberg S, Christiansen PE, Behnke K, et al. 1995. Paroxetine in the treatment of panic disorder: A randomised, double-blind, placebo-controlled study. British Journal of Psychiatry, 167: 374–379.

Oci TP, Llamas M, Evans L. 1997. Does concurrent drug intake affect the long-term outcome of group cognitive behaviour therapy in panic disorder with or without agoraphobia? Behaviour Research and Therapy, 35: 851–857.

Öhman A. 1986. Face the beast and fear the face: Animal and social fears as prototypes for evolutionary analyses of emotion. Psychophysiology, 23: 123–145.

Olfson M, Fireman B, Weissman MM, et al. 1997. Mental disorders and disability among patients in primary care practice. American Journal of Psychiatry, 154: 1734–1740.

Olfson M, Kessler RC, Berglund PA, et al. 1998. Psychiatric disorder onset and first treatment contact in the United States and Ontario. American Journal of Psychiatry, 155: 1415–1422.

O'Rourke D, Fahy TJ, Brophy J, et al. 1996. The Galway Study of Panic Disorder: III. Outcome at 5 to 6 years. British Journal of Psychiatry, 168: 462–469.

Öst L-G. 1987a. Applied relaxation: Description of a coping technique and review of controlled studies. Behaviour Research and Therapy, 25: 397–409.

Öst L-G. 1987b. Age of onset in different phobias, Journal of Abnormal Psychology, 96: 223–229.

Öst L-G. 1988. Applied relaxation vs. progressive relaxation in the treatment of panic disorder. Behaviour Research and Therapy, 26: 13–22.

Öst L-G. 1989. One-session treatment for specific phobias. Behaviour Research and Therapy, 27: 1–7.

Öst L-G. 1996. One-session group treatment of spider phobia. Behaviour Research and Therapy, 34: 707–715.

Öst L-G, Breitholtz E. 2000. Applied relaxation vs. cognitive therapy in the treatment of generalized anxiety disorder. Behaviour Research and Therapy, 38: 777–790.

Öst L-G, Fellenius J, Sterner U. 1991a. Applied tension, exposure in vivo, and tension-only in the treatment of blood phobia. Behaviour Research and Therapy, 29: 561–574.

Öst L-G, Ferebee I, Furmark T. 1997. One-session group therapy of spider phobia: Direct versus indirect treatments. Behaviour Research and Therapy, 35: 721–732.

Öst L-G, Hugdahl K. 1981. Acquisition of phobias and anxiety response patterns in clinical patients. Behaviour Research and Therapy, 19: 439–447.

Öst L-G, Johansson J, Jerremalm A. 1982. Individual response patterns and the effects of different behavioural methods in the treatment of claustrophobia. Behaviour Research and Therapy, 20: 445–460.

Öst L-G, Salkovskis PM, Hellström K. 1991b. One-session therapist-directed exposure vs. self-exposure in the treatment of spider phobia. Behavior Therapy, 22: 407–422.

Öst L-G, Sterner U. 1987. Applied tension: A specific behavioural method for treatment of blood phobia. Behaviour Research and Therapy, 25: 25–29.

O'Sullivan G, Noshirvani H, Marks I, et al. 1991. Six year follow-up after exposure and clomipramine therapy for obsessive compulsive disorder. Journal of Clinical Psychiatry, 52: 150–155.

Otto MW, Hinton D, Korbly NB, et al. 2003. Treatment of pharmacotherapy-refractory posttraumatic stress disorder among Cambodian refugees: A pilot study of combination treatment with cognitive-behavior therapy vs sertraline alone. Behaviour Research and Therapy, 41: 1271–1276.

Otto MW, Pollack MH, Sabatino SA. 1996. Maintenance of remission following cognitive behavior therapy for panic disorder: Possible deleterious effects of concurrent medication treatment. Behavior Therapy, 27: 473–482.

Otto MW, Pollack MH, Sachs GS, et al. 1992. Alcohol dependence in panic disorder patients. Journal of Psychiatric Research, 26: 29–38.

Otto MW, Pollack MH, Sachs GS, et al. 1993. Discontinuation of benzodiazepine treatment: Efficacy of cognitive-behavioral therapy for patients with panic disorder. American Journal of Psychiatry, 150: 1485–1490.

Otto MW, Tuby KS, Gould RA, et al. 2001. An effect-size analysis of the relative efficacy and tolerability of serotonin selective reuptake inhibitors for panic disorder. American Journal of Psychiatry, 158: 1989–1992.

Overbeek T, Schruers K, Vermetten E, et al. 2002. Comorbidity of obsessive-compulsive disorder and depression: Prevalence, symptom severity, and treatment effect. Journal of Clinical Psychiatry, 63: 1106–1112.

Page AC. 1994. Blood-injury phobia. Clinical Psychology Review, 14: 443–461.

Page AC, Bennett K, Carter O, et al. 1997. The Blood-Injection Symptom Scale (BISS): Assessing a structure of phobic symptoms elicited by blood and injections. Behaviour Research and Therapy, 35: 457–464.

Pande AC, Davidson JRT, Jefferson JW, et al. 1999. Treatment of social phobia with gabapentin: A placebo-controlled study. Journal of Clinical Psychopharmacology, 19: 341–348.

Papp LA, Klein DF, Gorman JM. 1993. Carbon dioxide hypersensitivity, hyperventilation, and panic disorder. American Journal of Psychiatry, 150: 1149–1157.

Pato MT, Zohar-Kadouch R, Zohar J, et al. 1988. Return of symptoms after discontinuation of clomipramine in patients with obsessive-compulsive disorder. American Journal of Psychiatry, 145: 1521–1525.

Pauls DL, Alsobrook JP, Goodman W, et al. 1995. A family study of obsessive-compulsive disorder. American Journal of Psychiatry, 152: 76–84.

Paunovic N. 2003. Prolonged exposure counterconditioning as a treatment for chronic posttraumatic stress disorder. Journal of Anxiety Disorders, 17: 479–499.

Perani D, Colombo C, Bressi S, et al. 1995. [18F]FDG PET study in obsessive-compulsive disorder: A clinical/metabolic correlation study after treatment. British Journal of Psychiatry, 166: 244–250.

Perna G, Bussi R, Allevi L, et al. 1999. Sensitivity to 35% carbon dioxide in patients with generalized anxiety disorder. Journal of Clinical Psychiatry, 60: 379–384.

Perse TL, Greist JH, Jefferson JW, et al. 1987. Fluvoxamine treatment of obsessive-compulsive disorder. American Journal of Psychiatry, 144: 1543–1548.

Pigott TA, Pato MT, Bernstein SE, et al. 1990. Controlled comparisons of clomipramine and fluoxetine in the treatment of obsessive-compulsive disorder: Behavioral and biological results. Archives of General Psychiatry, 47: 926–932.

Pilkonis PA, Zimbardo PG. 1979. The personal and social dynamics of shyness. In Izard CE, editor: Emotions in Personality and Psychopathology. New York: Plenum.

Pini S, Cassano GB, Simonini E, et al. 1997. Prevalence of anxiety disorder comorbidity in bipolar depression, unipolar depression and dysthymia. Journal of Affective Disorders, 42: 145–153.

Pini S, Dell'Osso L, Mastrocinque C, et al. 1999. Axis I comorbidity in bipolar disorder with psychotic features. British Journal of Psychiatry, 175: 467–471.

Pitman RK, van der Kolk BA, Orr SP, et al. 1990. Naloxone-reversible analgesic response to combat-related stimuli in posttraumatic stress disorder: A pilot study. Archives of General Psychiatry, 47: 541–544.

Pohl R, Yeragani VK, Balon R, et al. 1992. Smoking in patients with panic disorder. Psychiatry Research, 43: 253–262.

Pohl RB, Wolkow RM, Clary CM. 1998. Sertraline in the treatment of panic disorder: A double-blind multicenter trial. American Journal of Psychiatry, 155: 1189–1195.

Pollack MH, Otto MW, Worthington JJ, et al. 1998. Sertraline in the treatment of panic disorder: A flexible-dose multicenter trial. Archives of General Psychiatry, 55: 1010–1016.

Pollack MH, Simon NM, Worthington JJ, et al. 2003. Combined paroxetine and clonazepam treatment strategies compared to paroxetine monotherapy for panic disorder. Journal of Psychopharmacology, 17: 276–282.

Pollack MH, Worthington JJ, Otto MW, et al. 1996. Venlafaxine for panic disorder: Results of a double-blind, placebo-controlled study. Psychopharmacology Bulletin, 32: 667–670.

Pollack MH, Zaninelli R, Goddard A, et al. 2001. Paroxetine in the treatment of generalized anxiety disorder: Results of a placebo-controlled, flexible-dosage trial. Journal of Clinical Psychiatry, 62: 350–357.

Post RM, Weiss SR, Smith M, et al. 1997. Kindling versus quenching: Implications for the evolution and treatment of posttraumatic stress disorder. Annals of the New York Academy of Sciences, 821: 285–295.

Power KG, Simpson RJ, Swanson V, et al. 1990. A controlled comparison of cognitive-behavior therapy, diazepam, and placebo, alone and in combination, for the treatment of generalized anxiety disorder. Journal of Anxiety Disorders, 4: 267–292.

Prochaska JO. 1991. Prescribing to the stage and level of phobic patients. Psychotherapy, 28: 463–468.

Purdon C, Clark DA. 1994. Perceived control and appraisal of obsessional intrusive thoughts: A replication and extension. Behavioural and Cognitive Psychotherapy, 22: 269–285.

Quitkin FM, Harrison W, Stewart JW, et al. 1991. Response to phenelzine and imipramine in placebo nonresponders with atypical depression: A new application of the crossover design. Archives of General Psychiatry, 48: 319–323.

Rachman S. 1991. Neo-conditioning and the classical theory of fear acquisition. Clinical Psychology Review, 11: 155–173.

Rachman SJ. 1997. A cognitive theory of obsessions. Behaviour Research and Therapy, 35: 793–802.

Rachman SJ. 1998. A cognitive theory of obsessions: Elaborations. Behaviour Research and Therapy, 36: 385–401.

Rachman S, Hodgson RS. 1980. Obsessions and Compulsions. Englewood Cliffs, NJ: Prentice-Hall.

Rachman S, Lopatka C, Levitt K. 1988. Experimental analyses of panic: II. Panic patients. Behaviour Research and Therapy, 26: 33–40.

Radomsky AS, Rachman S. 1999. Memory bias in obsessive-compulsive disorder (OCD). Behaviour Research and Therapy, 37: 605–618.

Radomsky AS, Rachman S, Hammond D. 2001. Memory bias confidence and responsibility in compulsive checking. Behaviour Research and Therapy, 39: 813–822.

Radomsky AS, Rachman S, Teachman BA, et al. 1998. Why do episodes of panic stop? Journal of Anxiety Disorders, 12: 263–270.

Raguram R, Bhide AY. 1985. Patterns of phobic neurosis: A retrospective study. British Journal of Psychiatry, 147: 557–560.

Ramesh C, Yeragani VK, Balon R, et al. 1991. A comparative study of immune status in panic disorder patients and controls. Acta Psychiatrica Scandinavica, 84: 396–397.

Rapee RM. 1985. Distinctions between panic disorder and generalised anxiety disorder: Clinical presentations. Australian and New Zealand Journal of Psychiatry, 19: 227–232.

Rapee RM. 1991. Generalized anxiety disorder: A review of clinical features and theoretical concepts. Clinical Psychology Review, 11: 419–440.

Rapee RM. 1997. Potential role of childrearing practices in the development of anxiety and depression. Clinical Psychology Review, 17: 47–67.

Rapee RM, Craske MG, Barlow DH. 1990a. Subject-described features of panic attacks using self-monitoring. Journal of Anxiety Disorders, 4: 171–181.

Rapee RM, Heimberg RG. 1997. A cognitive-behavioral model of anxiety in social phobia. Behaviour Research and Therapy, 35: 741–756.

Rapee RM, Lim L. 1992. Discrepancy between self and observer ratings of performance in social phobics. Journal of Abnormal Psychology, 101: 727–731.

Rapee RM, Litwin EM, Barlow DH. 1990b. Impact of life events on subjects with panic disorder and on comparison subjects. American Journal of Psychiatry, 147: 640–644.

Rapee RM, Murrell E. 1988. Predictors of agoraphobic avoidance. Journal of Anxiety Disorders, 2: 203–217.

Raskin M, Peeke HVS, Dickman W, et al. 1982. Panic and generalized anxiety disorders: Developmental antecedents and precipitants. Archives of General Psychiatry, 39: 687–689.

Rasmussen SA. 1994. Obsessive compulsive spectrum disorders. Journal of Clinical Psychiatry, 55: 89–91.

Rasmussen SA, Eisen JL. 1988. Clinical and epidemiologic findings of significance to neuropharmacologic trials in OCD. Psychopharmacology Bulletin, 24: 466–470.

Rasmussen SA, Eisen JL. 1990. Epidemiology of obsessive-compulsive disorder. Journal of Clinical Psychiatry, 51 (Suppl. 2): 10–13.

Rasmussen SA, Eisen JL. 1991. Phenomenology of obsessive-compulsive disorder: Clinical subtypes, heterogeneity and coexistence. In Zohar J, Insel T, Rasmussen S, editors: Psychobiology of Obsessive-Compulsive Disorder. New York: Springer-Verlag, pp. 743–758.

Rasmussen SA, Eisen JL. 1992. The epidemiology and clinical features of obsessive-compulsive disorder. Psychiatric Clinics of North America, 15: 743–758.

Rasmussen S, Hackett E, DuBoff E, et al. 1997. A 2-year study of sertraline in the treatment of obsessive-compulsive disorder. International Clinical Psychopharmacology, 12: 309–316.

Rasmussen SA, Tsuang MT. 1986. DSM-III obsessive-compulsive disorder: Clinical characteristics and family history. American Journal of Psychiatry, 143: 317–322.

Rassin E, Merckelbach H, Muris P. 2000. Paradoxical and less paradoxical effects of thought suppression: A critical review. Clinical Psychology Review, 20: 973–995.

Rauch SL, Jenike MA 1993. Neurobiological models of obsessive-compulsive disorder. Psychosomatics, 34: 20–32.

Rauch SL, Jenike MA, Alpert NM, et al. 1994. Regional cerebral blood flow measured during symptom provocation in obsessive-compulsive disorder using oxygen 15-labeled carbon dioxide and positron emission tomography. Archives of General Psychiatry, 51: 62–70.

Rauch SL, van der Kolk BA, Fisler RE, et al. 1996. A symptom provocation study of posttraumatic stress disorder using positron emission tomography and script-driven imagery. Archives of General Psychiatry, 53: 380–387.

Redmond DE. 1979. New and old evidence for the involvement of a brain norepinephrine system in anxiety. In Fann WE, Karacan I, Pokorny AD, et al., editors: Phenomenology and Treatment of Anxiety. New York: Spectrum Press, pp. 153–203.

Regier DA, Boyd JH, Burke JD, et al. 1988. One-month prevalence of mental disorders in the United States based on five Epidemiologic Catchment Area sites. Archives of General Psychiatry, 45: 977–986.

Regier DA, Narrow WE, Rae DS. 1990. The epidemiology of anxiety disorders: The Epidemiologic Catchment Area (ECA) experience. Journal of Psychiatric Research, 24: 3–14.

Regier DA, Rae DS, Narrow WE, et al. 1998. Prevalence of anxiety disorders and their comorbidity with mood and addictive disorders. British Journal of Psychiatry, 173 (Suppl. 34): 24–28.

Reich J, Goldenberg I, Vasile R, et al. 1994. A prospective follow-along study of the course of social phobia. Psychiatry Research, 54: 249–258.

Reich J, Noyes R, Yates W. 1988. Anxiety symptoms distinguishing social phobia from panic and generalized anxiety disorders. Journal of Nervous and Mental Disease, 176: 510–513.

Reich J, Troughton E. 1988. Frequency of DSM-III personality disorders in patients with panic disorder: Comparison with psychiatric and normal control subjects. Psychiatry Research, 26: 89–100.

Reich J, Yates W. 1988. Family history of psychiatric disorders in social phobia. Comprehensive Psychiatry, 29: 72–75.

Reiss S, McNally RJ. 1985. Expectancy model of fear. In Reiss S, Bootzin RR, editors: Theoretical Issues in Behavioral Therapy. San Diego: Academic Press, pp. 107–121.

Reiss S, Peterson RA, Gursky DM, et al. 1986. Anxiety sensitivity, anxiety frequency and the prediction of fearfulness. Behaviour Research and Therapy, 24: 1–8.

Resick PA, Nishith P, Weaver TL, et al. 2002. A comparison of cognitive-processing therapy with prolonged exposure and a waiting condition for the treatment of chronic posttraumatic stress disorder in female rape victims. Journal of Consulting and Clinical Psychology, 70: 867–879.

Resick PA, Schnicke MK. 1992. Cognitive processing therapy for sexual assault victims. Journal of Consulting and Clinical Psychology, 60: 748–756.

Resnick H, Kilpatrick DG, Dansky BS, et al. 1993. Prevalence of civilian trauma and posttraumatic stress disorder in a representative national sample of women. Journal of Consulting and Clinical Psychology, 61: 984–991.

Resnick HS, Yehuda R, Pitman RK, et al. 1995. Effect of previous trauma on acute plasma cortisol level following rape. American Journal of Psychiatry, 152: 1675–1677.

Rickels K, Downing R, Schweizer E, et al. 1993. Antidepressants for the treatment of generalized anxiety disorder: A placebo-controlled comparison of imipramine, trazodone, and diazepam. Archives of General Psychiatry, 50: 884–895.

Rickels K, Pollack MH, Sheehan DV, et al. 2000. Efficacy of extended-release ven-lafaxine in nondepressed outpatients with generalized anxiety disorder. American Journal of Psychiatry, 157: 968–974.

Rickels K, Wiseman K, Norstad N, et al. 1982. Buspirone and diazepam in anxiety: A controlled study. Journal of Clinical Psychiatry, 43: 81–86.

Rickels K, Zaninelli R, McCafferty J, et al. 2003. Paroxetine treatment of generalized anxiety disorder: A double-blind, placebo-controlled study. American Journal of Psychiatry, 160: 749–756.

Riddle MA, Scahill L, King R, et al. 1990. Obsessive compulsive disorder in children and adolescents. Journal of the American Academy of Child and Adolescent Psychiatry, 29: 766–772.

Risse SC, Whitters A, Burke J, et al. 1990. Severe withdrawal symptoms after dis-continuation of alprazolam in eight patients with combat-induced posttrau-matic stress disorder. Journal of Clinical Psychiatry, 51: 206–209.

Robins LN, Helzer JE, Weissman MM, et al. 1984. Lifetime prevalence of specific psychiatric disorders in three sites. Archives of General Psychiatry, 41: 958–967.

Robins LN, Regier DA. 1991. Psychiatric Disorders in America. New York: Macmil-lan.

Rocca P, Fonzo V, Scotta M, et al. 1997. Paroxetine efficacy in the treatment of gen-eralized anxiety disorder. Acta Psychiatrica Scandinavica, 95: 444–450.

Rose S, Bisson J. 1998. Brief early psychological interventions following trauma: A systematic review of the literature. Journal of Traumatic Stress, 11: 697–710.

Rose S, Bisson J, Wessely S. 2003. A systematic review of single-session psycholog-ical interventions ("debriefing") following trauma. Psychotherapy and Psy-chosomatics, 72: 176–184.

Rosen GM. 2004. Litigation and reported rates of posttraumatic stress disorder. Per-sonality and Individual Differences, 36: 1291–1294.

Rosenbaum JF, Biederman J, Gersten M, et al. 1988. Behavioral inhibition in chil-dren of parents with panic disorder and agoraphobia: A controlled study. Archives of General Psychiatry, 45: 463–470.

Rosenbaum JF, Biederman J, Hirshfeld DR, et al. 1991. Further evidence of an asso-ciation between behavioral inhibition and anxiety disorders: Results from a family study of children from a non-clinical sample. Journal of Psychiatric Re-search, 25: 49–65.

Rosenbaum JF, Moroz G, Bowden CL. 1997. Clonazepam in the treatment of panic disorder with or without agoraphobia: A dose–response study of efficacy, safety, and discontinuance. Journal of Clinical Psychopharmacology, 17: 390–400.

Rosenberg DR, Keshavan MS, O'Hearn KM, et al. 1997. Frontostriatal measurement in treatment-naive children with obsessive-compulsive disorder. Archives of General Psychiatry, 54: 824–830.

Rosenberg DR, MacMaster FP, Keshavan MS, et al. 2000. Decrease in caudate glu-tamatergic concentrations in pediatric obsessive-compulsive disorder patients taking paroxetine. Journal of the American Academy of Child and Adolescent Psychiatry, 39: 1096–1103.

Roth D, Antony MM, Swinson RP. 2001. Interpretations for anxiety symptoms in social phobia. Behaviour Research and Therapy, 39: 129–138.

Roy-Byrne PP, Cowley DS, Greenblatt DJ, et al. 1990. Reduced benzodiazepine sen-sitivity in panic disorder. Archives of General Psychiatry, 47: 534–538.

Roy-Byrne PP, Geraci M, Uhde TW. 1986. Life events and the onset of panic disorder. American Journal of Psychiatry, 143: 1424–1427.

Russell JL, Kushner MG, Beitman BD, et al. 1991. Nonfearful panic disorder in neurology patients validated by lactate challenge. American Journal of Psychiatry, 148: 361–364.

Sachdev P, Hay P. 1995. Does neurosurgery for obsessive-compulsive disorder produce personality change? Journal of Nervous and Mental Disease, 183: 408–413.

Salkovskis PM. 1985. Obsessional-compulsive problems: A cognitive-behavioural analysis. Behaviour Research and Therapy, 23: 571–583.

Salkovskis PM. 1989. Cognitive-behavioural factors and the persistence of intrusive thoughts in obsessional problems. Behaviour Research and Therapy, 27: 677–682.

Salkovskis PM. 1996. Cognitive-behavioral approaches to the understanding of obsessional problems. In Rapee RM, editor: Current Controversies in the Anxiety Disorders. New York: Guilford Press, pp. 103–133.

Salkovskis PM. 1999. Understanding and treating obsessive-compulsive disorder. Behaviour Research and Therapy, 37 (Suppl. 1): S29–S52.

Salkovskis PM, Clark DM. 1993. Panic disorder and hypochondriasis. Advances in Behaviour Research and Therapy, 15: 23–48.

Salkovskis P, Shafran R, Rachman S, et al. 1999. Multiple pathways to inflated responsibility beliefs in obsessional problems: Possible origins and implications for therapy and research. Behaviour Research and Therapy, 37: 1055–1072.

Salvador-Carulla L, Segui J, Fernandez-Cano P, et al. 1995. Costs and offset effect in panic disorders. British Journal of Psychiatry, 166 (Suppl. 27): 23–28.

Salzman L. 1968. The Obsessive Personality: Origins, Dynamics, and Therapy. New York: Science House.

Sanavio E. 1988. Obsessions and compulsions: The Padua Inventory. Behaviour Research and Therapy, 26: 169–177.

Sanderson W, Rapee R, Barlow D. 1989. The influence of an illusion of control on panic attacks induced via inhalation of 5.5% carbon dioxide-enriched air. Archives of General Psychiatry, 46: 157–162.

Sanderson WC, Barlow DH. 1990. A description of patients diagnosed with DSM-III-R generalized anxiety disorder. Journal of Nervous and Mental Disease, 178: 588–591.

Sanderson WC, DiNardo PA, Rapee RM, et al. 1990. Syndrome comorbidity in patients diagnosed with a DSM-III-R anxiety disorder. Journal of Abnormal Psychology, 99: 308–312.

Sapolsky RM. 1995. Why stress is bad for your brain. Science, 273: 749–750.

Scheibe G, Albus M. 1994. Prospective follow-up study lasting 2 years in patients with panic disorder with and without depressive disorders. European Archives of Psychiatry and Clinical Neuroscience, 244: 39–44.

Scher CD, Stein MB. 2003. Developmental antecedents of anxiety sensitivity. Journal of Anxiety Disorders, 17: 253–269.

Schlenker B, Leary M. 1982. Social anxiety and self-presentation: A conceptualization and model. Psychological Bulletin, 92; 641–669.

Schneider F, Weiss U, Kessler C, et al. 1999. Subcortical correlates of differential classical conditioning of aversive emotional reactions in social phobia. Biological Psychiatry, 45: 863–871.

Schneier FR, Goetz D, Campeas R, et al. 1998. Placebo-controlled trial of moclobemide in social phobia. British Journal of Psychiatry, 172: 70–77.

Schneier FR, Heckelman LR, Garfinkel R, et al. 1994. Functional impairment in social phobia. Journal of Clinical Psychiatry, 55: 322–331.

Schneier FR, Johnson J, Hornig CD, et al. 1992. Social phobia: Comorbidity and morbidity in an epidemiological sample. Archives of General Psychiatry, 49: 282–288.

Schneier F, Liebowitz MR, Abi-Dargham A, et al. 2000. Low dopamine D2 binding potential in social phobia. American Journal of Psychiatry, 157: 457–459.

Schneier FR, Martin LY, Liebowitz MR, et al. 1989. Alcohol abuse in social phobia. Journal of Anxiety Disorders, 3: 15–23.

Schnurr PP, Friedman MJ, Foy DW, et al. 2003. Randomized trial of trauma-focused group therapy for posttraumatic stress disorder: Results from a Department of Veterans Affairs Cooperative Study. Archives of General Psychiatry, 60: 481–489.

Schnyder U, Moergeli H, Klaghofer R, et al. 2001. Incidence and prediction of posttraumatic stress disorder symptoms in severely injured accident victims. American Journal of Psychiatry, 158: 594–599.

Scholing A, Emmelkamp PMG. 1996. Treatment of generalized social phobia: Results at long-term follow-up. Behaviour Research and Therapy, 34: 447–452.

Schwartz JM, Stoessel PW, Baxter LR, et al. 1996. Systematic changes in cerebral glucose metabolic rate after successful behavior modification treatment of obsessive-compulsive disorder. Archives of General Psychiatry, 53: 109–113.

Schweizer E, Rickels K, Lucki I. 1986. Resistance to the anti-anxiety effect of buspirone in patients with a history of benzodiazepine use. New England Journal of Medicine, 314: 719–720.

Schweizer E, Rickels K, Weiss S, et al. 1993. Maintenance drug treatment of panic disorder: I. Results of a prospective, placebo-controlled comparison of alprazolam and imipramine. Archives of General Psychiatry, 50: 51–60.

Scrignar CB. 1984. Post-Traumatic Stress Disorder: Diagnosis, Treatment, and Legal Issues. New York: Praeger.

Seedat S, Stein MB. 2004. Double-blind, placebo-controlled assessment of combined clonazepam with paroxetine compared with paroxetine monotherapy for generalized social anxiety disorder. Journal of Clinical Psychiatry, 65: 244–248.

Seligman MEP. 1971. Phobias and preparedness. Behavior Therapy, 2: 307–320.

Sevy S, Papadimitriou G, Surmont W, et al. 1989. Noradrenergic function in generalized anxiety disorder, major depressive disorder, and healthy subjects. Biological Psychiatry, 25: 141–152.

Shafran R, Thordarson DS, Rachman S. 1996. Thought–action fusion in obsessive compulsive disorder. Journal of Anxiety Disorders, 10: 379–391.

Shalev AY. 2002. Acute stress reactions in adults. Biological Psychiatry, 51: 532–543.

Shalev AY, Bleich A, Ursano RJ. 1990. Posttraumatic stress disorder: Somatic comorbidity and effort tolerance. Psychosomatics, 31: 197–203.

Shalev AY, Freedman S, Brandes D, et al. 1997. Predicting PTSD in civilian trauma survivors: Prospective evaluation of self report and clinician administered instruments. British Journal of Psychiatry, 170: 558–564.

Shalev AY, Freedman S, Peri T, et al. 1998a. Prospective study of posttraumatic stress disorder and depression following trauma. American Journal of Psychiatry, 155: 630–637.

Shalev AY, Peri T, Canetti L, et al. 1996. Predictors of PTSD in injured trauma survivors: A prospective study. American Journal of Psychiatry, 153: 219–225.

Shalev AY, Sahar T, Freedman S, et al. 1998b. A prospective study of heart rate response following trauma and the subsequent development of posttraumatic stress disorder. Archives of General Psychiatry, 55: 553–559.

Shapira NA, Ward HE, Mandoki M, et al. 2004. A double-blind, placebo-controlled trial of olanzapine addition in fluoxetine-refractory obsessive-compulsive disorder. Biological Psychiatry, 55: 553–555.

Shapiro AK, Shapiro E. 1992. Evaluation of the reported association of obsessive-compulsive symptoms or disorder with Tourette's disorder. Comprehensive Psychiatry, 33: 152–165.

Shapiro D. 1965. Neurotic Styles. New York: Basic Books.

Shapiro F. 1995. Eye Movement Desensitization and Reprocessing: Basic Principles, Protocols, and Procedures. New York: Guilford Press.

Shavitt RG, Gentil V, Mandetta R. 1992. The association of panic/agoraphobia and asthma: Contributing factors and clinical implications. General Hospital Psychiatry, 14: 420–423.

Shear MK, Brown TA, Barlow DH, et al. 1997. Multicenter collaborative Panic Disorder Severity Scale. American Journal of Psychiatry, 154: 1571–1575.

Shear MK, Cooper AM, Klerman GL, et al. 1993. A psychodynamic model of panic disorder. American Journal of Psychiatry, 150: 859–866.

Sheehan DV, Ballenger J, Jacobson G. 1980. Treatment of endogenous anxiety with phobic, hysterical and hypochondriacal symptoms. Archives of General Psychiatry, 37: 51–59.

Sheehan D, Janavs J, Baker R, et al. 2000. The Worry–Anxiety–Tension Scale. Adapted from the M.I.N.I. International Neuropsychiatric Interview. Tampa FL: University of South Florida.

Sheeran T, Zimmerman M. 2002. Social phobia: Still a neglected anxiety disorder? Journal of Nervous and Mental Disease, 190: 786–788.

Shin LM, Kosslyn SM, McNally RJ, et al. 1997. Visual imagery and perception in posttraumatic stress disorder: A positron emission tomographic investigation. Archives of General Psychiatry, 54: 233–241.

Shin LM, McNally RJ, Kosslyn SM, et al. 1999. Regional cerebral blood flow during script-driven imagery in childhood sexual abuse-related PTSD: A PET investigation. American Journal of Psychiatry, 156: 575–584.

Shore JH, Tatum E, Vollmer WM. 1986. Psychiatric reactions to disaster: The Mt. St. Helen's experience. American Journal of Psychiatry, 143: 590–595.

Silove D, Manicavasagar V, O'Connell D, et al. 1993. Reported early separation anxiety symptoms in patients with panic and generalized anxiety disorders. Australian and New Zealand Journal of Psychiatry, 27: 489–494.

Silove D, Manicavasagar V, O'Connell D, et al. 1995. Genetic factors in early separation anxiety: Implications for the genesis of adult anxiety disorders. Acta Psychiatrica Scandinavica, 92: 17–24.

Silove D, Parker G, Hadzi-Pavlovic D, et al. 1991. Parental representations of patients with panic disorder and generalized anxiety disorder. British Journal of Psychiatry, 159: 835–841.

Simon NM, Safren SA, Otto MW, et al. 2002. Longitudinal outcome with pharmacotherapy in a naturalistic study of panic disorder. Journal of Affective Disorders, 69: 201–208.

Simpson HB, Gorfinkle KS, Liebowitz MR. 1999. Cognitive-behavioral therapy as an adjunct to serotonin reuptake inhibitors in obsessive-compulsive disorder: An open trial. Journal of Clinical Psychiatry, 60: 584–590.

Skoog G, Skoog I. 1999. A 40-year follow-up of patients with obsessive-compulsive disorder. Archives of General Psychiatry, 56: 121–127.

Skre I, Ontad S, Torgersen S, et al. 1993. A twin study of DSM-III-R anxiety disorders. Acta Psychiatrica Scandinavica, 88: 85–92.

Smail P, Stockwell T, Canter S, et al. 1984. Alcohol dependence and phobic anxiety states. British Journal of Psychiatry, 144: 53–57.

Smith K, Bryant RA. 2000. The generality of cognitive bias in acute stress disorder. Behaviour Research and Therapy, 38: 709–715.

Smith MA, Davidson J, Ritchie JC, et al. 1989. The corticotropin releasing hormone test in patients with posttraumatic stress disorder. Biological Psychiatry, 26: 349–355.

Solomon Z, Benbenishty R, Mikulincer M. 1991. The contribution of wartime, pre-war, and post-war factors to self-efficacy: A longitudinal study of combat stress reaction. Journal of Traumatic Stress, 4: 345–361.

Solomon Z, Kotler M, Shalev A, et al. 1989a. Delayed post-traumatic stress disorder. Psychiatry, 52: 128–136.

Solomon Z, Mikulincer M, Benbenishty R. 1989b. Locus of control and combat-related post-traumatic stress disorder: The intervening role of battle intensity, threat appraisal, and coping. British Journal of Clinical Psychology, 28: 131–144.

Southwick SM, Krystal JH, Bremner JD, et al. 1997. Noradrenergic and serotonergic function in posttraumatic stress disorder. Archives of General Psychiatry, 54: 749–758.

Southwick SM, Krystal JH, Morgan CA, et al. 1993. Abnormal noradrenergic function in posttraumatic stress disorder. Archives of General Psychiatry, 50: 266–274.

Spiegel DA, Bruce TJ. 1997. Benzodiazepines and exposure-based cognitive behavior therapies for panic disorder: Conclusions from combined treatment trials. American Journal of Psychiatry, 154: 773–781.

Spiegel DA, Bruce TJ, Gregg SF, et al. 1994. Does cognitive behavior therapy assist slow-taper alprazolam discontinuation in panic disorder? American Journal of Psychiatry, 151: 876–881.

Spinhoven P, Ros M, Westgeest A, et al. 1994. The prevalence of respiratory disorders in panic disorder, major depressive disorder and V-code patients. Behaviour Research and Therapy, 32: 647–649.

Staab JP, Grieger TA, Fullerton CS, et al. 1996. Acute stress disorder, subsequent posttraumatic stress disorder and depression after a series of typhoons. Anxiety, 2: 219–225.

Stahl SM, Gergel I, Li D. 2003. Escitalopram in the treatment of panic disorder: A randomized, double-blind, placebo-controlled trial. Journal of Clinical Psychiatry, 64: 1322–1327.

Stangier U, Heidenreich T, Peitz M, et al. 2003. Cognitive therapy for social phobia: Individual versus group treatment. Behaviour Research and Therapy, 41: 991–1007.

Starcevic V. 1992. Comorbidity models of panic disorder/agoraphobia and personality disturbance. Journal of Personality Disorders, 6: 213–225.

Starcevic V. 1995. Pathological worry in major depression: A preliminary report. Behaviour Research and Therapy, 33: 55–56.

Starcevic V. 1998. Treatment goals for panic disorder. Journal of Clinical Psychopharmacology, 18 (Suppl. 2): 19S–26S.

Starcevic V, Bogojevic G. 1999. The concept of generalized anxiety disorder: Between the too narrow and too wide diagnostic criteria. Psychopathology, 32: 5–11.

Starcevic V, Eric Lj, Kelin K, et al. 1994. The structure of discrete social phobias. European Journal of Psychiatry, 8: 140–148.

Starcevic V, Kellner R, Uhlenhuth EH, et al. 1992a. Panic disorder and hypochondriacal fears and beliefs. Journal of Affective Disorders, 24: 73–85.

Starcevic V, Kellner R, Uhlenhuth EH, et al. 1993a. The phenomenology of panic attacks in panic disorder with and without agoraphobia. Comprehensive Psychiatry, 34: 36–41.

Starcevic V, Kolar D, Latas M, et al. 2002. Panic disorder patients at the time of air strikes. Depression and Anxiety, 16: 152–156.

Starcevic V, Linden M, Uhlenhuth EH, et al. 2004. Treatment of panic disorder with agoraphobia in an anxiety disorders clinic: Factors influencing psychiatrists' treatment choices. Psychiatry Research, 125: 41–52.

Starcevic V, Uhlenhuth EH, Kellner R, et al. 1992b. Patterns of comorbidity in panic disorder and agoraphobia. Psychiatry Research, 42: 171–183.

Starcevic V, Uhlenhuth EH, Kellner R, et al. 1993b. Comorbidity in panic disorder: II. Chronology of appearance and pathogenic comorbidity. Psychiatry Research, 46: 285–293.

Stein DJ, Spadaccini E, Hollander E. 1995. Meta-analysis of pharmacotherapy trials for obsessive-compulsive disorder. International Clinical Psychopharmacology, 10: 11–18.

Stein DJ, Versiani M, Hair T, et al. 2002. Efficacy of paroxetine for relapse prevention in social phobia: A 24-week study. Archives of General Psychiatry, 59: 1111–1118.

Stein MB, Chartier MJ, Hazen AL, et al. 1998a. A direct-interview family study of generalized social phobia. American Journal of Psychiatry, 155: 90–97.

Stein MB, Forde DR, Anderson G, et al. 1997a. Obsessive-compulsive disorder in the community: An epidemiological study with clinical reappraisal. American Journal of Psychiatry, 154: 1120–1126.

Stein MB, Fuetsch M, Müller N, et al. 2001. Social anxiety disorder and the risk of depression: A prospective community study of adolescents and young adults. Archives of General Psychiatry, 58: 251–256.

Stein MB, Fyer AJ, Davidson JRT, et al. 1999a. Fluvoxamine treatment of social phobia (social anxiety disorder): A double-blind, placebo-controlled study. American Journal of Psychiatry, 156: 756–760.

Stein MB, Heuser IJ, Juncos JL, et al. 1990a. Anxiety disorders in patients with Parkinson's disease. American Journal of Psychiatry, 147: 217–220.

Stein MB, Jang KJ, Livesley WJ. 1999b. Heritability of anxiety sensitivity: A twin study. American Journal of Psychiatry, 156: 246–251.

Stein MB, Kean YM. 2000. Disability and quality of life in social phobia: Epidemiologic findings. American Journal of Psychiatry, 157: 1606–1613.

Stein MB, Koverola C, Hanna C, et al. 1997b. Hippocampal volume in women victimized by childhood sexual abuse. Psychological Medicine, 27: 951–959.

Stein MB, Liebowitz MR, Lydiard RB, et al. 1998b. Paroxetine treatment of generalized social phobia (social anxiety disorder): A randomized controlled trial. Journal of the American Medical Association, 280: 708–713.

Stein MB, McQuaid JR, Laffaye C, et al. 1999c. Social phobia in the primary care medical setting. Journal of Family Practice, 48: 514–519.

Stein MB, Tancer ME, Gelernter CS, et al. 1990b. Major depression in patients with social phobia. American Journal of Psychiatry, 147: 637–639.

Stein MB, Torgrud LJ, Walker JR. 2000. Social phobia symptoms, subtypes, and severity: Findings from a community survey. Archives of General Psychiatry, 57: 1046–1052.

Stein MB, Walker JR, Forde DR. 1994. Setting diagnostic thresholds for social phobia: Considerations from a community survey of social anxiety. American Journal of Psychiatry, 151: 408–412.

Stein MB, Walker JR, Hazen AL, et al. 1997c. Full and partial posttraumatic stress disorder: Findings from a community survey. American Journal of Psychiatry, 154: 1114–1119.

Stein MB, Yehuda R, Koverola C, et al. 1997d. Enhanced dexamethasone suppression of plasma cortisol in adult women traumatized by childhood sexual abuse. Biological Psychiatry, 42: 680 686.

Steketee G, Eisen J, Dyck I, et al. 1999. Predictors of course in obsessive-compulsive disorder. Psychiatry Research, 89: 229–238.

Stemberger RT, Turner SM, Beidel DC, et al. 1995. Social phobia: An analysis of possible developmental factors. Journal of Abnormal Psychology, 104: 526–531.

Stocchi F, Nordera G, Jokinen RH, et al. 2003. Efficacy and tolerability of paroxetine for the long-term treatment of generalized anxiety disorder. Journal of Clinical Psychiatry, 64: 250–258.

Stopa L, Clark DM. 1993. Cognitive processes in social phobia. Behaviour Research and Therapy, 31: 255–267.

Stopa L, Clark DM. 2000. Social phobia and interpretation of social events. Behaviour Research and Therapy, 38: 273–283.

Stravynski A, Lamontagne Y, Lavellee Y-J. 1986. Clinical phobias and avoidant personality disorder among alcoholics admitted to an alcoholism rehabilitation setting. Canadian Journal of Psychiatry, 31: 714–719.

Stravynski A, Marks I, Yule W. 1982. Social skills problems in neurotic Outpatients: Social skills training with and without cognitive modification. Archives of General Psychiatry, 39: 1378–1385.

Swedo SE. 1994. Sydenham's chorea: A model for autoimmune neuropsychiatric disorders. Journal of the American Medical Association: 272: 1788–1791.

Swedo SE, Leonard HL, Garvey M, et al. 1998. Pediatric Autoimmune Neuropsychiatric Disorders Associated with Streptococcus Infection (PANDAS): Clinical description of the first 50 cases. American Journal of Psychiatry, 155: 264–271.

Swedo SE, Leonard HL, Kiessling LS. 1994. Speculations on antineuronal antibody-mediated neuropsychiatric disorders of childhood. Pediatrics, 93: 323–326.

Swedo SE, Leonard HL, Kruesi MJ, et al. 1992. Cerebrospinal fluid neurochemistry in children and adolescents with obsessive-compulsive disorder. Archives of General Psychiatry, 49: 29–36.

Swedo SE, Rapoport JL, Leonard H, et al. 1989a. Obsessive compulsive disorder in children and adolescents: Clinical phenomenology of 70 consecutive cases. Archives of General Psychiatry, 46: 335–341.

Swedo SE, Schapiro MB, Grady CL, et al. 1989b. Cerebral glucose metabolism in childhood-onset obsessive-compulsive disorder. Archives of General Psychiatry, 46: 518–523.

Swoboda H, Amering M, Windhaber J, et al. 2003. The long-term course of panic disorder—An 11-year follow-up. Journal of Anxiety Disorders, 17: 223–232.

Szegedi A, Wetzel H, Leal M, et al. 1996. Combination treatment with clomipramine and fluvoxamine: Drug monitoring, safety, and tolerability data. Journal of Clinical Psychiatry, 57: 257–264.

Szeszko PR, Robinson D, Alvir JMJ, et al. 1999. Orbital frontal and amygdala volume reductions in obsessive-compulsive disorder. Archives of General Psychiatry, 56: 913–919.

Tarrier N, Pilgrim H, Sommerfield C, et al. 1999. A randomized trial of cognitive therapy and imaginal exposure in the treatment of chronic posttraumatic stress disorder. Journal of Consulting and Clinical Psychology, 67: 13–18.

Taylor S. 1995. Anxiety sensitivity: Theoretical perspectives and recent findings. Behaviour Research and Therapy, 33: 243–258.

Taylor S. 1996. Meta-analysis of CBTs for social phobia. Journal of Behavior Therapy and Experimental Psychiatry, 27: 1–9.

Taylor S, Koch WJ, McNally RJ. 1992. How does anxiety sensitivity vary across the anxiety disorders? Journal of Anxiety Disorders, 6: 249–259.

Taylor S, Thordarson DS, Maxfield L, et al. 2003. Comparative efficacy, speed, and adverse effects of three PTSD treatments: Exposure therapy, EMDR, and relaxation training. Journal of Consulting and Clinical Psychology, 71: 330–338.

Telch MJ, Agras WS, Taylor CB, et al. 1985. Combined pharmacological and behavioral treatment for agoraphobia. Behaviour Research and Therapy, 23: 325–335.

Telch MJ, Brouillard M, Telch CF, et al. 1989a. Role of cognitive appraisal in panic-related avoidance. Behaviour Research and Therapy, 27: 373–383.

Telch MJ, Lucas JA, Nelson P. 1989b. Nonclinical panic in college students: An investigation of prevalence and symptomatology. Journal of Abnormal Psychology, 98: 300–306.

Telch MJ, Lucas JA, Schmidt NB, et al. 1993. Group cognitive-behavioral treatment of panic disorder. Behaviour Research and Therapy, 31: 279–287.

Tesar GE, Rosenbaum JF, Pollack MH, et al. 1991. Double-blind, placebo-controlled comparison of clonazepam and alprazolam for panic disorder. Journal of Clinical Psychiatry, 52: 69–76.

Thayer JF, Friedman BH, Borkovec TD. 1996. Autonomic characteristics of generalized anxiety disorder and worry. Biological Psychiatry, 39: 255–266.

Thomas SE, Thevos AK, Randall CL. 1999. Alcoholics with and without social phobia: A comparison of substance use and psychiatric variables. Journal of Studies on Alcohol, 60: 472–479.

Thompson AH, Bland RC, Orn HT. 1989. Relationship and chronology of depression, agoraphobia, and panic disorder in the general population. Journal of Nervous and Mental Disease, 177: 456–463.

Thoren P, Asberg M, Cronholm B, et al. 1980. Clomipramine treatment of obsessive-compulsive disorder: I. A controlled clinical trial. Archives of General Psychiatry, 37: 1281–1285.

Thorpe SJ, Salkovskis PM. 1995. Phobic beliefs: Do cognitive factors play a role in specific phobias? Behaviour Research and Therapy, 33: 805–816.

Thyer B, Himle J. 1985. Temporal relationship between panic attack onset and phobic avoidance in agoraphobia. Behaviour Research and Therapy, 23: 607–608.

Tiffon L, Coplan JD, Papp LA, et al. 1994. Augmentation strategies with tricyclic or fluoxetine treatment in seven partially responsive panic disorder patients. Journal of Clinical Psychiatry, 55: 66–69.

Tiihonen J, Kuikka J, Rasanen P, et al. 1997. Cerebral benzodiazepine receptor binding and distribution in generalized anxiety disorder: A fractional analysis. Molecular Psychiatry, 2: 463–471.

Tiller JW, Biddle N, Maguire KP, et al. 1988. The dexamethasone suppression test and plasma dexamethasone in generalized anxiety disorder. Biological Psychiatry, 23: 261–270.

Tollefson GD, Rampey AH, Potvin JH, et al. 1994. A multicenter investigation of fixed-dose fluoxetine in the treatment of obsessive-compulsive disorder. Archives of General Psychiatry, 51: 559–567.

Tolin DF, Abramowitz JS, Brigidi BD, et al. 2003. Intolerance of uncertainty in obsessive-compulsive disorder. Journal of Anxiety Disorders, 17: 233–242.

Tolin DF, Lohr JM, Sawchuk CN, et al. 1997. Disgust and disgust sensitivity in blood-injection-injury and spider phobia. Behaviour Research and Therapy, 35: 949–953.

Toni C, Perugi G, Frare F, et al. 2000. A prospective naturalistic study of 326 panic-agoraphobic patients treated with antidepressants. Pharmacopsychiatry, 33: 121–131.

Torgersen S. 1983. Genetic factors in anxiety disorders. Archives of General Psychiatry, 40: 1085–1089.

Trower P, Yardley K, Bryant B, et al. 1978. The treatment of social failure: A comparison of anxiety-reduction and skills-acquisition procedures on two social problems. Behavior Modification, 2: 41–60.

True WR, Rice J, Eisen SA, et al. 1993. A twin study of genetic and environmental contributions to liability for posttraumatic stress symptoms. Archives of General Psychiatry, 50: 257–264.

Trull TJ, Nietzel MT, Main A. 1988. The use of meta-analysis to assess the clinical significance of behavior therapy for agoraphobia. Behavior Therapy, 19: 527–538.

Tucker P, Zaninelli R, Yehuda R, et al. 2001. Paroxetine in the treatment of chronic posttraumatic stress disorder: Results of a placebo-controlled, flexible-dosage trial. Journal of Clinical Psychiatry, 62: 860–868.

Turner SM, Beidel DC, Borden JW, et al. 1991. Social phobia: Axis I and II correlates. Journal of Abnormal Psychology, 100: 102–106.

Turner SM, Beidel DC, Cooley-Quille MR. 1995. Two-year follow-up of social phobics treated with social effectiveness therapy. Behaviour Research and Therapy, 33: 553–555.

Turner SM, Beidel DC, Dancu CV, et al. 1989. An empirically derived inventory to measure social fears and anxiety: The Social Phobia and Anxiety Inventory. Psychological Assessment, 1: 35–40.

Turner SM, Beidel DC, Townsley RM. 1990. Social phobia: Relationship to shyness. Behaviour Research and Therapy, 28: 497–505.

Turner SM, Beidel DC, Townsley RM. 1992. Social phobia: A comparison of specific and generalized subtypes and avoidant personality disorder. Journal of Abnormal Psychology, 101: 326–331.

Tyrer P. 1984. Classification of anxiety. British Journal of Psychiatry, 144: 78–83.

Tyrer P. 1985. Neurosis divisible? Lancet, I: 685–688.

Tyrer P. 1999. Anxiety: A Multidisciplinary Review. Singapore: World Scientific Publishing Company.

Tyrer P, Seivewright N, Ferguson B, et al. 1992. The general neurotic syndrome: A coaxial diagnosis of anxiety, depression and personality disorder. Acta Psychiatrica Scandinavica, 85: 201–206.

Uhde T, Boulenger J, Geraci H, et al. 1985. Longitudinal course of panic disorder. Progress in Neuropsychopharmacology and Biological Psychiatry, 9: 39–51.

Uhlenhuth EH, Balter MB, Ban TA, et al. 1999. International Study of Expert Judgment on Therapeutic Use of Benzodiazepines and Other Psychotherapeutic Medications: VI. Trends in recommendations for the pharmacotherapy of anxiety disorders, 1992–1997. Depression and Anxiety 9: 107–116.

Uhlenhuth EH, Balter MB, Mellinger GD, et al. 1983. Symptom checklist syndromes in the general population: Correlations with psychotherapeutic drug use. Archives of General Psychiatry, 40: 1167–1173.

Uhlenhuth EH, DeWit H, Balter MB, et al. 1988. Risks and benefits of long-term benzodiazepine use. Journal of Clinical Psychopharmacology, 8: 161–167.

Uhlenhuth EH, Matuzas W, Warner TD, et al. 2000. Do antidepressants selectively suppress spontaneous (unexpected) panic attacks? A replication. Journal of Clinical Psychopharmacology, 20: 622–627.

Uhlenhuth EH, Warner TD, Matuzas W. 2002. Interactive model of therapeutic response in panic disorder: Moclobemide, a case in point. Journal of Clinical Psychopharmacology, 22: 275–284.

Ullman SE, Filipas HH. 2001. Predictors of PTSD symptom severity and social reactions in sexual assault victims. Journal of Traumatic Stress, 14: 369–389.

Ursano RJ, Fullerton CS, Epstein RS, et al. 1999a. Peritraumatic dissociation and posttraumatic stress disorder following motor vehicle accidents. American Journal of Psychiatry, 156: 1808–1810.

Ursano RJ, Fullerton CS, Epstein RS, et al. 1999b. Acute and chronic posttraumatic stress disorder in motor vehicle accident victims. American Journal of Psychiatry, 156: 589–595.

Ustun TB, Sartorius N. 1995. Mental Illness in General Health Care: An International Study. Chichester: Wiley.

Vallejo J, Olivares J, Marcos T, et al. 1992. Clomipramine versus phenelzine in obsessive-compulsive disorder: A controlled clinical trial. British Journal of Psychiatry, 161: 665–670.

Van Ameringen MA, Lane RM, Walker JR, et al. 2001. Sertraline treatment of generalized social phobia: A 20-week, double-blind, placebo-controlled study. American Journal of Psychiatry, 158: 275–281.

Van Ameringen M, Mancini C, Styan G, et al. 1991. Relationship of social phobia with other psychiatric illness. Journal of Affective Disorders, 21: 93–99.

Van Ameringen M, Mancini C, Wilson C. 1996. Buspirone augmentation of selective serotonin reuptake inhibitors (SSRIs) in social phobia. Journal of Affective Disorders, 39: 115–121.

van Balkom AJLM, Bakker A, Spinhoven P, et al. 1997. A meta-analysis of the treatment of panic disorder with or without agoraphobia: A comparison of psychopharmacological, cognitive-behavioral, and combination treatments. Journal of Nervous and Mental Disease, 185: 510–516.

van Balkom AJ, de Haan E, van Oppen P, et al. 1998. Cognitive and behavioral therapies alone versus in combination with fluvoxamine in the treatment of obsessive-compulsive disorder. Journal of Nervous and Mental Disease, 186: 492–499.

van den Hout M, Arntz A, Hoekstra R. 1994. Exposure reduced agoraphobia but not panic and cognitive therapy reduced panic but not agoraphobia. Behaviour Research and Therapy, 32: 447–451.

van den Hout M, Kindt M. 2003. Phenomenological validity of an OCD-memory model and the remember/know distinction. Behaviour Research and Therapy, 41: 369–378.

van der Kolk BA, Boyd H, Krystal J, et al. 1984. Post-traumatic stress disorder as a biologically based disorder: Implications of the animal model of inescapable shock. In van der Kolk BA, editor: Post-Traumatic Stress Disorder: Psychological and Biological Sequelae. Washington, DC: American Psychiatric Press, pp. 123–134.

van der Kolk BA, Dreyfuss D, Michaels B, et al. 1994. Fluoxetine treatment in posttraumatic stress disorder. Journal of Clinical Psychiatry, 55: 517–522.

van der Kolk BA, McFarlane AC, Weiseath L, editors. 1996. Traumatic Stress: The Effects of Overwhelming Experience on Mind, Body, and Society. New York: Guilford Press.

van Dyck R, van Balkom AJLM. 1997. Combination therapy for anxiety disorders. In den Boer JA, editor: Clinical Management of Anxiety. New York: Marcel Dekker, pp. 109–136.

Van Emmerick AAP, Kamphuis JH, Hulsbosch AM, et al. 2002. Single session debriefing after psychological trauma: A meta-analysis. Lancet, 360: 766–771.

van Oppen P, De Haan E, Van Balkom AJLM, et al. 1995. Cognitive therapy and exposure in vivo in the treatment of obsessive compulsive disorder. Behaviour Research and Therapy, 33: 379–390.

van Velzen CJM, Emmelkamp PMJ, Scholing A. 2000. Generalized social phobia versus avoidant personality disorder: Differences in psychopathology, personality traits, and social and occupational functioning. Journal of Anxiety Disorders, 14: 395–411.

van Vliet IM, den Boer JA, Westenberg HGM. 1994. Psychopharmacological treatment of social phobia: A double-blind placebo-controlled study with fluvoxamine. Psychopharmacology, 115: 128–134.

Verburg K, Griez E, Meijer J, et al. 1995. Discrimination between panic disorder and generalized anxiety disorder by 35% carbon dioxide challenge. American Journal of Psychiatry, 152: 1081–1083.

Vermetten E, Vythilingam M, Southwick SM, et al. 2003. Long-term treatment with paroxetine increases verbal declarative memory and hippocampal volume in posttraumatic stress disorder. Biological Psychiatry, 54: 693–702.

Versiani M, Cassano G, Perugi G, et al. 2002. Reboxetine, a selective norepinephrine reuptake inhibitor, is an effective and well-tolerated treatment for panic disorder. Journal of Clinical Psychiatry, 63: 31–37.

Versiani M, Nardi AE, Mundim FD, et al. 1992. Pharmacotherapy of social phobia: A controlled study with moclobemide and phenelzine. British Journal of Psychiatry, 161: 353–360.

Villeponteaux VA, Lydiard RB, Laraia MT, et al. 1992. The effects of pregnancy on preexisting panic disorder. Journal of Clinical Psychiatry, 53: 201–203.

Von Korff M, Eaton WW, Keyl P. 1985. The epidemiology of panic attacks and panic disorder: Results of three community surveys. American Journal of Epidemiology, 122: 970–981.

Vrana SR, Cuthbert BN, Lang PJ. 1986. Fear imagery and text processing. Psychophysiology, 23: 247–253.

Vythilingum B, Stein DJ, Soifer S. 2002. Is "shy bladder syndrome" a subtype of social phobia? A survey of people with paruresis. Depression and Anxiety, 16: 84–87.

Wacker HR, Mullejans R, Klein KH, et al. 1992. Identification of cases of anxiety disorders and affective disorders in the community according to ICD-10 and DSM-III-R by using the Composite International Diagnostic Interview (CIDI). International Journal of Methods of Psychiatric Research, 2: 91–100.

Wade AG, Lepola U, Koponen HJ, et al. 1997. The effects of citalopram in panic disorder. British Journal of Psychiatry, 170: 549–553.

Walker EA, Gelfand AN, Gelfand MD, et al. 1995. Psychiatric diagnoses, sexual and physical victimization, and disability in patients with irritable bowel syndrome or inflammatory bowel disease. Psychological Medicine, 25: 1259–1267.

Walker EA, Roy-Byrne PP, Katon W, et al. 1990. Psychiatric illness and irritable bowel syndrome: A comparison with inflammatory bowel disease. American Journal of Psychiatry, 147: 1656–1661.

Walker JR, Van Ameringen MA, Swinson R, et al. 2000. Prevention of relapse in generalized social phobia: Results of a 24-week study in responders to 20 weeks of sertraline treatment. Journal of Clinical Psychopharmacology, 20: 636–644.

Wallace ST, Alden LE. 1997. Social phobia and positive social events: The price of success. Journal of Abnormal Psychology, 106: 416–424.

Warda G, Bryant RA. 1998a. Cognitive bias in acute stress disorder. Behaviour Research and Therapy, 36: 1177–1183.

Warda G, Bryant RA. 1998b. Thought control strategies in acute stress Disorder. Behaviour Research and Therapy, 36: 1171–1175.

Wardle J. 1990. Behaviour therapy and benzodiazepines: Allies or antagonists? British Journal of Psychiatry, 156: 163–168.

Wardle J, Hayward P, Higgitt A, et al. 1994. Effects of concurrent diazepam treatment on the outcome of exposure therapy in agoraphobia. Behaviour Research and Therapy, 32: 203–215.

Warshaw MG, Dolan RT, Keller MB. 2000. Suicidal behavior in patients with current or past panic disorder: Five years of prospective data from the Harvard/Brown Anxiety Research Program. American Journal of Psychiatry, 157: 1876–1878.

Warshaw MG, Fierman E, Pratt L, et al. 1993. Quality of life and dissociation in anxiety disorder patients with histories of trauma or PTSD. American Journal of Psychiatry, 150: 1512–1516.

Watson JB, Rayner R. 1920. Conditioned emotional reactions. Journal of Experimental Psychology, 3: 1–14.

Watt MC, Stewart SH, Cox BJ. 1998. A retrospective study of the learning history origins of anxiety sensitivity. Behaviour Research and Therapy, 36: 505–525.

Weiller E, Bisserbe JC, Boyer P, et al. 1996. Social phobia in general health care: An unrecognised undertreated disabling disorder. British Journal of Psychiatry, 168: 169–174.

Weiss DS, Marmar CR. 1996. The Impact of Event Scale—Revised. In Wilson JP, Keane TM, editors: Assessing Psychological Trauma and PTSD. New York: Guilford Press, pp. 399–411.

Weissman MM. 1993. Family genetic studies of panic disorder. Journal of Psychiatric Research, 27 (Suppl. 1): 69–78.

Weissman MM, Bland RC, Canino GJ, et al. 1994. The cross-national epidemiology of obsessive compulsive disorder. Journal of Clinical Psychiatry, 55 (Suppl. 3): 5–10.

Weissman MM, Klerman GL, Markowitz JS, et al. 1989. Suicidal ideation and suicide attempts in panic disorder. New England Journal of Medicine, 321: 1209–1214.

Weissman MM, Markowitz JS, Ouellette R, et al. 1990. Panic disorder and cardiovascular/cerebrovascular problems: Results from a community survey. American Journal of Psychiatry, 147: 1504–1508.

Wells A. 1994. Attention and the control of worry. In Davey GCL, Tallis F, editors: Worrying: Perspectives on Theory, Assessment and Treatment. New York: Wiley, pp. 91–114.

Wells A, Papageorgiou C. 1999. The observer perspective: Biased imagery in social phobia, agoraphobia, and blood/injury phobia. Behaviour Research and Therapy, 37: 653–658.

Wells A, Papageorgiou C. 2001. Social phobic interoception: Effects of bodily information on anxiety, beliefs and self-processing. Behaviour Research and Therapy, 39: 1–11.

Wenzlaff EM, Wegner DM. 2000. Thought suppression. Annual Review of Psychology, 51: 59–91.

Wessely S, 2003. In debate: Psychological debriefing is a waste of time. For. British Journal of Psychiatry, 183: 12–13.

Westra HA, Stewart SH. 1998. Cognitive behavioural therapy and pharmacotherapy: Complementary or contradictory approaches to the treatment of anxiety? Clinical Psychology Review, 18: 307–340.

Westra HA, Stewart SH, Conrad BE. 2002. Naturalistic manner of benzodiazepine use and cognitive behavioral therapy outcome in panic disorder with agoraphobia. Journal of Anxiety Disorders, 16: 233–246.

White WB, Baker CH. 1986. Episodic hypertension secondary to panic disorder. Archives of Internal Medicine, 146: 1129–1130.

Wiborg IM, Dahl AA. 1996. Does brief dynamic psychotherapy reduce the relapse rate of panic disorder? Archives of General Psychiatry, 53: 689–694.

Windle M, Windle RC, Scheidt DM, et al. 1995. Physical and sexual abuse and associated mental disorders among alcoholic inpatients. American Journal of Psychiatry, 152: 1322–1328.

Winfield I, George LK, Swartz M, et al. 1990. Sexual assault and psychiatric disorders among a community sample of women. American Journal of Psychiatry, 147: 335–341.

Winsberg ME, Cassic KS, Koran LM. 1999. Hoarding in obsessive-compulsive disorder: A report of 20 cases. Journal of Clinical Psychiatry, 60: 591–597.

Wittchen H-U, Carter RM, Pfister H, et al. 2000a. Disabilities and quality of life in pure and comorbid generalized anxiety disorder and major depression in a national survey. International Clinical Psychopharmacology, 15: 319–328.

Wittchen H-U, Fuetsch M, Sonntag H, et al. 2000b. Disability and quality of life in pure and comorbid social phobia: Findings from a controlled study. European Psychiatry, 15: 46–58.

Wittchen H-U, Kessler RC, Beeselo K, et al. 2002. Generalized anxiety and depression in primary care: Prevalence, recognition and management. Journal of Clinical Psychiatry, 63: 24–34.

Wittchen H-U, Stein MB, Kessler RC. 1999. Social fears and social phobia in a community sample of adolescents and young adults: Prevalence, risk factors and co-morbidity. Psychological Medicine, 29: 309–323.

Wittchen H-U, Zhao S, Kessler RC, et al. 1994. DSM-III-R generalized anxiety disorder in the National Comorbidity Survey. Archives of General Psychiatry, 51: 355–364.

Wlazlo Z, Schroeder-Hartwig K, Hand I, et al. 1990. Exposure in vivo vs. social skills training for social phobia: Long-term outcome and differential effects. Behaviour Research and Therapy, 28: 181–193.

Wolpe J. 1958. Psychotherapy by Reciprocal Inhibition. Stanford, CA: Stanford University Press.

Wolpe J, Lang PJA. 1964. A Fear Survey Schedule for use in behavior therapy. Behaviour Research and Therapy, 2: 27–30.

Wolpe J, Lazarus AA. 1966. Behavior Therapy Techniques. New York: Pergamon Press.

Wolpe J, Rowan VC. 1988. Panic disorder: A product of classical conditioning. Behaviour Research and Therapy, 26: 441–450.

Woodman CL, Noyes R, Black DW, et al. 1999. A 5-year follow-up study of generalized anxiety disorder and panic disorder. Journal of Nervous and Mental Disease, 187: 3–9.

Woody SR. 1996. Effects of focus of attention on social phobics' anxiety and social performance. Journal of Abnormal Psychology, 105: 61–69.

World Health Organization. 1992. The ICD-10 (International Classification of Diseases) Classification of Mental and Behavioural Disorders: Clinical Descriptions and Diagnostic Guidelines. Geneva: World Health Organization.

Wu JC, Buchsbaum MS, Hershey TG, et al. 1991. PET in generalized anxiety disorder. Biological Psychiatry, 29: 1181–1199.

Yehuda R, Boisoneau D, Lowy MT, et al. 1995. Dose-response changes in plasma cortisol and lymphocyte glucocorticoid receptors following dexamethasone administration in combat veterans with and without posttraumatic stress disorder. Archives of General Psychiatry, 52: 583–593.

Yehuda R, Levengood RA, Schmeidler J, et al. 1996. Increased pituitary activation following metyrapone administration in post-traumatic stress disorder. Psychoneuroendocrinology, 21: 1–16.

Yehuda R, Lowy MT, Southwick SM, et al. 1991. Increased lymphocyte glucocorticoid receptor number in posttraumatic stress disorder. American Journal of Psychiatry, 148: 499–504.

Yehuda R, McFarlane AC, Shalev AY. 1998a. Predicting the development of posttraumatic stress disorder from the acute response to a traumatic event. Biological Psychiatry, 44: 1305–1313.

Yehuda R, Schmeidler J, Wainberg M, et al. 1998b. Vulnerability to posttraumatic stress disorder in adult offspring of Holocaust survivors. American Journal of Psychiatry, 155: 1163–1171.

Yehuda R, Siever LJ, Teicher MH, et al. 1998c. Plasma norepinephrine and 3-methoxy-4-hydroxyphenylglycol concentrations and severity of depression in combat posttraumatic stress disorder and major depressive disorder. Biological Psychiatry, 44: 56–63.

Yehuda R, Southwick SM, Krystal JH, et al. 1993. Enhanced suppression of cortisol following dexamethasone administration in posttraumatic stress disorder. American Journal of Psychiatry, 150: 83–86.

Yehuda R, Southwick SM, Nussbaum G, et al. 1990. Low urinary cortisol excretion in PTSD. Journal of Nervous and Mental Disease, 178: 366–369.

Yellowlees PM, Alpers JH, Bowden JJ, et al. 1987. Psychiatric morbidity in patients with chronic airflow obstruction. Medical Journal of Australia, 146: 305–307.

Yellowlees PM, Haynor S, Potts N, et al. 1988. Psychiatric morbidity in patients with life-threatening asthma: Initial report of a controlled study. Medical Journal of Australia, 149: 246–249.

Yerkes RM, Dodson JD. 1908. The relation of strength of stimulus to rapidity of habit-formation. Journal of Comparative Neurology and Psychology, 18: 459–482.

Yonkers KA, Zlotnick C, Allsworth J, et al. 1998. Is the course of panic disorder the same in women and men? American Journal of Psychiatry, 155: 596–602.

Zaidi LY, Foy DW. 1994. Childhood abuse and combat-related PTSD. Journal of Traumatic Stress, 7: 33–42.

Zandbergen J, Bright M, Pols H, et al. 1991. Higher lifetime prevalence of respiratory diseases in panic disorder. American Journal of Psychiatry, 148: 1583–1585.

Zisook S, Braff DL, Click MA. 1985. Monoamine oxidase inhibitors in the treatment of atypical depression. Journal of Clinical Psychopharmacology, 5: 131–137.

Zisook S, Chentsova-Dutton YE, Smith-Vaniz A, et al. 2000. Nefazodone in patients with treatment-refractory posttraumatic stress disorder. Journal of Clinical Psychiatry, 61: 203–208.

Zitrin CM, Klein DF, Woerner MG. 1980. Treatment of agoraphobia with group exposure in vivo and imipramine. Archives of General Psychiatry, 37: 63–72.

Zitrin CM, Ross DC. 1988. Early separation anxiety and adult agoraphobia. Journal of Nervous and Mental Disease, 176: 621–625.

Zlotnick C, Shea MT, Rosen KH, et al. 1997. An affect-management group for women with posttraumatic stress disorder and histories of childhood sexual abuse. Journal of Traumatic Stress, 10: 425–436.

Zlotnick C, Warshaw M, Shea MT, et al. 1999. Chronicity in posttraumatic stress disorder (PTSD) and predictors of course of comorbid PTSD in patients with anxiety disorders. Journal of Traumatic Stress, 12: 89–100.

Zoellner LA, Foa EB, Bartholomew DB. 1999. Interpersonal friction and PTSD in female victims of sexual and nonsexual assault. Journal of Traumatic Stress, 12: 689–700.

Zohar J, Amital D, Miodownik C, et al. 2002. Double-blind placebo-controlled pilot study of sertraline in military veterans with posttraumatic stress disorder. Journal of Clinical Psychopharmacology, 22: 190–195.

Zohar J, Insel TR, Zohar-Kadouch RC, et al. 1988. Serotonergic responsivity in obsessive-compulsive disorder: Effects of chronic clomipramine treatment. Archives of General Psychiatry, 45: 167–172.

Index

Acrophobia, 194. *See also* Phobia of heights
Acute stress disorder, 3, 3*t*, 288, 295*t*, 296, 296*t*, 297, 307, 307*t*, 333–336. *See also* Posttraumatic stress disorder
Acute stress reaction, 4*t*
Adjustment disorders, 4, 4*t*
Agoraphobia. *See also* Avoidance; Panic disorder
  assessment of, 36–38, 201
  behavior therapy for, 89–90, 92, 92*t*, 93–95, 97–99, 101. *See also* Exposure-based therapy
  classification of, 2–3, 3*t*, 4*t*
  claustrophobia and, 44, 44*t*, 198–199, 199*t*, 205
  cognitive accounts of, 31*t*, 32, 66
  conceptualization of, 14, 25, 25*t*, 26, 26*t*, 27, 31
  controversies associated with, 6*t*, 29, 31
  couple therapy for, 95–96
  course of, 51
  demographic data for, 32, 47, 198, 199*t*
  dental phobia and, 197
  depression and, 32, 44*t*, 45
  developmental and childhood factors associated with, 68–69, 72. *See also* Behavioral inhibition; Childhood separation experiences; Separation anxiety
  diagnostic criteria for, 29, 37, 157*t*,
  help-seeking for, 47–48
  impairment caused by, 27
  marital therapy for, 95–96
  obsessive-compulsive disorder and, 44, 44*t*, 45
  onset of, 48, 198, 199*t*
  panic attacks and, 2, 6*t*, 14, 17, 17*t*, 25, 25*t*, 26, 26*t*, 27–29, 31, 31*t*, 37, 44, 51, 71, 160, 160*t*, 196–199, 199*t*, 200
  panic disorder and, 6*t*, 14–15, 29, 31, 31*t*, 32, 36–37, 47
  partner relationships and, 71–72, 95–96
  personality disorders and, 35
  phobia of driving and, 44, 44*t*, 196, 199–200, 205
  phobia of flying and, 25, 44, 44*t*, 196, 199–200
  phobia of heights and, 44, 44*t*, 200
  physical symptoms associated with, 27, 41, 160, 160*t*, 198, 199*t*

Anxiety management techniques;
Exposure-based therapy; Muscle
relaxation
behavioral model of, 314. *See also*
Classical conditioning
chronic, 290, 299, 302, 302*t*, 304, 306*t*,
330, 336, 341
classification of, 3, 3*t*, 4*t*, 6*t*
cognitive models of, 308*t*, 316–320, 341.
See also Dual representation theory;
Dysfunctional beliefs; Emotional
processing theory; Information
processing; Network model of
posttraumatic stress disorder;
Posttraumatic disorder and
memory disturbance;
Responsibility appraisals;
Traumatic memories
cognitive therapy for, 320, 337*t*, 339–
342
cognitive-behavioral therapy for,
318–319, 333, 335–337, 337*t*,
340–342. *See also* Cognitive
processing therapy; Stress
inoculation training
combat-related, 284–285, 285*t*, 300–301,
301*t*, 309–310, 313, 323*t*, 326, 328,
338, 340–342
combined treatment for, 321–322, 330,
343–344
complex, 289, 291
complications of, 277, 285, 292–293, 302,
302*t*, 304, 340
concentration camp experience and,
285–286, 286*t*, 289, 305
conceptualization of, 276–277, 278*f*
controversies associated with, 5, 6*t*
conversion disorder and, 283
course of, 288, 301–302, 302*t*, 303–304
demographic data for, 300–301, 301*t*
depression and. *See* Depression
developmental and childhood factors
associated with, 306*t*. *See also*
Childhood abuse; Childhood
separation experiences
diagnostic criteria for, 293–294
dissociative disorders and, 6*t*, 291, 295,
295*t*, 298
dissociative symptoms and, 282–284,
291, 296*t*, 305, 308*t*, 321. *See also*
Depersonalization; Derealization
early treatment for, 305, 321–323, 323*t*,
324, 333, 335–336

generalized anxiety disorder and. *See*
Generalized anxiety disorder
genetic aspects of, 309–310
group therapy for, 333, 342
help-seeking for, 321
impairment caused by, 280, 288, 302,
302*t*, 304
injuries and, 288, 288*t*, 307*t*, 340
litigation and, 277, 283, 288, 288*t*, 290,
298, 300, 340
malingering and, 295, 295*t*, 298, 300
medical conditions and, 303*t*, 304, 307*t*
memory disturbance and, 6*t*, 277,
282–283, 294, 308*t*, 313–314,
319–320, 327
model of alternate reprocessing and
avoidance for, 315–316
natural disasters and, 288–289, 300,
304–305
neuroendocrinological changes and. *See*
Cortisol; Hypothalamic-pituitary-
adrenal axis
neuroimaging studies of, 309*t*, 313–314.
See also Hippocampus; Limbic
system; Visual cortex
neurotransmitter systems associated
with, 311–312. *See also*
Norepinephrine system; Serotonin
system
obsessive-compulsive disorder and. *See*
Obsessive-compulsive disorder
onset of, 299
pain and, 284, 288, 288*t*, 291, 307*t*, 340
panic disorder and. *See* Panic disorder
partial, 289
personality changes and, 277, 289, 302,
302*t*, 341
personality disorders and, 289, 295*t*,
298, 306*t*
pharmacotherapy for, 311–313, 321–323,
323*t*, 324, 324*t*, 325, 325*t*, 326–327,
327*t*, 328–331, 331*t*, 332, 344. *See also*
Amitriptyline; Anticonvulsants;
Antipsychotics; Benzodiazepines;
Brofaromine; Buspirone; Carbamazepine; Clonidine; Cyproheptadine; Diphenhydramine;
Fluoxetine; Fluvoxamine; Hypnotics; Imipramine; Inositol; Lamotrigine; Lithium; Monoamine
oxidase inhibitors; Mood stabilizers; Nefazodone; Noradrenergic
suppressors; Olanzapine;